Secondary Neoplasias following Chemotherapy, Radiotherapy, and Immunosuppression

Contributions to Oncology
Beiträge zur Onkologie

Vol. 55

Series Editors

W. Queißer, Mannheim
W. Scheithauer, Wien

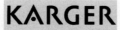

Basel · Freiburg · Paris · London · New York ·
New Delhi · Bangkok · Singapore · Tokyo · Sydney

Secondary Neoplasias following Chemotherapy, Radiotherapy, and Immunosuppression

Volume Editors

U. Rüther, Ludwigsburg
C. Nunnensiek, Reutlingen
H.-J. Schmoll, Halle/Saale

38 figures, 8 in color, 22 tables, 2000

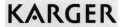

KARGER Basel · Freiburg · Paris · London · New York ·
New Delhi · Bangkok · Singapore · Tokyo · Sydney

Contributions to Oncology
Beiträge zur Onkologie

Library of Congress Cataloging-in-Publication Data

Secondary neoplasias following chemotherapy, radiotherapy and immunosuppression / volume editors,
U. Rüther, C. Nunnensiek, H.-J. Schmoll.
    p. ; cm. – (Contributions to oncology = Beiträge zur Onkologie; vol. 55)
  Includes bibliographical references and index.
  ISBN 380557116X (alk. paper)
  1. Carcinogenesis. 2. Metastasis. 3. Tumors. 4. Cancer – Chemotherapy – Complications. 5. Cancer –
Radiotherapy – Complications. 6. Immunosuppression – Complications. I. Rüther, U. (Ursula) II. Nunnensiek,
C. (Christa) III. Schmoll, H.-J. (Hans-Joachim) IV. Beiträge zur Onkologie ; Vol. 55.
  [DNLM: 1. Neoplasms, Second Primary – etiology. 2. Antineoplastic Agents – adverse effects.
3. Immunosuppressive Agents – adverse effects. 4. Neoplasms, Second Primary – prevention & control.
5. Radiotherapy – adverse effects. QZ 202 S445 2000]
RC268.5 .S42 2000
616.99'4071–dc21
                                                                              00-066398

Drug Dosage

> The authors and the publisher have exerted every effort to ensure that drug selection and dosage set forth
> in this text are in accord with current recommendations and practice at the time of publication. However,
> in view of ongoing research, changes in government regulations, and the constant flow of information
> relating to drug therapy and drug reactions, the reader is urged to check the package insert for each drug
> for any change in indications and dosage and for added warnings and precautions. This is particularly
> important when the recommended agent is a new and/or infrequently employed drug.

© Copyright 2000 by S. Karger GmbH, Postfach, D-79095 Freiburg, and S. Karger AG, P. O. Box, CH-1009
  Basel
  Printed in Germany on acid-free paper by Konkordia Druck GmbH, Bühl
  ISBN 3-8055-7116-X

Contents

Clinical Presentations

Emerging Therapies and Preventive Measures

Preface

Reports of secondary neoplasia developing after successful curative chemo- and/or radiotherapy for malignancies are increasing. Also of growing concern is the diagnostic and therapeutic problem of tumorigenesis during posttransplantation immunosuppressive therapy. With chapters contributed by internationally renowned researchers, this book discusses several aspects of this issue.

The first part covers the various causes of primary and secondary tumorigenesis and of neoplasia occurring during posttransplantation immunosuppressive therapy. As survival times lengthen and overall remission rates increase for patients with Hodgkin's disease, germ-cell tumors, non-Hodgkin's lymphomas or leukemia, the potential risk of developing therapy-associated secondary malignancy is becoming a focus of attention. What makes this problem even more relevant are the many breast and colon carcinoma patients who receive adjuvant chemotherapy after complete resection of the primary tumor or even of metastases. In addition, an increasing number of patients with chemosensitive disease are receiving high-dose chemotherapy with autologous peripheral-blood stem-cell transplantation.

Post chemotherapy, the most common secondary neoplasm is secondary acute myeloid leukemia, which develops primarily after treatment with alkylating agents or topoisomerase inhibitors. While secondary leukemia after alkylating-agent therapy often commences with a preleukemic phase of myelodysplasia, secondary leukemia associated with epipodophyllotoxin is acute, and lacks this preceding myelodysplasia. The correlating chapters in this book discuss in depth the risk of the individual cytostatic agents for inducing secondary malignoma, and include the aspects of cumulative dose dependency and chronology of administration.

Other chapters discuss the role of immunosurveillance and the immune system's recognition of tumors. In this area, our knowledge is constantly growing, in particular with respect to the molecular processes responsible for the changes on tumor cells and immune cells, the structure and function of a wide variety of surface receptors and ligands on these cells, lymphocytic signal transduction pathways, the characterization of murine tumor-specific transplantation antigens, and human tumor-associated antigens. Although far from complete, our understanding of cellular immune response to tumors has improved considerably, as has our understanding of how tumor cells escape detection by the immune system.

As more and more tumors develop during posttransplantation immunosuppressive therapy, today's findings on the underlying processes will lead to innovative changes in existing therapeutic concepts. Already, we must increasingly deal with aspects such as the antigenic characteristics of transformed cells, host-tumor interaction, molecular mechanisms of cell-dependent cytotoxicity, identification of components that generate and control effective immune response, induction of tolerance or of T-cell anergy, and immunologic effects of the host on the neoplastic growth of tumor cells. One therapeutic aspect is the modulation of the immune system or of tumor cells such that the latter can be more easily recognized and eliminated by immunoeffectors. In addition, this book covers the role and significance of herpesviruses in these areas.

The last part of this book discusses the prevention of secondary tumors and tumors occurring during immunosuppressive therapy. Here, the major substances for cytoprotection during chemo- and/or radiotherapy are presented. Also described are new vaccine strategies for treating varicella- and herpesvirus-associated tumors. These vaccines can be applied not only for treatment of infections, but are beginning to play an important role in tumor prevention as well. Of special interest is the chapter dealing with immunomodulatory therapy of posttransplantation lymphoproliferative disorders.

The authors repeatedly stress that early detection is a prerequisite for successful treatment of secondary neoplasms and neoplasms occurring during immunosuppression. Therefore, patients who are successfully treated for malignancy in particular require long-term follow-up including checks for therapy-associated late sequelae. However, this applies also to patients who, after organ transplantation, receive immunosuppressive therapy.

In closing, we can again only reiterate that our international group of authors underscores the importance of global collaboration if we are to find diagnostic and therapeutic solutions to these problems.

The editors wish to express their appreciation to Diane E. Crawford, who carefully and thoroughly translated and edited the manuscripts, and to Dr. Joachim Sick, Bene Meritus.

U. Rüther, Ludwigsburg
Ch. Nunnensiek, Reutlingen
H.-J. Schmoll, Halle/Saale

Rüther U, Nunnensiek C, Schmoll H-J (eds): Secondary Neoplasias following Chemotherapy, Radiotherapy, and Immunosuppression. Contrib Oncol. Basel, Karger, 2000, vol 55, pp 1–16

....

Basic Concepts of Tumor Biology

Alfred Nordheim[a], Bernhard Lüscher[b]

[a] Interfakultäres Institut für Zellbiologie, Abteilung für Molekularbiologie, Eberhard-Karls-Universität Tübingen
[b] Institut für Molekularbiologie, Medizinische Hochschule Hannover, Deutschland

Introduction

The cells that build up organisms, including human beings, exist in a tightly controlled equilibrium of growth and death, of proliferation and differentation. These equilibria are determined by genetic programs and are modulated by signals exerted by the extracellular environment. Mutations in the genome of a cell can drastically upset such equilibria, leading to disregulated proliferation patterns. Consequently, genomic changes – and the associated alterations in gene expression and function – form the basis of uncontrolled proliferation and subsequent tumor formation. Genomic changes often found in tumor cells include point mutations, deletions, insertions, amplifications, translocations, and viral integrations. Such mutagenic events can lead to the activation of cellular proto-oncogenes or the inactivaton of tumor suppressor genes (see below) [1]. Mutations in genes responsible for maintaining intact genomes and repairing genomic defects can lead to the accumulation of multiple genetic lesions. In fact, the progression of a premalignant cell to a tumorous, malignant cell is the consequence of a multi-step process leading to the accumulation of multiple lesions in the genome of one cell. Cells whose genetic stability is severely compromised can be removed from the pool of somatic cells by the process of apoptosis (programmed cell death). Therefore, apoptosis represents a safeguard mechanism for an organism to rid itself of dangerously mutated cells. Mutations reducing the efficiency of apoptotic execution can – in consequence – favor the survival of cells carrying tumorigenic genetic lesions.

Signal Transduction

Cellular activities are strongly determined by signals that trigger or terminate physiological processes. Cells communicate with each other via cell-cell interactions or via diffusable signaling molecules (e.g., growth factors, chemokines, hormones, etc.) [2]. Similarly, non-cellular signals, i.e. radiation, stress signals, or chemical and mechanical insults, also elicit signaling responses in target cells. Collectively, the intracellular processing of such signals determines to a large extent the physiologic state of a cell, including such diverse cellular activities as proliferation, growth arrest, differentiation, and cell death.

Cellular signal recognition and intracellular signal processing (signal transduction) can be remarkably specific, thereby ensuring very selective responses by individual cells to a given signal. Intracellular signal transduction often leads to very specific changes in gene expression profiles. This reflects the fact that extracellular signals can be specifically perceived at the extracellular compartment and processed across the plasma membrane and through the cytoplasm right into the cell nucleus. Signal processing inside cells is a truly complex system. Several functionally completely independent signal transduction cascades have been identified that convert an extracellular stimulus into an altered pattern of gene expression [1]. It is surprising that overlapping signal transduction cascades can fulfill regulatory functions regarding both cellular proliferation and differentiation. Accordingly, signaling mechanisms important for the development of an organism are relevant to the regulation and dysregulation of cell growth [2].

One of the best-studied examples of signal transduction is the Ras-MAPK signaling system, which interconnects several linear signal cascades into a complex network of signaling processes [3]. Once activated, the Ras-MAPK cascade triggers the enzymatic activation of a series of consecutively acting protein kinases (collectively called the 'mitogen-activated protein kinases') which transmit signals into the cell nucleus and direct the transcription of individual genes. The Ras-MAPK system deserves special mention here, since it involves several signaling molecules, such as Ras and Raf, which can strongly stimulate cellular transformation and tumor formation when rendered uncontrollable by mutagenic alteration. The components of this signaling system are promising drug targets for tumor therapy [4].

A second signaling pathway of interest is the Wg/Wnt-β-catenin pathway, which normally contributes to cellular growth control and developmental processes [5]. When deregulated, this pathway can promote colon cancer and melanoma development [6]. Important signaling components of this pathway include the Wnt receptor, APC protein ('adenomatous polyposis coli'), serine-threonine glycogen synthase kinase (GSK-3β), β-catenin protein, and Tcf-Lef transcription factor. In the non-stimulated state, this pathway has the active GSK-3β kinase contacting the APC/β-catenin complex in the cytoplasm. In this complex, β-catenin is phosphorylated by

GSK-3β and is thereby destined for degradation. In this process, APC helps maintain low levels of free β-catenin. Upon signal activation, GSK-3β kinase is inactivated, resulting in increased levels of free β-catenin. The latter then translocates to the nucleus and interacts with Tcf-Lef transcription factors, thereby stimulating the activation of target genes regulated by Tcf-Lef. In this manner, APC functions as a tumor suppressor gene and β-catenin acts as a proto-oncogene (see below).

Cell Cycle Control and Tumorigenesis

At any given time in an adult organism, the majority of cells is not proliferating; i.e., most cells are not going through the cell cycle. Some of these nonproliferating cells are differentiated to fulfill specific functions and can re-enter a proliferative phase under special circumstances. Other cells are in a quiescent or resting state (also called G_0, see below), and can be activated to re-enter the cell cycle upon specific signals that, in general, are provided by the environment. Cells can remain in a quiescent state for a considerable length of time. In multicellular organisms, the regulation of cellular proliferation is important for maintaining appropriate cell numbers of each individual cellular compartment. This is balanced by cell loss through apoptosis and necrosis (see below). Deregulation of these processes has been recognized as important for tumor development. The induction of cell-cycle progression, which ultimately leads to cell division leaving two genetically identical cells, is stringently controlled at multiple levels [7]. In particular, an equal, error-free distribution of genetic information during each cell division is critical for the survival of organisms.

Cell Cycle Phases, Cyclins and CDKs

The cell cycle is subdivided into five distinct phases (fig. 1). Early on, the S phase was recognized as the period during which DNA is replicated. In the M phase, or mitosis, the cell divides and the chromosomes are equally distributed to the two daughter cells. Thus, during these two cell cycle phases, events occur that are essential for maintaining genetic integrity. The G_1 and G_2 phases were originally defined as gaps between the M and S phases, with no obvious function attributed to them. However, evidence in the last 20 years has demonstrated important roles for both the G_1 and G_2 phases of the cell cycle. In addition, cells can reside in a G_0 phase in which no proliferative activities are maintained.

Essential decisions on cellular proliferation are made in the G_0/G_1 phases. In general, such decisions are dictated by extracellular cues which allow an organism to precisely control the number of cells that divide. This is crucial for maintaining appropriate cell numbers in a multicellular organism. These signals are generated by neighboring cells, the extracellular matrix, and diffusible molecules secreted by cells that may exist far from the target cell. These signals are integrated by correspond-

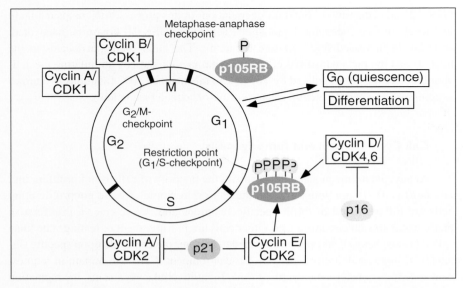

Fig. 1. Summary of the cell cycle and its regulatory elements. The five main phases of the cell cycle are indicated: M = mitosis, in which the cell divides; G_1 = Gap1, the cell is responsive to proliferation regulatory signals; S = DNA replication; G_2 = Gap2, the cell monitors DNA replication, preparation for mitosis; G_0 = resting or quiescent state, reduced metabolic activity, re-entering the cell cycle is possible upon stimulation by growth factors. Differentiation: Cells fulfill specialized functions and normally do not re-enter the cell cycle. Checkpoints have been recognized as molecular switches that regulate transitions between different phases of the cell cycle. Key regulators of the cell cycle are kinases that possess a cyclin as the regulatory subunit and a cyclin-dependent kinase (CDK) as the catalytic subunit. The activity of cyclin/CDK complexes is regulated by CDK inhibitors (CKI, i.e. p16 and p21). The regulatory protein pl05Rb is indicated as one CDK substrate.

ing receptors that regulate cellular behavior through interconnected signal transduction pathways (see above). These signals act mainly in the G_0/G_1 phase, and it is generally the sum of potentially diverse, or even antagonistic signals, that determines whether a cell will enter a proliferative cycle. Proliferative signals are required not only for quiescent cells to re-enter the cell cycle, but also to re-initiate the cell cycle after completion of mitosis. In addition to the presence of growth factors, a number of additional requirements must be fulfilled prior to progression from the G_1 into the S phase. For example, cells must reach a certain size, and the DNA must be undamaged. Thus, sufficient extracellular growth signals and appropriate cellular conditions are required for cell cycle progression.

Once cells have passed through G_1, growth factors are no longer necessary to complete the cell division cycle. Thus, the S phase, G_2, and mitosis will progress, in the absence of growth factors, without delay. Interestingly, cells that were deprived of growth factors in G_2 of the previous cell cycle will delay entry into the S phase of the next cell cycle in the presence of growth factors. This suggests that successive cell cycles are connected and that a cell builds up a 'memory' of the growth factor status of the previous cell cycle. At present, it is unclear how this is controlled at the molecular level.

Through mechanisms not fully understood, these signals stimulate the activation of specific kinases that appear to be key regulators [8]. These kinases are heterodimers of regulatory subunits, the cyclins; and catalytic subunits, the cyclin-dependent kinases (CDK). These cyclin/CDK complexes regulate transition from one cell cycle phase to the next by controlling checkpoints (for details see below). Several different cyclins and CDKs have been identified in recent years, most of which function in cell cycle control. In the G_1 phase, D-type cyclins (D1, D2, and D3), together with CDK4 and CDK6, are activated (fig. 1). For the G_1-S transition, the cyclin E/CDK2 complex is required, in addition to cyclin D/CDK4,6 complexes.

During S-phase DNA replication, a highly regulated process occurs that requires major metabolic activities. Some of these are initiated in the G_1 phase in preparation for efficient DNA replication. Of particular importance in the S phase are control mechanisms that prevent replication of DNA, so that DNA is replicated only once per cell cycle. Again, CDK complexes have regulatory functions in that they are important for establishing prereplication complexes and for preventing the formation of novel prereplication complexes on replicated DNA. Cyclin E/CDK2 complexes are thought to be important at the beginning of the S phase, whereas cyclin A/CDK2 is active during the S phase and in G_2.

The G_2 phase of the cell cycle is important for preparing the cell for mitosis, which is the culmination of the cellular proliferation cycle. One step in this preparation is to examine whether the DNA is fully replicated. Again, these control mechanisms impinge on the function of cyclin/CDK complexes that regulate the transition from G_2 into mitosis. In addition to cyclin A/CDK2 complexes, at the end of G_2, cyclin A/CDK1 and cyclin B/CDK1 are activated and function in stimulating mitosis.

The events that occur during mitosis, including the breakdown of the nuclear envelope, chromatin condensation, separation of the chromatides, and cytokinesis, are directly influenced by cyclin B-containing CDK complexes. Again, several checkpoints control progression into and through mitosis. Some of them have been recognized as vital to genetic stability and thus relevant to the control of tumorigenesis.

Regulation of the Kinases

Distinct cyclin/CDK complexes are activated during different phases of the cell cycle. This suggests a CDK-driven cell cycle with a cascade-like activation of the different complexes. Because these complexes are so important, their activities must be tightly controlled, and in fact, several regulatory mechanisms have been discovered. As the name indicates, cyclins are expressed in specific cell cycle-regulated patterns and thus restrict the activities of cyclin/CDK complexes to specific windows during the cell cycle. Regulation occurs at the level of expression of cyclin genes, which provides the basis for CDK activity.

The stability of cyclin proteins antagonizes their induced expression and provides a means of rapidly lowering protein levels. Degradation of cyclins is again tightly regulated and at least in some cases initiated by autophosphorylation. Such 'marked' cyclins are then ubiquitinated and proteolyzed by proteasomes. In addition, CDKs are targeted by phosphorylation/dephosphorylation reactions and by CDK inhibitors (CKI), adding additional levels of regulation to CDKs.

Of particular relevance for tumorigenesis are CKIs, since these molecules are frequently affected by mutations in human tumors [9, 10]. Two classes of CKIs exist. The first class includes p15, p16, p18 and p19, which are important in regulating the activities of cyclin-D-containing complexes. The second class includes p21, p27 and p57, which appear to affect cyclin E and cyclin A complexes, and, at least in vitro, cyclin D complexes as well. Several different conditions have been identified in which the regulation of such CKIs is important for efficient cell cycle regulation. p21 is a focus of interest because it also plays a role in cellular differentiation and in aging. Furthermore, it is a target gene of tumor suppressor p53, which is a central component of the DNA monitoring system of cells. The upregulation of p21 mediates, at least in part, inhibition of S-phase progression upon activation of p53. p27 plays a major role during the transition from resting cells to the G_1 and S phases. p16 is encoded from a locus that also codes for p19[ARF] by using an alternative exon 1 and an alternative reading frame, and is implicated in the regulation of the restriction point governing the G_1- to S-phase transition. Various signaling pathways appear to affect the expression of different CKIs, including growth-stimulatory signals that suppress CKI activity and growth-inhibitory signals that increase CKI function. Thus, CKIs are intimately associated with cellular growth control impinging on the activity of the central regulators of the cell cycle, the CDKs.

Substrates of CDKs

The findings summarized above demonstrate that cell cycle regulation is closely linked with the activities of CDKs and that these kinases are controlled by many different signaling pathways. To obtain greater insight into the mechanics of cell cycle control, it is important to identify the substrates of CDKs. Over the past 10 years, a number of CDK substrates have been identified. Some have been found to play a vital role at transitions from one cell cycle phase to the next, or to be involved in the regulation of checkpoints (see below). However, in many instances, details of the functional consequences for substrates of CDK phosphorylation are not understood.

Early on, it was found that a number of proteins are hyperphosphorylated during mitosis. Some of these proteins are modified directly by CDKs, while others appear to be substrates of kinases that are likely positioned downstream of CDKs.

Nuclear lamins and histones are substrates for CDKs, and their phosphorylation is important for the breakdown of the nuclear envelope and the condensation of chromatin, respectively. More recently, it has been shown that proteins that hold the chromatides together during metaphase are regulated by CKDs, an important function for maintaining genetic stability.

A major substrate in cell cycle control is the pl05Rb protein [10]. This tumor suppressor is a regulator of the restriction point in G_1 that integrates many regulatory signals important for S-phase entry. pl05Rb binds to transcription factors of the E2F class, which bind to DNA control elements that are found in a number of genes important for the S phase, including histone genes and cyclin A. Binding of pl05Rb to E2F blocks their transactivation domain, and recruits histone deacetylases, which are enzymes that can remove acetyl groups from histones and thus affect the organization of the chromatin of target genes. These functions of pl05Rb effectively inhibit the expression of E2F-regulated genes in G_1. Phosphorylation of pl05Rb by cyclin D- and possibly by cyclin E-containing complexes results in the release of pl05Rb from E2F and thus facilitates expression of E2F-regulated genes.

Checkpoints

The term 'checkpoint' was coined by yeast geneticists to define certain positions in the yeast cell cycle that are used to inspect the condition of a cell before it enters the next cell cycle phase [11, 12]. There is evidence of different checkpoints during the cell cycle. However, attention has mainly focused on the control of the G_1- to S- and the G_2- to M-phase transitions and, more recently, on the metaphase-to-anaphase transition. These checkpoints are positively regulated by cyclin/CDK complexes. Passage through these checkpoints can be inhibited by negatively regulating CDKs.

What is monitored at checkpoints? Often, it is the status of DNA, for DNA damage due to UV light, ionizing radiation and various chemicals activates both G_1-S and G_2-M checkpoints. Replication of damaged DNA may lead to the accumulation of mutations or to an uneven distribution of genetic information during mitosis. Furthermore, incomplete or incorrect alignment of mitotic chromatides, an additional source of uneven distribution of genetic material, activates the metaphase-to-anaphase checkpoint. These are alterations that contribute to the development and progression of tumors. Thus, cells have mechanisms that prevent damaged DNA from being replicated in the S phase, and that block cell division when DNA is damaged or when the chromatides are not properly aligned. Activation of the relevant checkpoints gives cells time to repair the damage. The regulation of checkpoints is therefore of immediate importance for maintaining genetic stability. If DNA damage is so extensive that successful repair is precluded, a dormant program of events is activated that leads to apoptosis. This is the ultimate and irreversible response to DNA damage and to other forms of cellular insult (see below), so that cellular suicide represents the cell's ultimate line of defense to prevent genetic instability.

Proto-Oncogenes and Tumor Suppressor Genes

Oncogenes and mutated variants of tumor suppressor genes can be collectively classified as cancer genes. These two types of growth control genes exert opposite effects on proliferation, as proven by the kind of mutations found in their respective genes in tumor cells: oncogenes are generated when mutations of their precursor genes, the proto-oncogenes, are activated. The products of tumor suppressor genes, on the other hand, are incapacitated by mutations. A comprehensive, highly recommendable treatise on genetic changes in the generation of cancer, i.e., on mutations in both proto-oncogenes and tumor suppressor genes, is provided by Vogelstein and Kinzler [7]. Tumor progression from a premalignant, benign neoplasm to a fully malignant and even metastatic form is understood to arise from several mutagenic events accumulating in a cell, and such mutations are found in both proto-oncogenes and tumor suppressor genes [13].

Oncogenes
Cellular genes whose products stimulate cell proliferation are closely regulated so that they do not stimulate cell division at inappropriate times. Mutation of such genes can render their products uncontrollable, leading to unregulated and tumorigenic cell proliferation. By definition, such a mutagenic event converts a cellular proto-oncogene into an activated oncogene [1]. These types of mutations clearly result in a gain-of-function phenotype and usually penetrate in a genetically dominant fashion. In tumor cells, many oncogenes and their corresponding oncoproteins have now been identified [1, 7]. Oncogenes often encode key regulatory molecules involved in signal transduction and gene regulation associated with the control of cell proliferation. Examples include growth factors (e.g., *v-sis, int 2, KS3*); growth factor receptors (e.g., *EGFR, v-fms*); nonreceptor tyrosine kinases (e.g., *c-src, bcr/abl*); membrane-associated G-proteins (e.g., *ras, gsp, gip*); the GEF family of proteins (e.g., *dbl, vav, ost*); serine/threonine kinases (e.g., *c-raf, c-mos, pim-1*), and transcription factors (e.g., *c-myc, N-myc, c-fos, c-myb, c-rel, c-ets*).

Tumor Suppressor Genes
Experiments fusing tumor cells and normal cells show that genetic information contributed by the normal cell causes the fused cells to lose their tumor characteristics. This tumor suppressor activity of normal cells obviously compensates for regulatory components of normal cell growth that were lost in the tumor cells. Tumor suppressor activity is genetically recessive; i.e., a single allele encoding the activity

usually suffices to maintain a normal cellular proliferation phenotype. This suggests that effective mutations in tumor suppressor genes are loss-of-function mutations. These must occur in both alleles of the tumor suppressor gene in order to substantially affect the proliferation control of a cell (Knudson's 'two-hit' theory) [14].

This concept was first developed for familial retinoblastoma, in which children rapidly develop multiple retinal tumors in both eyes (bilateral retinoblastoma) (cf. chapter 19 in Vogelstein and Kinzler [7]). Genetic predisposition for certain cancers is associated with heterozygosity (H) involving the alleles of a tumor suppressor gene.

The second mutagenic event, hitting the second allele, leads to loss of heterozygosity (LOH), promoting decontrolled cell proliferation. Many tumor suppressor genes have now been identified, as compiled in chapter 11 of Vogelstein and Kinzler [7]. Some examples are *RB1* (retinoblastoma, see below); *p53* (sarcomas, breast and brain tumors); *APC* (colon cancer); *WT-1* (nephroblastoma); *NF-1* (neurofibromas, sarcomas, gliomas); *NF-2* (schwannomas, meningiomas); *p16* (melanoma, pancreatic cancer); *E-cadherin* (metastatic cancers); *BRCA1* (breast and ovarian cancer), and *BRCA2* (breast cancer).

RB1, the Prototypical Tumor Suppressor Gene

The gene involved in the formation of retinoblastomas, the retinoblastoma gene *(RB1)* encoded on chromosome 13q, was the first tumor suppressor gene identified. Its gene product, the retinoblastoma protein (RB1 or pl05Rb), fulfills important functions in controlling gene activities during the cell cycle (see above). These functions are severely compromised when DNA tumor viruses infect cells and express viral oncoproteins, which bind to pl05Rb and its relatives [15], and selectively disrupt their activities. pl05Rb functions as a crucial relay between cellular signals controlling proliferation and the nuclear transcription machinery [15]. The interplay between pl05Rb and E2F transcription factors, which directly affects the transcriptional activity of target genes, determines growth arrest in G_1 or entry into the S phase of the cell cycle. Phosphorylation of pl05Rb by the CDKs, as indicated in figure 1, inhibits pl05Rb-E2F interactions, thereby permitting E2F to stimulate genes required for progression into the S phase. Activation of CKIs p16 and p21 counteracts this mechanism, thereby arresting growth when required. Since human cancer cells frequently display mutations in genes encoding pl05Rb, p16, cyclin D or CDK4, deregulated p105Rb's fundamental contribution to tumorigenesis is evident.

p53, the Most Versatile Tumor Suppressor Protein

Malfunction of tumor suppressor protein p53 is the most frequently observed molecular defect in tumor cells. More than 50% of all human neoplasms have a mutation in the p53 locus. Germline alterations of the p53 tumor suppressor gene located on chromosome 17pl3 have been observed in the majority of families suffering from Li-Fraumeni syndrome, a dominantly inherited autosomal disorder leading to bone and soft-tissue sarcoma at an early age. p53 activity has been linked to tumor suppression, cell cycle control, DNA repair, cell senescence, genomic stability and apoptotic cell death [16, 17]. This involvement in many different cellular processes is, in part, due to the ability of the p53 protein to fulfill several biochemical functions, including binding to RNA, sequence-specific recognition of DNA, activation and repression of transcription, and regulation of DNA replication. For example, transcriptional induction by p53 of the gene encoding the CKI p21 (fig. 1), a negative regulator of cyclin-dependent kinases, enables p53 to inhibit cell cycle progression before S-phase entry. p53 therefore acts as a guardian of the genome by enabling cells to repair damaged DNA before DNA replication – and thus before perpetuation of DNA changes (see below). If the damaged DNA cannot be repaired appropriately, p53 contributes to the extinction of such cells by initiating apoptosis. Mutations in the p53 gene render p53 protein derivatives unable to fulfill such protective functions.

DNA Repair and Mutator Genes

As indicated above, tumor formation is the result of multiple genetic lesions that accumulate in a cell. This reflects a fundamental problem; namely, the manner in which genetic information is stored. DNA is not an inert molecule, but is subject to both chemical and physical agents. These can affect: the expression and function of specific genes; the mechanics of DNA replication in the S phase; and the equal distribution of chromatides, in the M phase, to the two daughter cells. Thus, maintaining genetic stability is a vital task for every cell and organism. To protect the integrity of DNA and thus provide genetic stability, an intricate network of DNA repair systems evolved early. Major mechanisms for removing damage from DNA include mismatch repair (MMR), base excision repair (BER), nucleotide excision repair (NER) and double-strand break repair (DSBR). These repair systems, which at times have overlapping functions, are fundamental to genetic stability. Mutations in several components of these systems have been identified in human tumors, indicating that these molecules can function as cancer genes.

Mismatch Repair

DNA replication occurs with high fidelity. Mispairs and small unpaired regions that have escaped proofreading become substrates for mismatch repair [18, 19]. The process of postreplicative mismatch repair is well understood in *Escherichia coli*. It involves several factors associated with mismatch recognition (MutS protein); strand discrimination (MutH protein recognizes the 'old' DNA strand because it is methylated); exonucleolytic degradation of the strand carrying the error; resynthesis of the repair patch, and ligation. Similar systems operate in eukaryotes, but the process of mismatch repair is not as well understood there as in *E. coli*. Several homologues to the bacterial proteins have been isolated in humans (hMSH and hMLH for human MutS and MutL homologues, respectively), some of which are involved in the development of cancer. Germline mutations in some of the mismatch repair genes lead to a genetic predisposition for colon cancer, referred to as hereditary nonpolyposis colon cancer (HNPCC). This is one of the common cancer susceptibility syndromes that is inherited in an autosomal-dominant fashion [7, 13]. Cancer predisposition in most HNPCC kindreds is attributable to mutations in hMSH2 or in any of three hMLHs (hMLH1, hPMS1, hPMS2). These genetic defects result in a mutator phenotype with a high incidence of mutations in microsatellite repeat sequences, and thus generate genetic instability.

Base Excision Repair

Base excision repair fixes DNA damage that hydrolytic events (deamination or base loss), oxidative damage and methylation can spontaneously cause in a cell [18]. The key event in this process is the removal of base residues in their free form – generating apurinic or apyrimidinic sites – by DNA glycosylases. These enzymes are specific for particular lesions. Apurinic and apyrimidinic sites are removed by AP endonucleases and the gap is filled by DNA polymerase β. Since these spontaneous lesions are very frequent (several thousand modified bases/cell/day), complete loss of BER would be incompatible with life. Thus, back-up and alternative pathways exist that can repair such lesions. It is not clear whether mutations in BER genes are involved in the generation of human cancer.

Nucleotide Excision Repair

Nucleotide excision repair removes DNA lesions induced by UV, and by bulky chemical adducts stemming from treatment with certain chemotherapeutic agents [7, 20]. These alterations significantly distort the DNA helix, which appears to be the common denominator for recognition by the nucleotide excision repair system. The details of this repair mechanism are best understood for the UvrABC system in *E. coli*, with several distinct steps recognized. These involve damage recognition; incision of the damaged DNA strand on both sides of the lesion; removal of the damage-containing oligomer; gap-filling DNA synthesis, and ligation. Defects in nucleotide excision repair underlie the extreme photosensitivity and predisposition to skin cancer in patients with xeroderma pigmentosum (XP), a rare autosomal recessive disease. Seven XP complementation groups have been identified that represent distinct nucleotide excision repair genes, *XPA-G*.

Double-Strand Break Repair

Double-strand breaks are generated by endogenously produced radicals or by exogenous insults such as ionizing radiation (IR). Repair of double-strand breaks is of critical importance to prevent loss of chromosomal fragments, translocations, inversions and deletions [21]. These genetic alterations can lead to the activation of oncogenes or the inactivation of tumor suppressor genes. Thus, incorrect double-strand break repairs can induce neoplastic growth. Several pathways have evolved to repair double-strand breaks. Homologous recombination uses significant areas of DNA homology on the undamaged sister chromatid to repair double-strand breaks. Alternatively, DNA end-joining connects juxtaposed ends in a manner that requires little or no sequence homology. However, this process may not be error-free. Double-strand break repair through DNA end-joining is initiated by the recruitment and activation of the DNA-dependent protein kinase (DNA-PK) complex. It contains the catalytic subunit of DNA-PK (DNA-PK$_{CS}$) and the KU70 and KU80 proteins. Mutations in these proteins show increased sensitivity to IR, but also severe combined immunodeficiency, since the DNA-PK complex is also involved in immunoglobulin recombination. In addition, DNA-PK$_{CS}$-deficient mice show increased incidence of cancer, demonstrating the importance of this kinase in genetic stability.

Apoptosis

Cells have a built-in mechanism for destroying themselves, termed apoptosis. It is a programmed cell death process that ultimately leads to the fragmentation of cells into apoptotic bodies and their subsequent phagocytosis by neighboring cells. Apoptosis does not lead to the release of cellular content into the extracellular surroundings, so that an inflammatory response is not invoked. This is in contrast to cell death by necrosis, which is generally the result of mechanical insults or of poisoning of cells. Apoptosis has been recognized as (1) a major process during development and in homeostasis, and (2) responsible for sculpting tissue, maintaining the correct number of cells, and removing autoreactive immune cells. Dysregulation of either apoptosis or proliferation will affect homeostatic balance and can lead to neoplasia. At the molecular level, apoptosis is characterized by the activation of a cascade of proteases, the caspases. The activation of these enzymes results in the proteolytic cleavage of a distinct set of proteins and leads to various alterations typical for most apoptotic cells, including cell shrinking and blebbing, condensation of the nucleus and the chromatin, and DNA fragmentation [22–24].

Death Signaling

Apoptosis can be induced in cells by various stimuli. It is opposed by survival signals, but also by DNA repair processes. Several cell surface receptors (death receptors) have been identified that stimulate apoptosis upon binding of their ligand. These include receptors for Fas ligand, tumor necrosis factor (TNF) and TRAIL. Stimulation of these receptors by ligand binding results in the activation of the proteolytic enzyme caspase-8, which is present as a receptor-associated zymogen (fig. 2). Caspase-8 can then directly activate other caspases or stimulate the release of cytochrome c from mitochondria that is part of the activation scheme of caspase-9, which in turn can activate other caspases. An increasing number of caspase substrates are being identified that affect apoptosis [25]. Several structural proteins, including lamins, gelsolin, actin, as well as modulators of apoptosis such as Bcl-2, have been identified as caspase substrates. Furthermore, various kinases, including Mst1, MEKK-1, PAK65/PAK2, ppl25^{FAK} and CDKs, are activated by caspase cleavage and are involved in the apoptotic process, suggesting that signaling cascades are regulated during apoptosis. In addition, several transcriptional regulators are targeted by caspases, including NF-κB complexes, which are activated as a consequence of inactivating IκB, an inhibitor of NF-κB, by caspase-dependent cleavage. NF-κB can inhibit apoptosis, at least in part, by stimulating the expression of inhibitors of apoptosis (IAPs).

The Bcl-2 Family of Apoptosis Regulators

The *bcl-2* gene (for B-cell lymphoma/leukemia-2) was initially identified as the gene located on chromosome 18q21 that is at the breakpoint of the t(14;18) translocation found in the majority of B-cell follicular lymphomas. The role of Bcl-2 in tumorigenesis was unclear for some time, since this protein does not increase cellular proliferation, as is usually seen with most other oncoproteins. The finding that Bcl-2 stimulated cell survival defined a new category of oncogenes, and suggested that besides increased proliferation, the inhibition of cell death also contributed to tumorigenesis. Bcl-2 and related proteins affect apoptosis at least in part by regulating the release of cytochrome c from mitochondria. Several Bcl-2-related proteins have been identified in recent years. Some of them, such as Bcl-2 and Bcl-x$_L$, function anti-apoptotically, while others, such as Bcl-x$_S$, Bax, Bad and Bak, are proapoptotic.

Oncogenes and Apoptosis

Development of neoplasia is a multistep genetic process that requires the alterations of several cellular genes. Numerous oncoproteins have been shown to activate apoptosis [7]. This was demonstrated most clearly for c-Myc, a protein overexpressed in the majority of human tumors. c-Myc is a potent stimulator of cellular proliferation, but only in the presence of survival signals, since isolated overexpression of c-Myc results in apoptosis. Bcl-2 is one factor that inhibits Myc-induced apoptosis, and these two proteins cooperate efficiently in the generation of tumors in transgenic mice. These and other findings show strong synergistic activities of oncogenes that either stimulate proliferation or inhibit apoptosis. In addition, these studies give evidence of a safety mechanism that prevents uncontrolled proliferation upon activation of an oncogene. Cells which are driven through the cell cycle by an activated oncogene may require increased levels of survival factors, which are most likely not available under normal cellular circumstances. Such cells will thus switch from a proliferative to an apoptotic program.

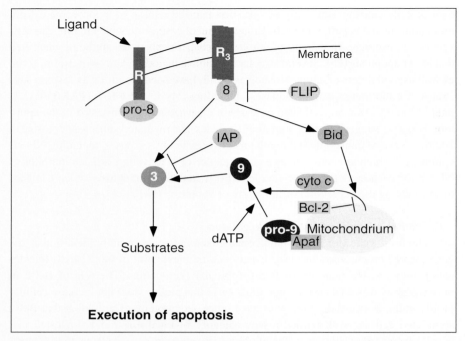

Fig. 2. Activation of caspases during receptor-mediated activation of apoptosis. Apoptosis can be triggered when death receptors such as Fas, TNFR, and TRAIL are activated by their respective ligands. This leads to a multimerization of receptor molecules and subsequently the activation of caspase-8, which binds directly or through mediator proteins to the receptors. Caspase-8 can directly activate downstream effector caspases or stimulate the release of cyctochrome c from mitochondria. This is necessary, together with dATP, to activate caspase-9, which is associated in its inactive form with mitochondria by binding to Apaf (apoptotic protease activating factor). Caspase-9 can then stimulate effector caspases. These cleave multiple substrates, triggering the alterations associated with the apoptotic process. Multiple levels of regulation target this cascade-like activation process of caspases and thus regulate apoptosis. Some regulatory events are indicated. The activation of caspase-8 is inhibited by FLIP (Flice inhibitory protein), which binds competitively to the receptor or to receptor-associated adaptor molecules. IAPs (inhibitors of apoptosis) are another class of caspase inhibitors that can block the activity of caspase-3 and caspase-7 by direct binding. Bcl-2 and other antiapoptotic members of the Bcl-2 family inhibit the release of cytochrome c. Proapoptotic members of the Bcl-2 family interfere with the function of antiapoptotic members.

Studies on viral oncogenes also demonstrate a close association between proliferation and apoptosis in the regulation of cellular behavior. The E7 protein of oncogenic papillomaviruses, which are implicated in anogenital carcinomas, stimulates S-phase progression by inhibiting the function of the pl05Rb tumor suppressor. Similar to c-Myc, the overexpression of E7 alone induces apoptosis, which is mediated, at least in part, by the p53 tumor suppressor. Papillomaviruses encode a second oncoprotein, E6, that targets p53 for degradation and thus inhibits p53-dependent cell cycle arrest and apoptosis. Similarly, adenoviruses encode the E1A oncoprotein that interferes with pl05Rb function while the E1B 55-kDa gene product inhibits p53. In addition, the E1B 19-kDa protein encodes a Bcl-2 homologue. These two examples demonstrate that viruses have evolved to express genes that interfere with the two main cellular processes, proliferation and apoptosis, thereby promoting neoplastic growth.

Immunosuppression and Tumor Formation: A New Suspicion

As the focus of this book outlines, long-term treatment of transplant patients with immunosuppressive drugs like cyclosporine A (CsA) can increase a patient's risk of contracting cancer. While this is thought to be a consequence of the patient's suppressed immune system, recent data indicate that immunosuppressive drugs not only compromise immune defense against spontaneously arising tumor cells, but may also directly contribute to tumor formation. This latter mechanism is mediated by CsA selectively affecting gene expression in cells of the body. Two recent studies add new facets to this concept. In one case, CsA was shown to induce expression of the gene encoding the transforming growth factor β molecule (TGF-β) [26]. This signaling molecule promotes the spread and invasion of tumor cells, thereby potentially contributing to tumor progression. In a second study, CsA was shown to inhibit the transcriptional induction of the *pol β* gene, which encodes the DNA repair enzyme DNA polymerase β [27]. In primary human blood cells, treatment with CsA reduced *pol β* gene expression at both the mRNA and protein levels. Pol β is the major enzyme in a base excision repair pathway responsible for correction of DNA damage induced by depurination. The hypothesis was advanced that CsA-mediated inhibition of the biosynthesis of DNA repair enzymes could result in enhanced mutation frequencies leading to cancer-promoting genetic lesions.

References

1   Hunter T: Oncoprotein networks. Cell 1997;88:333–346.
2   Alberts B, Bray D, Johson A, Lewis J, Raff M, Roberts K, Walter P: Essential Cell Biology. New York, Garland Publishing, 1998.
3   Treisman RT: Regulation by MAP kinases. Curr Opin Cell Biol 1996;8:205–215.
4   Sebolt-Leopold JS, Dudley DT, Herrera R, Van Becelaere K, Wiland A, Gowan RC, Tecle H, Barrett SD, Bridges A, Przybranowski S, Leopold WR, Saltiel AR: Blockade of the MAP kinase pathway suppresses growth of colon tumors in vivo. Nat Med 1999;5:810–816.
5   Eastman Q, Grosschedl R: Regulation of LEF-1/TCF transcription factors by Wnt and other signals. Curr Opin Cell Biol 1999;11:233–240.

6   Peifer M: p-Catenin as oncogene: The smoking gun. Science 1997;275:1752–1753.
7   Vogelstein B, Kinzler KW: The Genetic Basis of Human Cancer. New York, McGraw-Hill, 1998.
8   Morgan DO: Cyclin-dependent kinases: Engines, clocks, and microprocessors. Annu Rev Cell Dev Biol 1997;13:261–291.
9   Sherr CJ, Roberts JM: CDK inhibitors: Positive and negative regulators of G_1-phase progression. Genes Dev 1999;13:1501–1512.
10 Sherr CJ: Cancer cell cycles. Science 1996;274:1672–1677.
11 Elledge SJ: Cell cycle checkpoints: Preventing an identity crisis. Science 1996;274: 1664–1672.
12 Russell P: Checkpoints on the road to mitosis. Trends Biochem Sci 1998;23:399–402.
13 Fearon ER, Vogelstein B: A genetic model for colorectal tumorigenesis. Cell 1990;61: 759–767.
14 Knudsons AG: Mutation and cancer – statistical study of retinoblastoma. Proc Natl Acad Sci USA 1971;68:820–823.
15 Mulligan G, Jacks T: The retinoblastoma gene family: Cousins with overlapping interests. Trends Genet 1998;14:223–229.
16 Levine AJ: p53, the cellular gatekeeper for growth and division. Cell 1997;88:323–331.
17 Mowat MRA: p53 in tumor progression: Life, death, and everything. Adv Cancer Res 1998;74:25–48.
18 Wood RD: DNA repair in eukaryotes. Annu Rev Biochem 1996;65:135–167.
19 Jiricny J: Replication errors: Cha(lle)nging the genome. EMBO J 1998;17:6427–6436.
20 de Laat WL, Jaspers NGJ, Hoeijmakers JHJ: Molecular mechanism of nucleotide excision repair. Genes Dev 1998;13:768–785.
21 Kanaar R, Hoeijmakers JHJ, van Gent DC: Molecular mechanisms of DNA double-strand break repair. Trends Cell Biol 1998;8:483–489.
22 Wyllie AH: The genetic regulation of apoptosis. Curr Opin Genet Dev 1995;5:97–104.
23 Thompson CB: Apoptosis in the pathogenesis and treatment of disease. Science 1995;267:1456–1462.
24 Martin SJ: Apoptosis and Cancer: An Overview. Basel, Karger Landes Systems, 1998.
25 Cryns V, Yuan J: Proteases to die for. Genes Dev 1998;12:1551–1570.
26 Hojo M, Morimoto T, Maluccio M, Asano T, Morimoto K, Lagman M, Shimbo T, Suthanthiran M: Cyclosporine induces cancer progression by a cell-autonomous mechanism. Nature 1999;397:530–534.
27 Ahlers C, Kreideweiß S, Nordheim A, Rühlmann A: Cyclosporin A inhibits Ca^{++}-mediated upregulation of the DNA repair enzyme DNA polymerase β in human PBMCs. Eur J Biochem 1999;264:1–9.

Prof. Dr. Alfred Nordheim, Abteilung und Lehrstuhl für Molekularbiologie, Eberhard-Karls-Universität Tübingen, Auf der Morgenstelle 15, D–72076 Tübingen (Germany)
Tel. +49 7071 29-78898, Fax -5359, E-mail alfred.nordheim@uni-tuebingen.de

Prof. Dr. B. Lüscher, Institut für Mikrobiologie, Medizinische Hochschule Hannover, Carl-Neuberg-Str. 1, D–30625 Hannover (Germany)
Tel. +49 511 532-4585, Fax -4283, E-mail Luscher.Bernhard@mh-hannover.de

Rüther U, Nunnensiek C, Schmoll H-J (eds): Secondary Neoplasias following Chemotherapy, Radiotherapy, and Immunosuppression. Contrib Oncol. Basel, Karger, 2000, vol 55, pp 17–35

....

Herpesviruses in Secondary Tumorigenesis

Fritz Schwarzmann, Hans Wolf

Insitut für Medizinische Mikrobiologie und Hygiene, Universität Regensburg, Deutschland

Introduction

The World Health Organization estimates that 15–20% of malignancies involve infectious agents. In terms of their molecular analysis, most of the relevant data collected have been for virus-associated disease. In fact, viral involvement in tumorigenesis was suspected for communicable leukemia in chickens as far back as the early 1900s. Later, this hypothesis was verified for papillomaviruses in rabbits and for retroviruses, where molecular analysis of the retroviral genomes showed that the transforming regions were not specific for the viruses. They were found to come from cellular genomes and were seen only very rarely in natural isolates. These regions encoded for proteins whose properties had been altered by various mutations in the tumor cells.

These alterations were significant enough to disrupt control of the cell cycle – even independently of altered intensity or kinetics of expression. This, in turn, benefited cell growth. The genes mutated in this manner were then absorbed at random into the genomes of retroviruses undergoing retroviral replication. It was discovered, moreover, that expression of these sequences, termed oncogenes, was not essential for these viruses to proliferate.

The same appears to apply to *human* tumorigenesis: The direct transduction of such oncogenes seems to play only a subordinate role in the development of malignancy in humans. Even so, knowledge of this function was a prerequisite to learning how cells transform. In the meantime, thanks to the molecular biological analysis of various tumors and transforming retroviruses, many of the homologous cellular, unaltered genes have been identified that are key to regulation of the cell cycle and cell differentiation (table 1). We now know that deregulation, mutation, deletion or func-

Table 1. Selected categories of retroviral oncogenes

	Oncogenes	Retrovirus
Growth factors	Sis	Simian sarcoma virus
Signal receptors and tyrosine kinases	ErbB	Avian erythroblastosis virus
	Fms	Feline sarcoma virus
Tyrosine kinases, membrane-associated	Src	Rous sarcoma virus
	Abl	Abelson murine leukemia virus
G proteins	Ras	Rat sarcoma virus
Protein kinases in cytoplasm	Mos	Moloney murine sarcoma virus
Nuclear proteins and transcription factors	Jun	ASV17
	Fos	FBJ murine osteosarcoma virus
Hormone receptors	ErbA	AEV-ES4

tional deactivation of these genes are important steps in transforming a benign cell that has been immortalized by virus into a malignant tumor cell.

The viruses known to be associated with human malignancy do not evince any genes comparable to the oncogenes described above. However, some have proteins that cause the cell cycle to be overridden – either via other mechanisms or through interaction with cellular regulator proteins (table 2). In contrast to oncogenes of cellular origin, these viral factors are essential for the replication of these viruses. Such viral factors include the regulatory proteins E6 and E7 of the papillomaviruses, and the Epstein-Barr virus' latent membrane protein 1 (LMP-1), which is localized in the membrane of the infected cell.

Two cellular control proteins of the cell cycle, retinoblastoma tumor suppressor protein pRB (p105) and protein p53 [Levine, 1990; Weinberg, 1991], are the best-researched targets of modulation by human pathogenic viruses. These proteins exert a complex influence on cell cycle control. Like the oncogenes described above, they were discovered during molecular biological analysis of tumors. There, they are often deleted, or appear in mutated forms.

The infectious viral agents that use these effects on the cell cycle to their own advantage usually persist in the organism for long periods. It follows that they must be able to draw on mechanisms enabling them, in the infected cells, to replicate the viral genome – but without synthesis of infectious successor viruses. Only thus will they live on in the daughter cells after the host cells divide. This is facilitated either by (1) integration of the viral genomes into the genetic information of the host cell, or (2) by more or less cell-synchronous extrachromosomal replication. In addition, lytic viral replication in the induced cells must normally be inhibited before cells can transform.

Table 2. Viral oncogenic proteins

Virus	Cancer type	Target cells	Viral gene product	Cellular target genes
HTLV-1	Adult T-cell leukemia/lymphoma	T cells	Tax	↑CREB/CREM ↑ NF-κB, SRE
HPV	Various carcinomas	Epithelial cells	E6	↓ p53
			E7	↓ p105/pRB ↑ cyclins A/E ↓ p21/p27
EBV	Burkitt's lymphoma	B cells	BZLF-1	↓ p53
	Hodgkin's lymphoma T-cell lymphomas Immunoblastic lymphomas	B cells T cells B cells	LMP-1	↑ A20, bcl-2 ↑ NF-κB
	Nasopharyngeal carcinoma	Epithelial cells	v-bcl-2	↓ bax
HBV	Hepatocellular carcinoma	Hepatocytes	HBx	↑ c-fos, c-myc, IGF-II, ICAM-I
HCV	Hepatocellular carcinoma	Hepatocytes		
HHV-8	Kaposi's sarcoma Multicentric Castleman's disease	Spindle cells B cells	ORF72	↑ CDK6 ↓ p16, p21, p27
	Primary effusion lymphoma	B cells	vFLIP	↓ FLICE
			ORF16	↓ bax
			ORFK9/vIRF	↓ IFN

To avoid being eliminated by the organism, the persisting infectious agents must also prevent the immune system from recognizing infected cells. The agents consequently restrict expression of their viral genes to a level far below that of the productive phase of viral proliferation. Some viruses inhibit presentation of infectious-agent-specific proteins on antigen-presenting cells. They may, for example, inhibit proteolytic processing, the loading of MHC molecules with antigens, or their transport to the cell surface [Banks and Rouse, 1992]. Other viral proteins directly modulate the cellular (e.g., cytolytic T cells and NK cells) and humoral immune response. Other viruses counteract the apoptosis the infected cell induces in its response to cell cycle disruption. Viruses may also work against interferon-mediated antiviral and antiproliferative mechanisms. When coupled with an unceasing stimulation of cell proliferation, these mechanisms enable malignant cells to escape detection and elimination.

Epstein-Barr Virus (EBV)

In 1964, Epstein and Barr used the electron microscope to study a culture of African Burkitt's lymphoma cells, and became the first to detect EBV [Epstein and Barr, 1964]. Later, EBV was identified as the agent of infectious mononucleosis, a self-limiting lymphoproliferative disorder when first contracted from the virus. It is caused, on the one hand, by the proliferation of EBV-infected B cells. This, in turn, escalates proliferation of reactive, primarily (up to 70%) EBV-specific T cells. In the course of resolution, most virally infected cells are eliminated, but latent EBV persists in quiescent memory B cells for the rest of the host's life [Qu and Rowe, 1992; Decker et al., 1996; Miyashita et al., 1995; Babcock et al., 1998, 1999]. At certain sites in the body, such as in the parotid gland [Wolf et al., 1984] or in esophagopharyngeal lympho-epithelial tissue [Sixbey et al., 1984; Tao et al., 1995a, b], lytic viral replication and production of infectious viral particles continue during the life-long phase of persistence. These infectious particles are then excreted in saliva [Yao et al., 1985a, b].

EBV-Associated Tumors

EBV has been linked to a number of malignancies (table 3). Nevertheless, despite certain cases where a virus is known to be associated with a tumor, the virus' role in pathogenesis is not irrefutable until it has been detected in the tumor cells and proven essential to the cell's transformation. Using in situ hybridization, EBV was proven to accompany nasopharyngeal carcinoma regularly [Wolf et al., 1973]. Interestingly, the fully undifferentiated nonkeratinized form of nasopharyngeal carcinoma is 100% EBV-positive, although EBV infection need not necessarily result in genesis of such tumors, nor of other, nonmalignant diseases. Rather, the virus persists in most persons with intact immune systems asymptomatically for the rest of their lives.

EBV-associated diseases involving proliferation of the infected cells develop where immunologic control of the virally infected cells is insufficient. Under these conditions, the number of viremic cells in peripheral blood increases. The latest findings show that immunosuppressed cases in which proliferative illness has not yet developed usually involve latently infected, quiescent B cells [Babcock et al., 1999]. In these cases, however, EBV's ability to immortalize B cells (that is, to spur their endless proliferation) frequently generates polyclonal, initially benign, proliferations – that later develop into oligoclonal and monoclonal malignant diseases.

Because tumorigenesis is a multistep process, it is possible that viruses play a crucial role only in certain stages. For instance, in a compromised immune system, EBV might raise the number of EBV-positive proliferating cells such that additional mutations – some of which would be caused by differentiation – would lead to a malignant phenotype. This phenotype would be determined primarily by cellular genes.

Experimental models have been developed far enough here to explain even hit-and-run mechanisms. These are mechanisms behind the complete disappearance, in

Table 3. EBV-associated malignancies

Disease	Association with EBV
Associated with lytic infection	
Infectious mononucleosis	
Chronic active infections	100%
AIDS-related hairy leukoplakia	
Associated with primarily latent infection and proliferation	
of the infected cells	
Immunoblastic lymphomas	70–100%
T-cell lymphomas	40–100%
Burkitt's lymphoma	
Endemic	>95%
Nonendemic	15–25%
Nasopharyngeal carcinoma (well-differentiated)	
High-risk areas	100%
Rest of the world	100%
Hodgkin's disease, various forms	40–90%

tumor cells, of the genes specific for the infectious agent. Such models have helped to show that although the role of EBV in tumorigenesis is not yet fully understood, the virus appears to contribute directly by altering cell cycle regulation and the immune system's detection of infected cells.

Posttransplant Lymphoproliferative Disorders

After organ transplantation with subsequent immunosuppression or after bone marrow transplantation with T-cell depletion, a number of lymphoproliferative disorders may occur. For example, recipients not infected by EBV until after organ or bone marrow transplantation are especially at risk of contracting EBV-associated lymphoproliferation. The same holds true for EBV-positive recipients who experience lasting reactivation of active lytic viral proliferation [Ho et al., 1985, 1988; Randhawa et al., 1990; Randhawa and Yousem, 1990].

Posttransplantation lymphoproliferative disorders can be divided morphologically and molecularly into three groups [Knowles, 1995]: (1) plasmocytic hyperplasia, or diffuse reactive plasma cell hyperplasia, is a polyclonal disorder. Studies of the EBV genomes in infected cells disclosing a heterogeneous number of terminal repeat sequences in the region of the circularized ends of the genomes point towards multiple infectious events. This, in turn, indicates polyclonality of the cell population. As a rule, no mutations of known oncogenes or tumor suppressor genes are to be detected. (2) Polymorphous B-cell hyperplasia, or polyclonal B-cell lymphoma, is oligoclonal or monoclonal, and can be traced to one, or only a few, events of immortalization. Further mutations in oncotropic cellular genes are not demonstrable here. Immunoblastic lymphomas and multiple myelomas are monoclonal. (3) Also, mutations are very frequently found, such as in the gene for c-myc, n-ras or bcl-6, as are various forms of trisomy (chromosomes 9 or 11) [Lyons and Liebowitz, 1998]. These disorders are usually progressive. Without therapy, polyclonal benign plasmocytic hyperplasia develops into a monoclonal malignant immunoblastic lymphoma.

In all three categories described above, EBV-associated lymphoproliferative disorders after organ transplantation usually express completely all 12 possible viral gene products expressed during latency. This indicates that the viral genes are necessary for immortalization and proliferation of the cells.

AIDS-Associated Non-Hodgkin's Lymphoma (AIDS-NHL)

AIDS-NHLs are usually of B-cell origin [Ziegler et al., 1984; Caligiuri et al., 1987]. As is the case after organ transplantation, polyclonal forms will develop into oligoclonal and monoclonal ones without therapy. In addition, AIDS patients very often evince CNS immunoblastic lymphomas. In contrast to the situation for immunosuppression after organ transplantation, AIDS-NHL is not as distinctly associated with EBV [Hamilton Dutoit et al., 1991a, b; Pedersen et al., 1991; Shiramizu et al., 1992]. This indicates that EBV is only one of several possible pathogenic factors triggering lymphoproliferative disorders.

EBV-Associated T-Cell Lymphomas

T cells are not the primary targets of EBV. Nevertheless, various T-cell lymphomas are clearly associated with EBV [Lee et al., 1996]. These include T-cell lymphocytosis in conjunction with a virus-associated hemophagocytic syndrome; nasal T-cell lymphomas, and peripheral T-cell lymphomas with an angioimmunoblastic lymphadenopathic appearance. In contrast to lymphoproliferative disorders after organ transplantation and in AIDS-NHL, not all of the viral genes of latency that are possible are actually expressed. Instead, only a restricted group is expressed (EBNA-1, LMP-1 and LMP-2; Lat-II), as is the case for nasopharyngeal carcinoma.

Leiomyosarcoma

Only rarely have immunosuppressed children been reported with smooth muscle tumors [Lee et al., 1995; McClain et al., 1995]. In these cases, too, only viral genes of latency are expressed (EBNA-1, EBNA-2, LMP-2A; Lat-II).

Additional EBV-Associated Malignancies

There are certain other malignancies that are often or always associated with EBV. Secondary to primary infectious mononucleosis, they are thus termed secondary disorders of EBV. These are endemic Burkitt's lymphoma, various forms of

Hodgkin's lymphoma, and nasopharyngeal carcinoma [Lee et al., 1996]. These disorders, however, are not in the category of secondary neoplasms following iatrogenic immunosuppression.

Molecular Pathogenesis

Latent Infection

EBV can infect B lymphocytes latently and induce their unrestricted proliferation and growth (immortalization). During latency, the virus expresses up to 12 viral genes. These regulate viral gene expression, influence regulation of the cell cycle, and affect the immune system's ability to detect infected cells. The pattern of viral expression depends on cell type and differentiation (table 4). For example, in quiescent B cells, only membrane protein LMP-2 and EBER genes are produced (Lat-0). But in cultures of latently infected B cells (lymphoblastoid cell lines) and in periph-

Table 4. Latency of Epstein-Barr virus

Type of latency	EBNA promoter usage	Expressed gene products	Tissue or cell types
Lat-0	Qp	LMP-2A	Small resting PBL from healthy seropositives
Lat-I	Qp	EBNA-1 EBERs BARF-0 transcripts	Burkitt's lymphoma biopsy and freshly established LCL
Lat-II	Qp	EBNA-1 EBERs BARF-0 transcripts + LMP-1, LMP-2B, LMP-2A (Lat-IIa)	Nasopharyngeal carcinoma Hodgkin's lymphoma
		+EBNA-2 (Lat-IIb)	Smooth muscle tumor
Lat-III	Wp < 24 h	EBNA-1 to 6	LCL, PBL from infectious mononucleosis patients
	Cp > 24 h	LMP-1, LMP-2B, LMP-2A EBERs BARF-0 transcripts	Passaged BL cell lines Immunoblastic lymphoma

eral blood B cells, all 12 genes of the latency period are synthesized (Lat-III) during initial infection by the virus. An even more restricted and characteristic pattern of expression is found with nasopharyngeal carcinoma and Hodgkin's lymphoma (Lat-II), as well as in biopsies of Burkitt's lymphoma (Lat-I).

Expression of the latent gene products leads to immortalization of the infected B cells and to unrestricted growth in culture. Even so, these latently infected immortal cells differ from tumor cells in that the body's immune system can detect and destroy them. Unlike true tumor cells, these lymphoblastoid cells cannot generate lymphomas or tumors in thymus-aplastic nude mice. Of the maximum of 12 viral genes that EBV expresses during latency, 6 are essential for immortalization in vitro (EBNA-1, 2, 3A, 3C, 5 and LMP-1).

This is why all of the genes and gene products that help immortalize B cells in vivo and which enable these cells to persist in a functioning immune system are important in the pathogenesis of EBV-associated tumor disease.

Stimulation of the Cell Cycle and Inhibition of Apoptosis

EBV can infect both quiescent and proliferating B cells. By deploying various viral proteins, the virus disrupts the cell cycle and inhibits apoptosis of the infected cell (fig. 1). Surface molecule CD21, which is the receptor for complement factor C3d, is also the receptor for EBV on B and T cells. The virus binds to CD21 via membrane protein gp350/250. This interaction between gp350/250 and CD21 initially activates quiescent B cells, which enables expression of viral genes [Guy et al., 1986; Hurley and Thorley-Lawson, 1988; Sinclair et al., 1994].

The first viral gene products demonstrable in latently infected cells are EBNA-2 and EBNA-5 [Hitt et al., 1989; Rooney et al., 1989; Alfieri et al., 1991]. EBNA-2 is a regulatory transactivator protein. Its expression directly or indirectly increases several cellular (CD21, CD23, c-frg) and viral (LMP-1, LMP-2, EBNA-1) proteins. Here, the EBNA-2 protein does not bind directly to the target promoters, but indirectly, by interacting with cellular transcription factor RBPjk (CBF-1) [Henkel et al., 1994]. In the early phase of infection of B cells, EBNA-5 and EBNA-2 together cause cell cycle transition from quiescent phase G_0 to phase G_1 [Sinclair et al., 1994]. This shift into the G_1 phase correlates with the upregulation of the expression of cyclin D2. In the G_1 phase, cyclin D2 is associated with cyclin-dependent kinase cdk4. When cyclin D2 binds to pRb, it induces pRB's hyperphosphorylation and the subsequent transition from the G_1 to the S phase of the cell cycle. In its hypophosphorylated form, retinoblastoma suppressor protein pRb is associated with transcription factors E2F-1, -2, -3 and DP. Hyperphosphorylation releases both of the transcription factors. They then stimulate the genes which enable transition into the S phase of the cell cycle [reviewed in Weinberg, 1995].

How EBNA-5 works is, for the most part, unknown. In vitro experiments have shown that EBNA-5 interacts with pRb and p53 [Jiang et al., 1991]. Other DNA

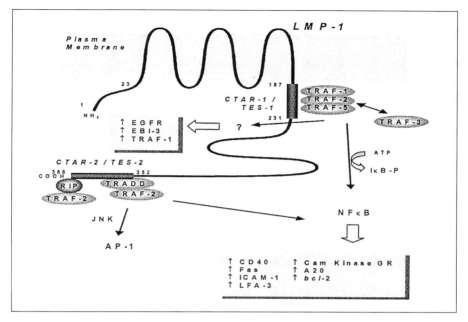

Fig. 1. The EBV LMP-1 works like a constitutively activated CD40 receptor. Its transactivating and transforming properties are mediated by domains CTAR/TES-1 and -2 (carboxy-terminal activation region/transforming effector site) in the carboxy-terminal region of the protein. These factors interact directly with several cellular factors (TRAF1, 2, 3, 4, 5, TRADD, and RIP), which are also bound by structurally and functionally related proteins such as TNF receptor and CD40. Target genes are regulated by activation of transcription factors NF-κB, AP-1, or other, unknown, factors. In epithelial cells, expression of EGFR is induced via the CTAR-1 domain.

viruses such as papilloma-, adeno-, and papovaviruses (SV40) also encode for proteins which interact with both p53 (E1B, T-Ag, E6) and pRb (E1A, T-Ag, E7) and which thus regulate the function of both factors for the cell cycle. Interaction with EBNA-5 has not yet been found to have any functional significance.

LMP-1 is a key membrane protein expressed in immortalized B cells and in some EBV-positive tumors (fig. 2). A shortened form may be found in lytically infected cells and in infectious virus particles. LMP-1 was the first EB-viral protein for which transforming properties were demonstrated [reviewed in Knecht et al., 1997]. In cell culture, LMP-1 can transform immortalized rodent cells and delay epithelial cell differentiation. LMP-1 is not expressed in Burkitt's lymphoma. In those cases, chromosomal translocations (c-myc site on chromosome 8q24 and immunoglobulin genes on chromosomes 2, 8 and 22) alter regulation of cellular genes (c-myc). This altered regulation results in the malignant transformation in Burkitt's lymphoma and derived cells. Apparently, viral factors are not involved here. A better grasp of the mechanism at work is described in de Thè [1993].

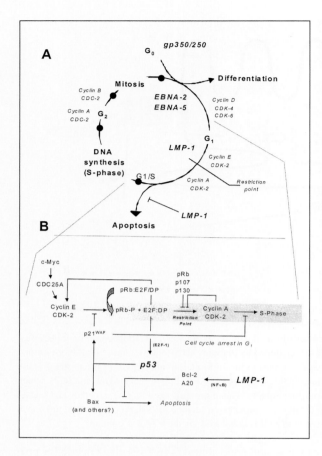

Fig. 2. **A** EBV proteins modulate the replicative cycle and inhibit apoptosis of the latently infected cells. **B** EBV's latent membrane protein 1 inhibits p53-mediated apoptosis via induction of bcl-2 and A20. p53, a cellular protein, intervenes in the cell cycle at two key positions. First, it induces $p21^{WAF}$, an inhibitor of cyclin-dependent kinase 2 (CDK-2). The resulting inhibition of CDK-2 blocks the hyperphosphorylation of pRB and of related factors p107/p130. This, in turn, inhibits release of transcription factors E2F and DP. The cell cycle is thereby arrested at the restriction point and at the G_1/S control point. Second, by inducing bax, p53 induces apoptosis. Viral membrane protein LMP-1 inhibits p53-mediated apoptosis via induction of cellular antiapoptotic factors bcl-2 and A20. LMP-1, on the other hand, has no affect on $p21^{WAF}$-mediated functions.

Epidemiologic studies do indicate, however, EBV involvement in nasopharyngeal carcinogenesis [Zeng et al., 1982, 1983] and in Burkitt's lymphoma [de Thè et al., 1978], since considerably elevated EBV titers precede these diseases. Early presence of EBV in conjunction with, for example, malarially induced overproliferation of B cells could foster the chromosomal translocations typical of Burkitt's lymphoma [de Thè, 1993].

At the molecular level, LMP-1 belongs to the family of TNF receptor-like proteins (TNF receptor, CD40, lymphotoxin receptor). After interacting with their extracellular ligands (TNF, CD40 ligand, lymphotoxin), these cellular receptor molecules aggregate in the membrane into multimers. Via a further protein interaction with intracellular protein kinases, they set off a signal cascade. LMP-1, however, differs from the above-mentioned receptor molecules because it does not need this extracellular interaction to aggregate in the membrane and to bind protein kinases

[Mosialos et al., 1995]. LMP-1 is therefore a constitutively active receptor whose function correlates with that of the activated CD40 receptor [Kilger et al., 1998]. Both membrane proteins can substitute for one another as activators of B cells.

LMP-1 works by interacting with cellular cytoplasmic factors which also bind to the proteins of the family of TNF receptor proteins [Mosialos et al., 1995] (fig. 2). Causing this interaction are two areas in the carboxy-terminal region of the protein which interact with different factors: CTAR/TES-1 and -2 (carboxy-terminal activation region / transformation effector site) [Huen et al., 1995; Mitchell and Sugden, 1995]. A conserved PXQXT/S motif in the CTAR-1 region is the binding site for various factors of the TRAF family (TNF receptor-associated factor). Direct binding of TRAF1, 2 and 5 leads to expression of transcription factor NF-κB [Brodeur et al., 1997; Devergne et al., 1998; Mosialos et al., 1995; Sandberg et al., 1997]. TRAF3, on the other hand, appears to act as a negative regulatory factor that impedes binding of the other TRAFs.

The CTAR-2 region, which also acts via activation of NF-κB, is mediated, on the other hand, by the binding of TRADD (TNF receptor 1-associated death domain protein) and RIP (Fas receptor interacting protein). These, in turn, interact with TRAF2 [Eliopoulos et al., 1999a, b]. Direct or indirect recruiting of TRAF2 leads to activation of NIK and IκB kinase, phosphorylation of IκB, and finally to activation of NF-κB. It is via this recruitment that both CTAR domains are involved in the up-regulation of activation markers CD40, ICAM-1, LFA-3 and Fas. NF-κB, however, also induces expression of a calcium/calmodulin-dependent protein kinase, camkinase GR [Mosialos et al., 1994], interleukin (IL)-6, and a 40-kDa-sized IL-12-like factor [Devergne et al., 1996]. NF-κB additionally induces expression of the two antiapoptotic proteins A20 and bcl-2 [Henderson et al., 1991; Laherty et al., 1992; Murray et al., 1988; Wang et al., 1990a, b].

The CTAR-1 region also induces expression of TRAF1, an EBV-induced protein, EBI3, as well as the receptor for epidermal growth factor EGFR in epithelial cells. The CTAR-2 domain activates transcription factor AP-1 via c-Jun-N-terminal kinase (JNK) or via a stress-activated protein kinase [Eliopoulos et al., 1999a, b].

A major difference between LMP-1 and the TNF receptor is that LMP-1 cannot trigger apoptosis, while TNFR can, even though both proteins bind FADD. The reason may be that LMP-1's FADD binding site in its CTAR/TES-2 domain is markedly smaller than that of TNFR's. It is hypothesized that CTAR/TES-2 interacts with only one part of the functional FADD domain [Izumi et al., 1999]. This would mean that LMP-1 triggers only those actions which stimulate cell proliferation, but not those that induce apoptosis, as is the case when FADD binds to TNFR.

Not only can LMP-1 activate the cell cycle, it can also actively inhibit cell apoptosis. Its molecular target here is the p53 protein, which can negatively regulate the cell cycle in two ways [review in Lundberg and Weinberg, 1999] (fig. 2B): (1) p53 can respond to damage to DNA by triggering increased expression of p21 and mdm-2, which both have an inhibitory effect on the cyclin-dependent protein kinases (CDK) during the G_1 phase. This arrests the cell cycle in the G_1 phase – an action which LMP-1 is unable to block. (2) However, p53 protein can also induce cell apoptosis. LMP-1, in turn, can upregulate bcl-2 and A20 [Henderson et al., 1991; Laherty et al., 1992], two proteins which act antiapoptotically. A20 disrupts apoptosis in epithelial cells [Fries et al., 1996]; and A20 and bcl-2 disrupt it in B cells (fig. 2B).

EBNA-1 protein is expressed in every EBV-infected proliferating cell, and therefore in every EBV-positive tumor cell. Although its role is not as clearly understood [reviewed in Lee et al., 1996], EBNA-1 is known to be involved in cell immortalization and thus indirectly in cell transformation, since it safeguards the replication of the viral genome and its distribution among the daughter cells. In addition, EBNA-1 can regulate transcription and expression of the other EBNA proteins. A few years ago, experiments on transgenic mice directly demonstrated EBNA-1's transforming ability – although such proof has thus far been limited to the mouse model [Wilson et al., 1996].

Modulation of the Immune System

Unlike tumor cells, immortalized B cells in vivo can be detected and eliminated by the immune system. However, a few genes and proteins of the latent period possess properties that impede immune system detection of infected cells. EB-viral transcripts EBER-1 and EBER-2, two short, untranslated transcripts of polymerase III, are structurally similar to RNAs VA-1 and VA-2 in adenovirally infected cells. EBER-1 and -2 were therefore assumed to inhibit the antiviral and antiproliferative effects of interferon. In vitro it was observed that by binding to interferon-induced protein kinase DAI/PKR, EBER-1 prevents autophosphorylation of the enzyme. This can inhibit interferon's activity [Sharp et al., 1993]. However, investigations involving recombinant EBVs without EBER genes showed, at least in cell culture, unrestricted growth of infected cells and lytic proliferation of the recombinant viruses. The possibility of a correlating function in vivo cannot be excluded. Thus, the role of the EBER transcripts in EBV latency and in transforming infected cells in vivo remains unexplained [reviewed in Clemens, 1994].

Cytolytic T cells and antibody-dependent cellular cytotoxic mechanisms can detect EB-virally infected tumor cells. A viral homologue with IL-10 (vIL-10, reading frame BCRF-1) is almost completely homologous functionally with cellular IL-10 [Hsu et al., 1990; Rousset et al., 1992]. IL-10 is secreted by type Th-2 T-helper cells. It directs the organism's immune reaction away from a cellular cytolytic response by its cytolytic T cells, and towards an antibody response.

Finally, multiple repetition of a glycine-alanine motif renders viral protein EBNA-1, which is expressed in every EBV-infected proliferating cell, unfit for processing by proteasomes. As a consequence, EBNA-1 cannot be presented to the cellular immune system in conjunction with MHC class 1 molecules [Levitskaya et al., 1995]. And since expression of the viral genes is in general severely restricted, it is harder for EBV-specific cytolytic T cells to detect and eliminate them.

Human Herpesvirus 8 (HHV-8)
HHV-8 and Kaposi's Sarcoma (KS)

In 1994, Chang et al., using PCR (polymerase chain reaction), were the first to detect, in KS, the nucleic acid of a herpesvirus strongly homologous with EBV and HVS [Chang et al., 1994]. This came to be designated KS-associated herpesvirus (KSHV) or HHV-8. The classical form of KS is frequently found in older males in the Mediterranean region, the Middle East and Eastern Europe. It also appears endemically in certain regions of Africa. Recently, a third form was discovered that correlates with the appearance of AIDS. About 20% of all AIDS patients develop KS. Of these AIDS patients, homosexual men contract KS significantly more often than do heterosexual drug addicts, hemophiliacs, or persons who contracted AIDS through heterosexual contact. This is why KS was assumed to be transmitted sexually. Substantiating this hypothesis were the results of subsequent tests: 90% of all KS biopsies and 15% of all non-KS biopsies gained from AIDS patients were HHV-8-positive, while in control biopsies from persons without KS or HIV, HHV-8 was not detected. Regarding the classical form of KS, the frequency of occurrence of HHV-8 correlated with that of KS. In PCR tests in the United States and Northern Europe, 0% of those examined were found to have HHV-8; and using serologic methods, 0–3%. In Italy and Africa, on the other hand, about 10% were found positive using PCR, and 6–53% using serologic methods.

These molecular biologic and serologic investigations clearly point towards a causal relationship between HHV-8 and development of KS. Accordingly, detection of HHV-8 in peripheral blood cells is a marker for imminent KS. Persons who developed KS were found to have undergone HHV-8 seroconversion a few weeks before.

Sexual intercourse appears to be the main method of transmission of AIDS-associated KS. A study of children in Eastern and Southern Africa, however, showed significant infiltration of children aged 2–12 years. Here, the incidence of KS correlates with evidence of HBV infection. Since HBV is transmitted not only by blood contact but also sexually and perinatally, perinatal transmission is most likely the main route here. The virus has also been detected in saliva and buccal mucosa, indicating additional transmission pathways.

Other Tumors Associated with HHV-8

HHV-8 appears to be involved in two additional lymphoproliferative disorders: primary effusion lymphoma (body cavity-based lymphoma) and multicentric Castelman's disease.

Molecular Pathogenesis

HHV-8 targets endothelial and spindle cells, B and T cells, macrophages and certain epithelial tissues. Long-term cultivation of HHV-8-positive cells is possible with PEL, and often demonstrates simultaneous EBV infection. These cells are latently infected by HHV-8, and the genome is circular and episomal. Only a few genes are expressed during this latency period [Schulz, 1998].

Viral reading frame ORF72 homologizes with cellular cyclin D2. D-type cyclins are the link between the receptor-activated signal cascades and the cell cycle. When D-type cyclins interact with cyclin-dependent kinases CDK4 and CDK6, transcription factors E2F and DP are induced, and thereafter cyclins E and A. This launches the phase of DNA synthesis. Viral cyclin D can interact with CDK6 and thereby override control of the cell cycle. Under these circumstances, the vcyclin-CDK6 functional complex cannot be inhibited by the usual CDK inhibitors – p16, p21 and p27.

The cell responds to nonphysiologic stimulation of its cycle by initiating apoptosis. Viruses able to override the cell cycle, such as papillomaviruses, EBV or HHV-8, have developed mechanisms to block apoptosis of the infected cell. vFLIP is a viral inhibitor of FLICE, a mediator of cellular apoptosis. Two domains of vFLIP evince homology with death effector domains (DED) of the cellular proteins FADD (MORT1) and FLICE. After interaction of the fas-receptor/CD95 molecule or of the TNF receptors with their extracellular ligands, these domains mediate interaction between factors FADD and FLICE. This usually leads to apoptosis. vFLIP, however, inhibits activation of FLICE and thus that of apoptosis.

Several other viral genes homologous with cellular factors have been identified that are involved in regulation of the cell cycle or of the immune response. These include glycosylated transmembrane proteins with transforming properties (orfK1); viral homologues with various cytokines, such as IL-6 (vIL-6, orfK2), IL-8 receptor (orf74), MIP-1α (vMIP-I, orfK6; vMIP-II, orfK4); a viral homologue with bcl-2 (orf16), and possibly a viral inhibitor of interferon (vIRF, orfK9) [as in Schulz, 1998].

Diagnosis, Therapy and Prevention of HHV-8-Associated Tumors

Seroepidemiologic studies have established a definite causal relationship between HHV-8 infection and development of KS. Direct proof of HHV-8 in peripheral blood cells (using PCR), as well as indirect serologic evidence via HHV-8-specific antibodies, can indicate imminent development or presence of KS.

Therapy of KS traditionally entails tumor removal through excision or cryotherapy. For HIV-associated KS, a three-prong therapy primarily targeting HIV has proven useful. Vaccine for HHV-8 has yet to be developed.

References

Alfieri C, Birkenbach M, Kieff E: Early events in Epstein-Barr virus infection of human B lymphocytes. Virology 1991;181: 595–608 [Erratum: Virology 1991;185:946].

Babcock GJ, Decker LL, Freeman RB, Thorley-Lawson, DA: Epstein-Barr virus-infected resting memory B cells, not proliferating lymphoblasts, accumulate in the peripheral blood of immunosuppressed patients. J Exp Med 1999;190:567–576.

Babcock GJ, Decker LL, Volk M, Thorley-Lawson DA: EBV persistence in memory B cells in vivo. Immunity 1998;9:395–404.

Banks TA, Rouse BT: Herpesviruses – immune escape artists? Clin Infect Dis 1992;14:933–941.

Brodeur SR, Cheng G, Baltimore D, Thorley-Lawson DA: Localization of the major NF-κB-activating site and the sole TRAF3 binding site of LMP-1 defines two distinct signaling motifs. J Biol Chem 1997;272:19777–19784.

Caligiuri M, Murray C, Buchwald D, Levine H, Cheney P, Peterson D, Komaroff AL, Ritz J: Phenotypic and functional deficiency of natural killer cells in patients with chronic fatigue syndrome. J Immunol 1987;139:3306–3313.

Chang Y, Cesarman E, Pessin MS, Lee F, Culpepper J, Knowles DM, Moore PS: Identification of herpesvirus-like DNA sequences in AIDS-associated Kaposi's sarcoma. Science 1994;266: 1865–1869.

Clemens MJ: Functional significance of the Epstein-Barr virus-encoded small RNAs. Epstein Barr Virus Rep 1994;5:107–111.

De Thè G: The etiology of Burkitt's lymphoma and the history of the shaken dogmas. Blood Cells 1993;19:667–673.

De Thè G, Geser A, Day NE, Tukei PM, Williams EH, Beri DP, Smith PG, Dean AG, Bronkamm GW, Feorino P, Henle W: Epidemiological evidence for causal relationship between Epstein-Barr virus and Burkitt's lymphoma from Ugandan prospective study. Nature 1978;274: 756–761.

Decker LL, Klamen LD, Thorley-Lawson DA: Detection of the latent form of Epstein-Barr virus DNA in the peripheral blood of healthy individuals. J Virol 1996;70:3286–3289.

Devergne O, Hummel M, Koeppen H, Le Beau MM, Nathanson EC, Kieff E, Birkenbach M: A novel interleukin-12 p40-related protein induced by latent Epstein-Barr virus infection in B lymphocytes. J Virol 1996;70:1143–1153 [Erratum: J Virol 1996;70:2678].

Devergne O, McFarland EC, Mosialos G, Izumi KM, Ware CF, Kieff E: Role of the TRAF binding site and NF-κB activation in Epstein-Barr virus latent membrane protein 1-induced cell gene expression. J Virol 1998;72:7900–7908.

Eliopoulos AG, Blake SM, Floettmann JE, Rowe M, Young LS: Epstein-Barr virus-encoded latent membrane protein 1 activates the JNK pathway through its extreme C terminus via a mechanism involving TRADD and TRAF2. J Virol 1999a;73:1023–1035.

Eliopoulos AG, Gallagher NJ, Blake SM, Dawson CW, Young LS: Activation of the p38 mitogen-activated protein kinase pathway by Epstein-Barr virus-encoded latent membrane protein 1 coregulates interleukin-6 and interleukin-8 production. J Biol Chem 1999b;274:16085–16096.

Epstein MA, Barr YM: Virus particles in cultured lymphoblasts from Burkitt's lymphoma. Lancet 1964;i:702–703.

Fries KL, Miller WE, Raab-Traub N: Epstein-Barr virus latent membrane protein 1 blocks p53-mediated apoptosis through the induction of the A20 gene. J Virol 1996;70:8653–8659.

Guy GR, Gordon J, Walker L, Michell RH, Brown G: Redistribution and activation of protein kinase C during mitogenesis of human B lymphocytes. Biochem Biophys Res Commun 1986; 135:146–153.

Hamilton Dutoit SJ, Delecluse HJ, Raphael M, Lenoir G, Pallesen G: Detection of Epstein-Barr virus genomes in AIDS related lymphomas: Sensitivity and specificity of in situ hybridisation compared with Southern blotting. J Clin Pathol 1991a;44:676–680.

Hamilton Dutoit SJ, Pallesen G, Franzmann MB, Karkov J, Black F, Skinhoj P, Pedersen, C: AIDS-related lymphoma. Histopathology, immunophenotype, and association with Epstein-Barr virus as demonstrated by in situ nucleic acid hybridization. Am J Pathol 1991b;138:149–163.

Henderson S, Rowe M, Gregory C, Croom Carter D, Wang F, Longnecker R, Kieff E, Rickinson A: Induction of bcl-2 expression by Epstein-Barr virus latent membrane protein 1 protects infected B cells from programmed cell death. Cell 1991;65:1107–1115.

Henkel T, Ling PD, Hayward SD, Peterson MG: Mediation of Epstein-Barr virus EBNA2 transactivation by recombination signal-binding protein J κ. Science 1994;265:92–95.

Hitt MM, Allday MJ, Hara T, Karran L, Jones MD, Busson P, Tursz T, Ernberg I, Griffin BE: EBV gene expression in an NPC-related tumour. EMBO J 1989;8:2639–2651.

Ho M, Jaffe R, Miller G, Breinig MK, Dummer JS, Makowka L, Atchison RW, Karrer F, Nalesnik MA, Starzl TE: The frequency of Epstein-Barr virus infection and associated lymphoproliferative syndrome after transplantation and its manifestations in children. Transplantation 1988;45:719–727.

Ho M, Miller G, Atchison RW, Breinig MK, Dummer JS, Andiman W, Starzl TE, Eastman R, Griffith BP, Hardesty RL: Epstein-Barr virus infections and DNA hybridization studies in post-transplantation lymphoma and lymphoproliferative lesions: The role of primary infection. J Infect Dis 1985;152:876–886.

Hsu DH, de Waal Malefyt R, Fiorentino DF, Dang MN, Vieira P, de Vries J, Spits H, Mosmann TR, Moore KW: Expression of interleukin-10 activity by Epstein-Barr virus protein BCRF1. Science 1990;250:830-832.

Huen DS, Henderson SA, Croom-Carter D, Rowe M: The Epstein-Barr virus latent membrane protein-1 mediates activation of NF-κB and cell surface phenotype via two effector regions in its carboxy-terminal cytoplasmic domain. Oncogene 1995;10:549–560.

Hurley EA, Thorley-Lawson DA: B cell activation and the establishment of Epstein-Barr virus latency. J Exp Med 1988;168:2059–2075.

Izumi KM, McFarland EC, Ting AT, Riley EA, Seed B, Kieff ED: The Epstein-Barr virus oncoprotein latent membrane protein 1 engages the tumor necrosis factor receptor-associated proteins TRADD and receptor-interacting protein (RIP) but does not induce apoptosis or require RIP for NF-κB activation. Mol Cell Biol 1999;19:5759–5767.

Jiang WQ, Szekely L, Wendel-Hansen V, Ringertz N, Klein G, Rosen A: Co-localization of the retinoblastoma protein and the Epstein-Barr virus-encoded nuclear antigen EBNA-5. Exp Cell Res 1991;197:314–318.

Kilger E, Kieser A, Baumann M, Hammerschmidt W: Epstein-Barr virus-mediated B-cell proliferation is dependent upon latent membrane protein 1, which simulates an activated CD40 receptor. EMBO J 1998;17:1700–1709.

Knecht H, Berger C, al-Homsi AS, McQuain C, Brousset P: Epstein-Barr virus oncogenesis. Crit Rev Oncol Hematol 1997;26:117–135.

Knowles DM, Cesarman E, Chadburn A, Frizzera G, Chen J, Rose EA, Michler RE: Correlative morphologic and molecular genetic analysis demonstrates three distinct categories of post-transplantation lymphoproliferative disorders. Blood 1995;85:552–565.

Laherty CD, Hu HM, Opipari AW, Wang F, Dixit VM: The Epstein-Barr virus LMP1 gene product induces A20 zinc finger protein expression by activating nuclear factor κ B. J Biol Chem 1992;267:24157–24160.

Lee ES, Locker J, Nalesnik M, Reyes J, Jaffe R, Alashari M, Nour B, Tzakis A, Dickman PS: The association of Epstein-Barr virus with smooth-muscle tumors occurring after organ transplantation. N Engl J Med 1995;332:19–25.

Lee SP, Thomas WA, Blake NW, Rickinson AB: Transporter (TAP)-independent processing of a multiple membrane-spanning protein, the Epstein-Barr virus latent membrane protein 2. Eur J Immunol 1996;26:1875–1883.

Levine AJ: The p53 protein and its interactions with the oncogene products of the small DNA tumor viruses. Virology 1990;177:419–426.

Levitskaya J, Coram M, Levitsky V, Imreh S, Steigerwald-Mullen PM, Klein G, Kurilla MG, Masucci MG: Inhibition of antigen processing by the internal repeat region of the Epstein-Barr viral nuclear antigen-1. Nature 1995;375:685–688.

Lundberg AS, Weinberg RA: Control of the cell cycle and apoptosis. Eur J Cancer 1999;35:531–539.

Lyons SF, Liebowitz DN: The roles of human viruses in the pathogenesis of lymphoma. Semin Oncol 1998;25:461–475.

McClain KL, Leach CT, Jenson HB, Joshi VV, Pollock BH, Parmley RT, DiCarlo FJ, Chadwick EG, Murphy SB: Association of Epstein-Barr virus with leiomyosarcomas in children with AIDS. N Engl J Med 1995;332:12–18.

Mitchell T, Sugden B: Stimulation of NF-κB-mediated transcription by mutant derivatives of the latent membrane protein of Epstein-Barr virus. J Virol 1995;69:2968–2976.

Miyashita EM, Yang B, Lam KM, Crawford DH, Thorley Lawson DA: A novel form of Epstein-Barr virus latency in normal B cells in vivo. Cell 1995;80:593–601.

Mosialos G, Birkenbach M, Yalamanchili R, VanArsdale T, Ware C, Kieff E: The Epstein-Barr virus transforming protein LMP1 engages signaling proteins for the tumor necrosis factor receptor family. Cell 1995;80:389–399.

Mosialos G, Hanissian SH, Jawahar S, Vara L, Kieff E, Chatila TA: A Ca^{2+}/calmodulin-dependent protein kinase, CaM kinase-Gr, expressed after transformation of primary human B lymphocytes by Epstein-Barr virus (EBV) is induced by the EBV oncogene LMP1. J Virol 1994;68:1697–1705.

Murray RJ, Wang D, Young LS, Wang F, Rowe M, Kieff E, Rickinson AB: Epstein-Barr virus-specific cytotoxic T-cell recognition of transfectants expressing the virus-coded latent membrane protein LMP. J Virol 1988;62:3747–3755.

Pedersen C, Gerstoft J, Lundgren JD, Skinhoj P, Bottzauw J, Geisler C, Hamilton Dutoit SJ, Thorsen S, Lisse I, Ralfkiaer E, et al: HIV-associated lymphoma: Histopathology and association with Epstein-Barr virus genome related to clinical, immunological and prognostic features. Eur J Cancer 1991;27:1416–1423.

Qu L, Rowe DT: Epstein-Barr virus latent gene expression in uncultured peripheral blood lymphocytes. J Virol 1992;66:3715–3724.

Randhawa PS, Markin RS, Starzl TE, Demetris AJ: Epstein-Barr virus-associated syndromes in immunosuppressed liver transplant recipients. Clinical profile and recognition on routine allograft biopsy. Am J Surg Pathol 1990;14:538–547.

Randhawa PS, Yousem SA: Epstein-Barr virus-associated lymphoproliferative disease in a heart-lung allograft. Demonstration of host origin by restriction fragment-length polymorphism analysis. Transplantation 1990;49:126–130.

Rooney C, Howe JG, Speck SH, Miller G: Influence of Burkitt's lymphoma and primary B cells on latent gene expression by the nonimmortalizing P3J-HR-1 strain of Epstein-Barr virus. J Virol 1989;63:1531–1539.

Rousset F, Garcia E, Defrance T, Peronne C, Vezzio N, Hsu DH, Kastelein R, Moore KW, Banchereau J: Interleukin-10 is a potent growth and differentiation factor for activated human B lymphocytes. Proc Natl Acad Sci USA 1992;89:1890–1893.

Sandberg M, Hammerschmidt W, Sugden B: Characterization of LMP-1's association with TRAF1, TRAF2, and TRAF3. J Virol 1997;71:4649–4656.

Schulz TF: Kaposi's sarcoma-associated herpesvirus (human herpesvirus-8). J Gen Virol 1998;79: 1573–1591.

Sharp TV, Schwemmle M, Jeffrey I, Laing K, Mellor H, Proud CG, Hilse K, Clemens MJ: Comparative analysis of the regulation of the interferon-inducible protein kinase PKR by Epstein-Barr virus RNAs EBER-1 and EBER-2 and adenovirus VAI RNA. Nucleic Acids Res 1993; 21:4483–4490.

Shiramizu B, Herndier B, Meeker T, Kaplan L, McGrath M: Molecular and immunophenotypic characterization of AIDS-associated, Epstein-Barr virus-negative, polyclonal lymphoma. J Clin Oncol 1992;10:383–389.

Sinclair AJ, Palmero I, Peters G, Farrell PJ: EBNA-2 and EBNA-LP cooperate to cause G0 to G1 transition during immortalization of resting human B lymphocytes by Epstein-Barr virus. EMBO J 1994;13:3321–3328.

Sixbey JW, Nedrud JG, Raab Traub N, Hanes RA, Pagano JS: Epstein-Barr virus replication in oropharyngeal epithelial cells. N Engl J Med 1984;310:1225–1230.

Tao Q, Ho FC, Loke SL, Srivastava G: Epstein-Barr virus is localized in the tumour cells of nasal lymphomas of NK, T or B cell type. Int J Cancer 1995a;60:315–320.

Tao Q, Srivastava G, Chan AC, Chung LP, Loke SL, Ho FC: Evidence for lytic infection by Epstein-Barr virus in mucosal lymphocytes instead of nasopharyngeal epithelial cells in normal individuals. J Med Virol 1995b;45:71–77.

Wang F, Gregory C, Sample C, Rowe M, Liebowitz D, Murray R, Rickinson A, Kieff E: Epstein-Barr virus latent membrane protein (LMP1) and nuclear proteins 2 and 3C are effectors of phenotypic changes in B lymphocytes: EBNA-2 and LMP1 cooperatively induce CD23. J Virol 1990a;64:2309–2318.

Wang F, Tsang SF, Kurilla MG, Cohen JI, Kieff E: Epstein-Barr virus nuclear antigen 2 transactivates latent membrane protein LMP1. J Virol 1990b;64:3407–3416.

Weinberg RA: Tumor suppressor genes. Science 1991;254:1138–1146.

Weinberg RA: The molecular basis of oncogenes and tumor suppressor genes. Ann NY Acad Sci 1995;758:331–338.

Wilson JB, Bell JL, Levine AJ: Expression of Epstein-Barr virus nuclear antigen-1 induces B cell neoplasia in transgenic mice. EMBO J 1996;15:3117–3126.

Wolf H, Haus M, Wilmes E: Persistence of Epstein-Barr virus in the parotid gland. J Virol 1984;51: 795–798.

Wolf H, zur Hausen H, Becker V: EB viral genomes in epithelial nasopharyngeal carcinoma cells. Nature New Biol 1973;244:245–247.

Yao QY, Rickinson AB, Epstein MA: A re-examination of the Epstein-Barr virus carrier state in healthy seropositive individuals. Int J Cancer 1985a;35:35–42.

Yao QY, Rickinson AB, Epstein MA: Oropharyngeal shedding of infectious Epstein-Barr virus in healthy virus-immune donors. A prospective study. Chin Med J (Engl) 1985b;98:191–196.

Zeng Y, Zhang LG, Li HY, Jan MG, Zhang Q, Wu YC, Wang YS, Su GR: Serological mass survey for early detection of nasopharyngeal carcinoma in Wuzhou City, China. Int J Cancer 1982; 29:139–141.

Zeng Y, Zhong JM, Li LY, Wang PZ, Tang H, Ma YR, Zhu, JS, Pan WJ, Liu YX, Wei ZN: Follow-up studies on Epstein-Barr virus IgA/VCA antibody-positive persons in Zangwu County, China. Intervirology 1983;20:190–194.

Ziegler JL, Bragg K, Abrams D, Beckstead J, Cogan M, Volberding P, Baer D, Wilkinson L, Rosenbaum E, Grant K: High-grade non-Hodgkin's lymphoma in patients with AIDS. Ann N Y Acad Sci 1984;437:412–419.

PD Dr. Fritz Schwarzmann, Institut für Medizinische Mikrobiologie und Hygiene,
Franz-Josef-Strauß-Allee 11, D–93053 Regensburg (Germany)
E-mail Fritz.Schwarzmann@gmx.de

Rüther U, Nunnensiek C, Schmoll H-J (eds): Secondary Neoplasias following Chemotherapy, Radiotherapy, and Immunosuppression. Contrib Oncol. Basel, Karger, 2000, vol 55, pp 36–61

....

Carcinogenicity of Cytostatic Agents – Secondary Malignancy after Chemotherapy

W. Haussmann

Kliniken Landkreis Sigmaringen GmbH, Sigmaringen, Deutschland

Many pharmaceutical substances have mutagenic potential, as demonstrated by posttherapeutic studies on agents such as intercalating antibiotics or nitroimidazole derivatives like metronidazole, nimorazole or tinidazole.

In nitroimidazoles, mutagenicity stems from their mechanism of action: in predominantly anaerobic environments, reduction of the nitro group leads to formation of reactive intermediate products and hence destruction of essential cell components. Breaks in DNA strands and uncoiling of the double helix have been reported [1].

Of special note are the oncogenic and mutagenic characteristics of cytostatic agents, medications that can cause the same disorders they are intended to fight. To a varying degree, probably all cytostatic agents are potentially mutagenic, carcinogenic and teratogenic [1]. This is why pregnancy should be avoided not only during chemotherapy, but also for the first 2 years thereafter. Specialized literature must therefore state that their administration has led to chromosomal aberrations and that mutagenicity has been observed in cell cultures and animal tests. Information on carcinogenicity must state that certain tumors have been triggered, at least in animal tests. In addition, some cytostatic agents contain an immunosuppressive component which renders the organism unable to eliminate mutated cells sufficiently. This probably promotes secondary tumorigenesis after chemotherapy [2–5].

Ironically, it is the increase in survival time and overall remission rate after radio- and/or chemotherapy that has led to therapy-related secondary malignancy developing years after primary therapy. Aggravating this problem is that some secondary malignancies do not respond to the cytostatic agents effective for the corresponding de novo tumors, but require a completely different kind of therapy [6]. This dilemma has led some authors to conclude that the best 'therapy' of a cytostatically induced secondary tumor is its avoidance.

Not only chemotherapy is a risk. Experience has shown that radiotherapy can also induce tumors, with chemo- and/or radiotherapy-associated secondary malignancies usually occurring 5–10 years after the end of primary tumor therapy [7, 8]. For *radiotherapy,* there is no clear-cut dosage threshold for avoiding carcinogenesis. Here, it is primarily *solid secondary tumors* that develop; there are far fewer reports of secondary leukemia [9]. After *chemotherapy,* on the other hand, secondary malignancies are mainly *secondary acute myeloid leukemias (AML)* [10, 11]. Most of these secondary leukemias appear in the first 10 years after chemotherapy, especially after *alkylating agents or nitrosourea derivatives.* Of the alkylating agents, melphalan is thought to be the most leukemogenic [12–17].

As to tumorigenicity, the cumulative dose of the cytostatic agent probably plays a more important role than time. Also increasing risk are age over 40 years, the combination of chemotherapy and radiotherapy, and other risk factors such as *smoking, sex, Epstein-Barr virus, warts, sunshine,* etc. [18–22]. Complicating individual substance risk assessment is the administration of multiple cytostatic agents (polychemotherapy) and/or radiotherapy in addition [23].

Based on their characteristics, secondary malignancies, especially secondary leukemias, can be divided into *two types: Secondary leukemia after administration of alkylating agents* usually occurs about 5–7 years after chemotherapy; while secondary malignoma after therapy with *topoisomerase II inhibitors, such as etoposide or epipodophyllotoxin, can* arise as early as 2–3 years after therapy [24–26]. Therapy-associated leukemia after etoposide or epipodophyllotoxin therapy progresses acutely; that is, without prodromal myelodysplasia, while secondary leukemia after alkylating agents is preceded by a phase of preleukemic myelodysplasia [27]. The prognosis for secondary leukemia after alkylating agent administration is less favorable than for acute secondary leukemia after therapy with topoisomerase II inhibitors. In any case, whether occurring after alkylating agent or epipodophyllotoxin therapy, *secondary lymphatic leukemias* account for only about 5% of such cases [28].

Also pointing towards two different pathomechanisms for secondary malignancies, and thus towards the above division into two groups, is that chromosomal damage varies according to the cytostatic agent used. For example, secondary leukemia after administration of alkylating agents is associated with mutations in *chromosomes 5 and 7.* With secondary leukemia associated with topoisomerase II inhibitors, however, translocations have been reported affecting *chromosome 11* (11q23) [29, 30].

The cumulative 10-year incidence of secondary leukemia varies greatly, depending on the underlying disease. For example, after curative treatment for Hodgkin's disease, incidence is cited at 1.5–10%, and peaks about 4–8 years after therapy [31–33]. Compared to the normal population, relative risk is about 20–40 [34, 35].

By contrast, the ABVD regimen appears to incur a relatively low risk of leuke-mogenicity, while the MOPP regimen incurs the highest, which correlates with the methyl-CCNU dose. This risk is apparently about twice as high for patients aged 40–50 years than for younger patients.

Patients surviving ovarian carcinoma have a relative risk of about 12% of devel-oping leukemia, with chlorambucil and melphalan posing the greatest risk [15, 36–38]. Thiotepa, cyclophosphamide and treosulfan also appear to increase the risk of secondary leukemia.

Testicular cancer patients have a 3- to 8-fold risk over that of the normal popu-lation. Here, it is postulated that the risk engendered by etoposide in particular depends on cumulative dose. Studies have shown that the cumulative 10-year inci-dence of secondary leukemia in postchemotherapy female breast cancer patients was maximally 1.5%, and thus higher than that of the surgery-only group.

The following pharmaceutical substances have been found to incur the greatest risk for patients' developing secondary leukemia:

1. Alkylating Agents

It is probable that leukemogenicity is a class effect of the *alkylating agents,* and that leukemia may appear even years after treatment with any of the following alky-lating agents:

(a) *Nitrogen mustard and its derivatives:*

Chlormethine = nitrogen mustard	Mustargen[®]
Chlorambucil	Leukeran[®]
Busulfan	Myleran[®]
Melphalan	Alkeran[®]

(b) *Oxazaphosphorines:*

Cyclophosphamide	Endoxan[®], Cyclostin[®]
Ifosfamide	Holoxan[®]
Trofosfamide	Ixoten[®]

(c) *Nitrosourea derivatives:*

Nimustine (ACNU)	ACNU[®]
Carmustine (ACNU)	BiCNU[®], Carmubris[®]
(Methyl-)CCNU = Lomustine	Cecenu[®], Lomeblastin[®]
Bendamustine	Ribomustin[®]

(d) *Aziridine/ethyleneimine derivatives:*

Thiotepa	Thiotepa[®]

(e) *Others:*

Treosulfan	Ovastat[®].

Because they can react chemically with many different cell components and in every stage of the cell cycle, these alkylating agents exert phase-unspecific cytotoxicity. When mitosis under the influence of these agents is observed under the microscope, these substances are seen to act similarly to ionizing radiation, so that they are sometimes called radiomimetics.

2. *Alkaloids/Podophyllin and Podophyllotoxin Derivatives*
   Etoposide   Vepesid®, Etopophos®
   Teniposide   VM-26®.

3. *Platinum Derivatives*
   Cisplatin   Cisplatin®, Platinex®
   Carboplatin   Carboplat®, Ribocarbo®.

While there are incidence data on podophyllin derivatives and on antibiotics, the incidence of secondary malignancy associated with the antimetabolitic and alkaloid classes of substances is unknown. Nor are data available on hormones (antiandrogens, aromatase inhibitors or GnRH analogs).

Characteristics and Mechanisms of Action

1. Alkylating Agents

(a) Nitrogen Mustard Derivatives
Chlormethine/N-Lost
Formula:

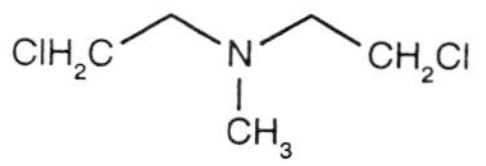

Chlormethine, also called mustine, Mustargen and nitrogen mustard, was developed and used during the First World War as a mustard gas weapon. Victim autopsies revealed not only severe irritation of the skin and respiratory system, but also damage to all highly proliferative cells. These observations led to the decision to use nitrogen mustard as a cytostatic agent. By synthesizing various derivatives and reducing their basicity via N oxide formation or acylation, the agent's toxicity was lessened and it became suitable for chemotherapy.
Chemically, chlormethine is 2,2'-dichloro-N-methyldiethylamine and thus the 'mother substance' of all alkylating agents derived from it, such as busulfan, melphalan and chlorambucil, as well as of the oxazaphosphorines cyclophosphamide, ifosfamide and trofosfamide. Like all substances derived therefrom, chlormethine is

a phase-unspecific cytotoxic substance that can interact with many different cell components during any phase of the cell cycle. After activation to carbocations, all nitrogen mustard derivatives react with DNA guanine. By generating single- and double-stranded cross-links, they cause multiple DNA mutations, thus inhibiting DNA replication and mitosis.

Chlorambucil (CBL)
Formula:

C_2H_4Cl

ClH_4C_2—N—

CO_2H

Like melphalan, chlorambucil is an aromatic derivative of nitrogen mustard which has two alkylating centers in the molecule. Chemically, it is the covalent binding of the cytotoxic part of nitrogen mustard to phenylbutyric acid. As an aromatic derivative, chlorambucil reacts much more slowly than the highly reactive methyl derivative of nitrogen mustard, so that it is not hydrolyzed during stomach passage. This makes it suitable for oral administration.

Like all aliphatic fatty acids, chlorambucil undergoes ß-oxidation after resorption and is reduced to the nitrogen mustard derivative of phenylacetic acid (phenylacetic acid mustard). As with melphalan, and especially in a slightly acidic environment, cleavage of a chlorine ion produces a highly reactive cyclical ethyleneimmonium ion [39, 40]. This ion can covalently bind to various nucleophiles such as amino, sulfhydryl, hydroxy and carboxyl groups, as well as with purines, pyrimidines and phosphates [41, 42].

In particular, it is the highly alkaline nitrogen on position 7 of DNA guanine that undergoes alkylation. Because of the molecule's bifunctionality, it forms the basis for inter- and intrahelical cross-links. This alkylation of guanine destabilizes the imidazole ring, facilitating an opening of the guanine ring system.

These chemical cross-links within the DNA strand and between the DNA strands, and, possibly, the alkylation of enzymes and structure proteins, inhibit replication, proliferation and production of new malignant cells [43]. Studies have also proven that chlorambucil interacts with histones and other proteins in DNA as well [44, 45].

Of special note is that when DNA synthesis is suppressed, RNA synthesis simultaneously increases by up to 50% due to the blockade of the G2 cell cycle.

Furthermore, alkylating agents like chlorambucil may have an immunologic mechanism of action, as indicated by reports of chlorambucil-induced apoptosis of CLL cells [46]. The phagocytosis caused by macrophages and monocytes probably results from chlorambucil-induced alteration of tumor cell permeability [47].

Specialized literature on chlorambucil states that it causes chromosomal aberrations in humans, and lymphatic and myeloid leukemia [48]. Over 90% of these leukemias are acute and of nonlymphocytic origin. Of these, the AMLs alone account for 55% of secondary malignancies. This is why the risk of contracting leukemia must be carefully weighed against the therapeutic benefits expected – especially where children are concerned, and for nonmalignant disorders such as juvenile chronic arthritis.

Busulfan (BUS)
Formula:

H_3C-O_2S —O— $\diagup\diagdown\diagup\diagdown$ —O— SO_2CH_3

Busulfan is a cytostatic, bifunctional alkylating agent. Chemically, it is 1,4-butanediol dimethanesulfonate. Its mechanism of action is based on alkylation of RNA and DNA (cycle-specific, S/G2 phase), in which the single DNA strands are alkylated by covalent binding to alkyl groups. It is postulated that busulfan also alkylates structure proteins and enzymes [49]. As a bifunctional alkylating agent, busulfan first supplants the highly alkaline nitrogen in position 7 of DNA guanine, establishing the basis for further nucleophilic substitution on a second guanine molecule. Given the bifunctional structure of busulfan, intra- or interhelical cross-linking of DNA strands seems likely, but has not yet been proven [50, 51].

Once cross-linking reaches a certain extent, regular transcription is no longer possible, nor, indirectly, is translation. This disrupts, and may even completely suppress, cell proliferation and protein synthesis. Also, busulfan esterifies the phosphate bridges of DNA, which may be an additional mechanism arresting the cell cycle [52, 53].

Busulfan's effect depends on its concentration, and is subject to type 2 (sn2) nucleophilic substitution. Busulfan is almost certainly much less aggressive than nitrogen mustard compounds, including chlorambucil and melphalan. Even so, we must assume that thiol or amino groups are the intracellular points of attack for busulfan [54].

Once attacked, some damaged DNA can be fixed by repair mechanisms, although damage remaining at the time of synthesis will disrupt replication. The extent of this disruption determines whether the tumor cell will simply grow more slowly, or be killed. Proliferating cells exposed to the alkylating agent immediately before synthesis will therefore be damaged more heavily than cells in the G0 phase (resting phase) at that time [55].

Busulfan is particularly cytotoxic to proliferating bone marrow, including bone marrow stem cells. Its selective impact on granulocytopoiesis, especially in small doses, is not yet fully understood. At higher doses, busulfan also suppresses thrombocytes, lymphocytes and the erythrocytic cell line. This relatively selective impact on granulocytes and lymphocytes is probably due to busulfan's pronounced lipophilia [56,

57]. Granulocytes and lymphocytes appear to be especially permeable for busulfan, although neither a receptor nor a transport mechanism appears to be involved here.

In vivo mutagenicity studies on rodents and humans have documented various chromosomal aberrations from busulfan in both gametes and somatic cells. Based on short-term tests, busulfan was classified as a potential carcinogen, with the WHO concluding that treatment with busulfan can lead to cancer. Long-term therapy in particular has given rise to various histologic and cytologic mutations, including extensive dysplasia of cervical, bronchial and other epithelia, which in some cases have evinced precancerous lesions [58–60]. There are also reports of various malignant tumors developing [61–64], and specialized literature on busulfan states that it (like other alkylating substances) is leukemogenic. Long-term follow-up studies show an increased incidence of acute leukemia, but no increase in the incidence of solid tumors [65–67].

Melphalan (L-PAM, MPL)
Formula:

Melphalan is a bifunctional molecule consisting of phenylalanine (an amino acid) and nitrogen mustard. It is the levorotatory form of phenylalanine mustard (L-PAM), the phenylalanine derivative from mustard gas. When developed, it was hoped that this derivative would selectively target melanoma cells, since phenylalanine is a key component in melanin synthesis.

Melphalan is most effective in slightly acidic environments. Cleavage of a chloride ion produces a highly reactive cyclical ethyleneimmonium ion that covalently binds to the widest variety of nucleophilic groups [68]. The aromatic substitute on nitrogen mustard, phenylalanine, reduces the substance's aggressiveness. This reduced toxicity is advantageous, however, because melphalan takes effect only after diffusing throughout the organism without prior irreversible covalent binding to blood components.

Melphalan primarily alkylates the highly alkaline nitrogen atom on position 7 of guanine's purine ring system. Because of its bifunctionality, melphalan thus bound can still undergo further binding, resulting in intra- and interhelical cross-linking of DNA strands. In addition, it is postulated that other bases, such as adenine, are alkylated, as well as phosphates of the DNA strand [69–71].

After quaternization of guanine's N-7, guanine can base pair with thymidine, which would otherwise not take place. The guanine molecule is then destabilized and the imidazole ring of guanine subsequently opened. These processes, together with cross-linking of DNA strands, inhibit transcription and thus translation [72]. This, in turn, inhibits enzyme systems of cellular metabolism such as pyruvate oxidases, choline oxidases, urease, dehydrogenase, cholinesterase, hyaluronidases and phosphatases [73]. Together, these actions are responsible for the cytotoxicity of melphalan, which culminates in the blockade of the S and G2 phases of the cell cycle [74]. These effects may even be irreparable [75].

Specialized literature on melphalan states that, like other alkylating agents, this substance can cause leukemia, a risk which must be weighed against possible benefits of melphalan therapy. Animal tests have proven its mutagenicity, and some human patients treated with melphalan have developed chromosomal aberrations.

(b) Oxazaphosphorines

Cyclophosphamide (CTX)
Formula:

$$\text{(ring: O–P(=O)–NH–CH}_2\text{CH}_2\text{CH}_2\text{)} \quad P-N \begin{cases} C_2H_4Cl \\ C_2H_4Cl \end{cases}$$

Cyclophosphamide is also a derivative of the highly toxic nitrogen mustard, which was originally developed and used as a gas weapon. It is a synthetic derivative of mechlorethamine, and its toxicity was reduced by altering the third substituent on nitrogen. Further development led to substances of the oxazaphosphorine group, such as cyclophosphamide, ifosfamide, and trofosfamide.

Cyclophosphamide is so stable that it can be administered orally. It is first metabolically converted into the active form: in vivo, this substance is metabolized by microsomal liver enzymes (in particular, by cytochrome P_{450}) in the presence of oxygen and NADPH/H+ into 4-hydroxycyclophosphamide and aldophosphamide. 4-Hydroxycyclophosphamide and aldophosphamide are in equilibrium.

Enzyme action on 4-hydroxycyclophosphamide results in ketocyclophosphamide. The tautomers 4-hydroxycyclophosphamide and aldophosphamide undergo a partially spontaneous and partially enzymatic conversion into active and inactive metabolites such as phosphoramide mustard and acrolein.

Out of open-ringed aldophosphamide develops the most strongly alkylating compound, N, N-bis(2-chlorethyl)phosphoric acid. This takes place through cleavage of acrolein, but without enzymatic action. Carboxyphosphamide and 4-oxocyclophosphamide, additional metabolites, have little or no cytotoxicity, while phosphoramide mustard and acrolein are toxic. Acrolein is not an antineoplast but does cause urotoxic side effects [76].

The cytostatic effect of the active metabolites is mainly based on alkylation of DNA, primarily in a blockade of the late S and early G2 phases. This results in

DNA- and DNA-protein cross-linking, and, depending on the cycle, single- and double-stranded breaks [77–79].

The deactivation of cyclophosphamide plus the simultaneous reduction of the glutathione system influence not only the choice of oncologic treatment, but also repair and detoxification measures, and thus the genesis of secondary tumors.

Cyclophosphamide's mutagenic potential has been demonstrated in many in vitro and in vivo tests. It has been found to cause chromosomal aberrations in humans, and tumorigenicity in rats and mice [80]. Cyclophosphamide is therefore potentially carcinogenic and should be administered only with appropriate safety measures. On the basis of epidemiologic studies, cyclophosphamide therapy must be assumed capable of causing secondary tumors in humans [81–84].

Also limiting the use of cyclophosphamide is its tendency to cause hemorrhagic cystitis by releasing toxic catabolic products (acrolein) in the efferent urinary tract. Mesna (sodium 2-mercaptoethane sulfonate) detoxifies these catabolic products in the kidneys by producing a renally excretable, nontoxic addition product with acrolein, making higher doses of cyclophosphamide possible. Supplementing cyclophosphamide with mesna may prevent the later development of bladder tumors, which most likely also stem from acrolein.

Ifosfamide
Formula:

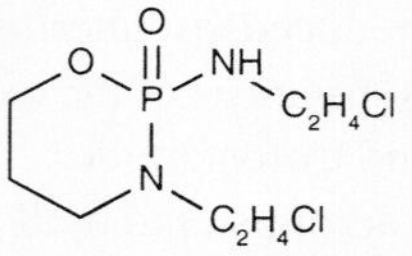

Like trofosfamide and cyclophosphamide, ifosfamide is a derivative of nitrogen mustard, but is much less toxic. Its metabolism and efficacy differ considerably from cyclophosphamide's, nor does ifosfamide accumulate as heavily, making it is less toxic to bone marrow. Ifosfamide is used primarily to treat cyclophosphamide-resistant solid tumors.

Ifosfamide, an oxazaphosphorine, is primarily used to therapy lung carcinoma. Metabolically, it is activated to 4-hydroxyifosfamide [85], and this unstable substance is in turn converted into isophosphoramide mustard, an alkylating substance which damages DNA through multifunctional adducts and inter- and intrahelical cross-linkage [86]. Alkylation primarily attacks nitrogen on position 7 of guanine, and the resulting cross-linkage of DNA is much more stable than that generated by cyclophosphamide [87].

Specialized literature states that secondary tumors or their precursors may develop after ifosfamide administration. Such late malignancy is probable, given the irreversible damage to DNA such as cross-linkage and links with proteins [88].

There is a higher risk of developing urinary tract tumors and myelodysplastic mutations, including acute leukemias.

Trofosfamide
Formula:

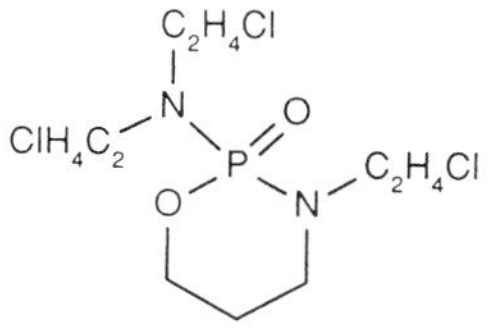

Like cyclophosphamide and ifosfamide, trofosfamide is derived from nitrogen mustard, and was developed to circumvent the latter's acute toxicity. In vitro, trofosfamide is mainly inactive, but after activation in the liver is carcinolytic for a wide variety of tumors. As with all nitrogen mustard derivatives, trofosfamide's cytotoxic property stems from its ability to generate mitosis- and proliferation-inhibiting intra- and interhelicular DNA cross-links. Like all alkylating substances, including cyclophosphamide and ifosfamide, trofosfamide interferes in the cell's G2 phase and, at higher dosages, in the S phase as well.

(c) Nitrosourea Derivatives

Nimustine
Formula:

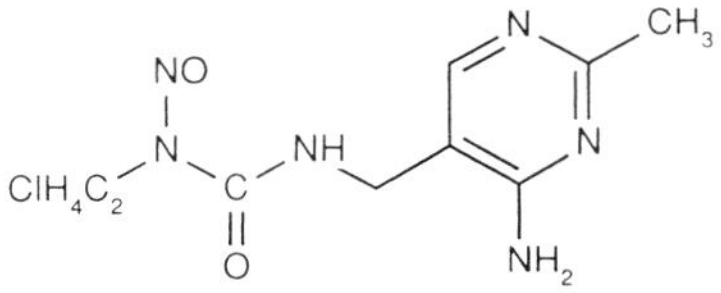

Nimustine is a nitrosourea derivative developed in 1974 by Arakawa and colleagues. As a hydrochloride, it is both lipid- and water-soluble. Playing the key role in the carcinolytic activity of nimustine is the metabolism, during which DMPP and hydroxylated compounds are produced, and, as alkylating components, active cations such as $ClCH_2CH_2$. Via alkylation and carbamoylation reactions, nimustine disrupts DNA synthesis. Here, according to Green et al. [89], the central structures of the nucleosomes (core particles) in particular are alkylated. After incubation with nimustine, cells in the S and G2 + M phases accumulate [90, 91]. Nimustine kills HeLa cells, especially in the G1 and G2 + M phases, whereas cells in the S phase are resistant [92]. Therapy combining nimustine and other cytostatic agents can be expected to lead to immunosuppressive reactions.

Carmustine (BCNU)

Formula:

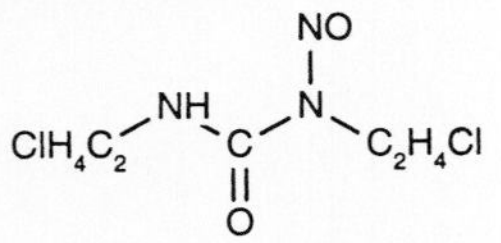

Carmustine [1,3-bis(2-chloroethyl)-1-nitrosourea] was one of the first nitrosourea derivatives, and as such was gained from methylnitrosoguanidine. The bifunctionality of its two chloroethyl groups makes carmustine a bifunctional alkylating agent, and thus able to generate intra- and interhelicular DNA cross-links [93–96]. Considerably faster and more prevalent than the DNA-DNA links, however, is the cross-linkage between DNA and protein generated by carmustine. These result in longer inhibition of DNA synthesis [97–99].

Especially resistant to carmustine are cells evincing high O6-alkyltransferase activity, for they can eliminate DNA monoadducts. Studies have also shown that carmustine can inhibit DNA repair mechanisms, carbamoylation of proteins [100, 101], and cellular absorption of nucleic acid bases [102]. It is unclear whether carmustine's effect is cell-cycle-dependent, although it appears to be most cytotoxic during the G1 and early S phases.

Like all nitrosourea derivatives, carmustine is highly lipophilic, and thus penetrates the central nervous system well [103].

Specialized literature on carmustine states that in dosages similar to those used clinically, this substance is carcinogenic in rats and mice.

Lomustine (CCNU) and Semustine (Methyl-CCNU)

Formulae:

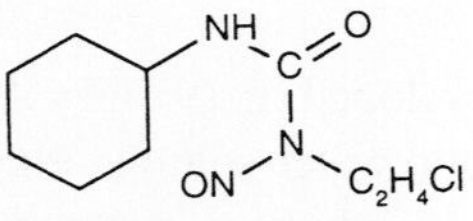

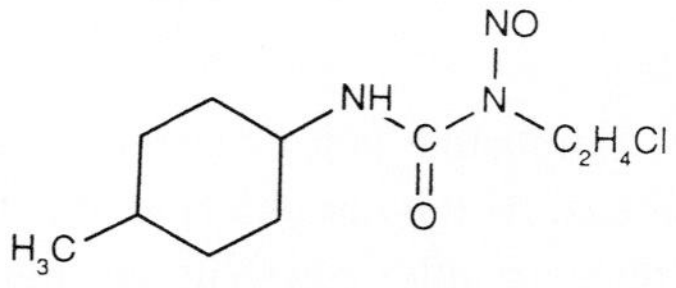

In 1950, the United States' National Cancer Institute launched a large-scale screening program for developing new cytostatic agents and testing them on murine leukemic cells.

In 1960, the first reports that N'-nitro-N-nitrosoguanidine was active against these leukemic cells spurred the development of many nitrosourea derivatives, including BCNU, CCNU and methyl-CCNU.

Chemically, lomustine is 1-(2-chloroethyl)-3-cyclohexyl-1-nitrosourea. Methyl-CCNU differs from CCNU only in the methylation in position 4 on the cyclohexane ring. It is thus considerably more lipophilic than CCNU and crosses the blood-brain barrier well, achieving much higher cerebral concentrations [104].

As with all nitrosourea derivatives, CCNU works by alkylation and by inhibiting various vital enzyme processes. The production of monohydroxylated derivatives, such as chloroethyldiazoniumhydroxide, gives CCNU its alkylating characteristics, while production of isocyanate is at the root of its carbamoylating properties. It is predominantly the lysine remnants on cellular proteins that undergo carbamoylation [105].

Apparently, the first step in alkylation is the transfer of the chloroethyl group from chloroethylnitrosourea onto the oxygen on position 6 of guanine. This is followed by intramolecular condensation and production of an intermediate 1-O6-ethanoguanine, which reacts with nitrogen on position 3 of cytosine [106]. Under the influence of CCNU, DNA and RNA strands are alkylated (phase-unspecifically, for resting G0 cells are also affected) and cross-linked, which inhibits proliferation of the correlating damaged cells [107–109]. Inhibition of repair mechanisms is also under discussion [110]. There are many reports on the leukemogenic potential of lomustine [111, 112].

Bendamustine
Formula:

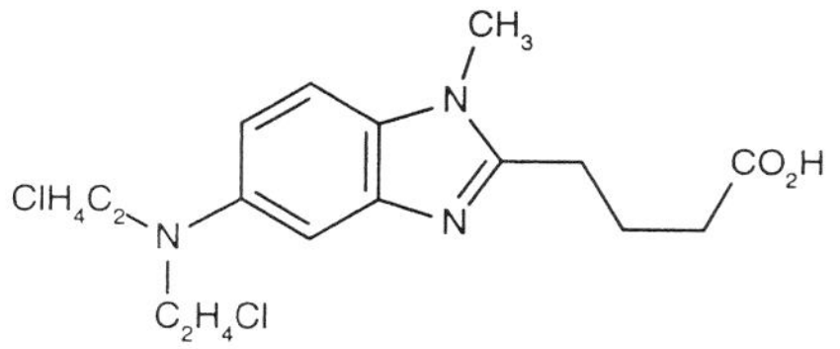

Bendamustine was synthesized in the early 1960s at the Institute for Microbiology and Experimental Therapy in Jena, Germany. From 1971 to 1991, it was produced by Jenapharm and marketed under the product name of Cytostasan®. Since 1991, bendamustine has been marketed as Ribomustin® by Ribosepharm.

Bendamustine is an antineoplastic, bifunctional alkylating agent derived from nitrogen mustard. It is hepatically metabolized and primarily eliminated renally. The nitrogen mustard group is bound to a benzimidazole ring at position 5. In position 1, the benzimidazole ring is substituted with a methyl group. Structurally, bendamustine is a benzimidazolyl-alkan carbonic acid that is fairly water-soluble. Cross-reactions with other alkylating agents have not been reported.

The objective of this synthesis was to combine unnatural amino acids or modified nucleic acid bases with the nitrogen mustard group, which is known for its antineoplastic properties. The goal was a synthetic substance with less toxicity than usual for the nitrogen mustard group, but with an altered amino acid whose amino group would be bound to a heterocyclic ring system (benzimidazole), a system which is chemically related to the purine ring system [113, 114].

The original objective of developing a cytostatic agent with both alkylating and purine antagonistic or amino acid antagonistic characteristics was not reached.

Apparently, the antineoplastic effect of bendamustine comes solely from the alkylating nitrogen mustard group, for none of the derivatives of the benzimidazole carrier molecule evince cytostatic qualities.

The antineoplastic and cytocidal effects of bendamustine result from the alkylation-induced cross-linking of single- and double-stranded DNA. Preclinical tests on human carcinoma cell lines show that production of bendamustine-associated DNA adducts (alkylation of guanine in position N7) correlates significantly with the individual IC_{50} of the cell lines. Alkylation disrupts the messenger function of DNA and DNA synthesis. There is also cross-linking among proteins, as well as between DNA and proteins [115].

It has also been demonstrated that bendamustine-induced breaks in DNA double strands repair more slowly than those induced by other alkylating agents such as melphalan, cyclophosphamide and BCNU.

It is not known whether the benzimidazole ring possesses additional antimetabolitic properties. Thus far, there are only phase-1 study findings that β-hydroxybendamustine produced during metabolism is also alkylative and thus cytotoxic.

Bendamustine induces chromosomal aberrations and is mutagenic in cell culture and animal experiments [116]. After its administration, lung tumors and mammary carcinomas were detected in mice, so that bendamustine is also classified as carcinogenic [117].

(d) Aziridine/Ethyleneimine Derivatives

Thiotepa
Formula:

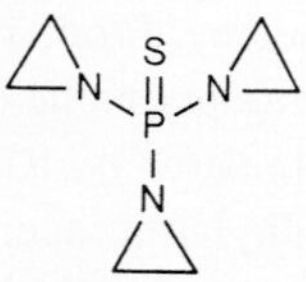

Like triethylenemelamine and trenimon, thiotepa belongs to the group of aziridines. This substance group was developed when it was found that the nitrogen mustard derivatives produce reactive aziridine intermediates prior to alkylation.

Thiotepa's mechanism of action probably resembles that of nitrogen mustard, with the aziridine rings opening spontaneously. Reactivity of these rings is based on the pressure of the three-member ring systems. Thiotepa is less reactive than nitrogen mustard, although its reactivity increases when pH values decline [118].

The cytotoxicity of thiotepa and its active metabolites results from alkylation of macromolecules via inhibition of nucleic acid synthesis, of protein synthesis, and of various enzymes. Inhibition of glycolysis has also been reported [119].

Thiotepa's main metabolite, TEPA (triethylenephosphoramide), is formed by oxidative desulfurization and is also considered reactive. In the liver, thiotepa converts into TEPA, which is then also found in plasma and urine [120]. Just 5 min after injection of thiotepa, its main metabolite, TEPA, is already detectable in plasma. After 2 h, relatively high plasma concentrations of thiotepa and TEPA are detectable, although TEPA concentrations are higher thereafter.

TEPA itself also has antitumor characteristics. Due to its relevant level in plasma, TEPA is thought to act at least partially as the prodrug of thiotepa. It is likely that other active metabolites besides TEPA play a role because there is more alkylating activity in urine than can be accounted for by the concentrations of TEPA and thiotepa [121]. Studies have also shown that thiotepa decomposes in urine, although alkylating activity continues. This indicates that other alkylating metabolites have been produced [122].

The activity of thiotepa itself is strongly subject to the intracellular level of thiol. Sensitivity to thiotepa increases considerably when the intracellular level of thiol sinks [123].

(e) Others

Treosulfan (TREO)
Formula:

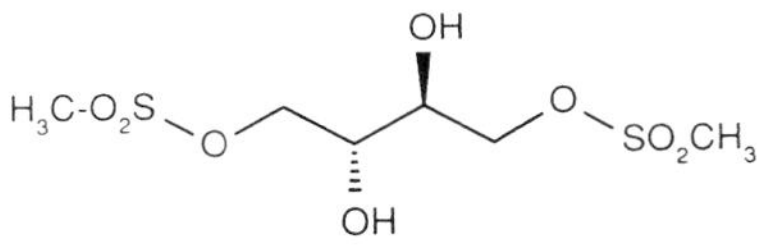

Treosulfan, a bifunctional alkylating agent, is L-threitol-1,4-bis-methanesulfonate. It differs structurally from busulfan due to the introduction of two hydroxyl groups, and also has a different mechanism of action. Via an Sn2 reaction, busulfan reacts, through its methanesulfonyloxy groups, directly with the nucleophile (for example, N-7 of guanine). In contrast, treosulfan (in the physiologic environment of pH 7.4 and 37 °C) is nonenzymatically converted into the active mono- and diepoxides (1,2-epoxy-3,4-butandiol-4-methanesulfonate and L-di-epoxybutane). Cleavage of one molecule each of methanesulfonic acid results in epoxide formation [118]. These reactive epoxides are thought to catalyze alkylation; i.e., they can bind to biologic macromolecules. Treosulfan itself is pharmacologically inert and is thus a prodrug for the alkylating epoxides [124].

Epoxides are similar to the aziridines (see the sections on nitrogen mustard and thiotepa), and probably alkylate in a similar manner. Like busulfan and the aziridines, the epoxides also alkylate via an Sn2 reaction [119, 125].

The mechanism of action is thus based on the conversion of treosulfan into mono- or di-epoxides, which bifunctionally alkylate, causing single- or double-stranded DNA cross-links and hence chromosomal breakage during the S/G2 phases [126].

Treosulfan does not evince significant nonhematologic toxicity, making it suitable for high-dosage chemotherapy regimens with autologous stem cell transplantation. In 1.4% of the cases of long-term oral administration of treosulfan, acute non-lymphatic leukemia was observed [15]. Like other alkylating agents, treosulfan is potentially mutagenic, so that women of child-bearing age should in any case avoid pregnancy during treosulfan therapy [127].

2. Podophyllin Derivatives / Podophyllotoxin Alkaloids

Etoposide (VP-16)
Formula:

Etoposide, also termed VP-16 and VP-16-213, is epipodophyllotoxin or ethylidene lignan P, and thus a semisynthetic epipodophyllotoxin derived from the root of *Podophyllum peltatum* [128]. Its chemical name is 4'-demethyl-epipodophyllotoxin 9-(4,6-O-(R)-ethylidene-β-D-glucopyranoside). Sandoz Laboratories first isolated and synthesized the substance from *Podophyllum embodi*, a plant indigenous to India. Its phosphate, etoposide phosphate (Etopophos®), is rapidly hydrolyzed to the active metabolite, etoposide [129].

Etoposide's cytotoxic effect is phase-specific – primarily during the G2 phase – although some activity is also seen in the late S phase [130]. Etoposide basically inhibits DNA repair enzymes (topoisomerase II), which leads to single- and double-stranded breaks in DNA [131]. This principle also accounts for etoposide's phase specificity, since topoisomerase activity, and thus condensation and decondensation of the superhelices, is not detectable in cells in the resting phase. The substance is antineoplastic and cytocidal, and in high concentrations, cytocidal for cells in the resting phase as well [132]. This cytotoxicity is based not only on interaction with the DNA repair enzyme topoisomerase II, but also on the intra-cellular formation of free radicals. Etoposide's inhibition of topoisomerase II is energy-intensive, so that dosage and length of administration are critical factors [133].

Etoposide itself does not react directly with DNA, but rather 'stabilizes' the DNA-topoisomerase II complex. This suppresses normal topoisomerase II activity and blocks cell proliferation in the G2 phase [134].

Also described are chromosomal breaks under the influence of etoposide, and chromatid exchange reactions. Inhibition of nucleoside transport has been observed, although only with high concentrations of etoposide, and it is unclear whether this effect contributes to cytotoxicity [135].

Specialized literature on etoposide states that both in vitro and in vivo tests show gene and chromosomal mutations. These findings point towards mutagenicity in humans as well [136]. Even though etoposide has not undergone animal tests for carcinogenicity, the above-mentioned proven genotoxicity points towards carcinogenic potential [137, 138]. Etoposide has also demonstrated immunosuppressive potential, which may enhance proliferation of malignant cells [139–142].

Teniposide
Formula:

Teniposide, also called VM-26 and thenylidene lignan, is a semisynthetic podophyllotoxin gained from the root of *P. peltatum* [143]. Podophyllin resin derivatives have been used medicinally for about 250 years, and their cytotoxic effect had already been described by 1861 [144]. For example, podophyllin is administered as a topical oily solution for condyloma acuminata [145]. Chemically, teniposide is 4'-demethyl-epipodophyllotoxin 9-(4,6-O-(R)-2-thenylidene-β-D-glucopyranoside).

Like etoposide, teniposide inhibits topoisomerase II, the repair enzyme responsible for the formation of the super helix [146, 147]. Teniposide does not bind directly to DNA, but rather prevents DNA ligase activity in the nucleus by forming a DNA-topoisomerase II complex. This causes protein-associated double-stranded breaks in DNA, thus inhibiting the cell cycle [148]. Teniposide acts phase-specifically, and because only topoisomerase II is active here, affects only the late S and early G2 phases. Like etoposide, teniposide is antineoplastic, and because it produces free radicals, cytocidal. In high concentrations, it is cytocidal even for cells in the resting phase [130].

Specialized literature states that both in vitro and in vivo tests with teniposide have induced mutations in genes and chromosomes. A mutagenic effect on humans may therefore be assumed. In addition, canine tests have demonstrated teniposide's potential carcinogenicity. On the basis of these results, as well as its DNA-damaging effect and proven genotoxicity, teniposide must be assumed to have carcinogenic potential. Moreover, teniposide causes immunosuppression, which probably favors malignant-cell proliferation and thus secondary tumorigenesis [139, 149].

3. Platinum Derivatives

Cisplatin/Carboplatin
Formulae:

$$\begin{array}{cc} H_3N & Cl \\ & \diagdown Pt \diagup \\ H_3N & Cl \end{array}$$

In 1969, cisplatin, the first heavy-metal complex to be developed for its antineoplastic effect, was proven to inhibit growth of graft tumors [150]. Structurally, as *cis*-diammine-dichloroplatinum, cisplatin is a planar complex containing a central bivalent atom of platinum surrounded by two chlorine atoms and two ammonia molecules in the *cis* position. The correlating trans-tautomers have little or no antineoplastic activity.

Carboplatin is an analog preparation and, like cisplatin, a planar heavy-metal complex with a dicarboxy chelate system and two amine ligands in the *cis* position (*cis*-diammine[1,1-cyclobutane-dicarboxylato(2-)-0,0']). Substitution of chloride ions by the dicarboxylate ligand renders carboplatin more stable than cisplatin.

Clinical use has shown carboplatin's antineoplastic activity to be comparable to that of cisplatin, although carboplatin's nonhematologic side effects are much less pronounced [151]. This is due less to the *kind* of side effects of carboplatin than to the degree of severity [152]. On the other hand, carboplatin's damage to bone marrow is more severe and protracted than cisplatin's. Carboplatin was approved for malignant tumor therapy in Germany in 1988. The effects of cisplatin and carboplatin resemble those of the alkylating compounds, and their mechanism of action correlates with that of the bifunctional alkylating agents [153]. The first step is displacement of the ammonia ligands by water. Electrophile aquo complexes then develop intracellularly, and react with the nucleophile centers of DNA. Both chlorine ligands can then be replaced by nucleophiles.

The main point of attack is the highly alkaline nitrogen on position 7 of DNA guanine. Cross-links form between the neighboring DNA strands, between DNA and protein, and especially between adjacent guanine remnants within DNA strands. The mechanism of action is thus phase-independent, just like for the nitrogen mustard derivatives. But unlike nitrogen mustard derivatives, the platinum bonds lead primarily to cross-links of single strands [154].

The formation of cross-links inhibits cell division, affecting in particular the S phase and rapidly proliferating cells, such as malignant cells. The cytotoxic effect of platin medications is nevertheless not phase-specific, for it also impacts G0 (resting phase) cells [155].

Carboplatin and cisplatin do not differ qualitatively in their mechanisms of effect, but rather pharmacokinetically. For example, carboplatin is less reactive than cisplatin, and reacts more slowly to DNA, but is preferred for patients whose reduced renal function does not tolerate cisplatin [156, 157].

Until a few years ago, it was primarily alkylating agents and nitrosourea derivatives that were reported to be associated with secondary tumorigenesis. These have recently been joined, however, by similar reports involving platinum derivatives [136, 158]. The *New England Journal of Medicine,* for example, has published a study on 28,000 women who were administered platinum-derivative chemotherapy for ovarian carcinoma [159]. The study found that the incidence of secondary malignancy correlated closely with the total platinum dosage. Women who had received a total of < 500 mg had a twofold risk of developing leukemia, while risk was eightfold for women with total dosages of ≥ 1,000 mg.

Despite the side effects here – which apply to all cytostatic agents – the authors emphasized that the data should not serve to restrict administration of platinum derivatives, for treating ovarian carcinoma with platinum derivatives has raised the 5-year survival rate from 40% to 60–70%. Again, the risk must always be weighed against expected therapeutic benefit. The data in the above-mentioned study should simply give the oncologist cause to reconsider dosage levels of platinum derivatives.

References

1   Curtis RE, Hankey BF, Myers MH, Young JL Jr: Risk of leukemia associated with the first course of cancer treatment: An analysis of the surveillance, epidemiology, and end results program experience. J Natl Cancer Inst 1984;72:531–544.
2   Starzl TE, Nalesnik MA, Porter KA, Ho M, Iwatsuki S, Griffith BP, Rosenthal JT, HakalaTR, Shaw BW Jr, Hardesty RL, et al: Reversibility of lymphomas and lymphoproliferative lesions developing under cyclosporine-steroid therapy. Lancet 1984;1:583–587.
3   Maize JC: Skin cancer in immunosuppressed patients. JAMA 1977;237:1857–1858.
4   Kinlen LJ, Sheil AG, Peto J, Doll R: Collaborative United Kingdom-Australasian Study of cancer in patients treated with immunosuppressive drugs. Br Med J 1979;2:1461–1466.
5   Li PKT, Nicholls MG, Lai KN: The complications of newer transplant antirejection drugs: Treatment with cyclosporin a, OKT3, and FK506. Adverse Drug React Acute Poisoning Rev 1990;9:123–155.

6   Neugut Al, Robinson E, Nieves J, Murray T, Tsai WY: Poor survival of treatment-related acute non-lymphocytic leukemia. JAMA 1990;264:1006–1008.

7   Casciato DA, Scott JL: Acute leukemia following prolonged cytotoxic agent therapy. Medicine (Baltimore) 1979;58:32–47.

8   Meadows AT, Robison LL, Neglia JP, Sather H, Hammond D: Potential long-term toxic effects in children treated for acute lymphoblastic leukemia. N Engl J Med 1989;321: 1830–1831.

9   Tucker MA, D'Angio GJ, Boice JD Jr, Strong LC, Li FP, Stovall M, Stone BJ, Green DM, Lombardi F, Newton W, et al: Bone sarcomas linked to radiotherapy and chemotherapy in children. N Engl J Med 1987;317:588–593.

10   Michels SD, McKenna RW, Arthur DC, Brunning RD: Therapy-related acute myeloid leukemia and myelodysplastic syndrome: A clinical and morphologic study of 65 cases. Blood 1985;65:1364–1372.

11   Williams CJ: Leukaemia and cancer chemotherapy. Br Med J 1990;301:73–74.

12   Dorr FA, Coltman CA Jr: Second cancers following antineoplastic therapy. Curr Probl Cancer 1985;9:1–43.

13   Lien EJ, Ou XC: Carcinogenicity of some anticancer drugs and survey. J Clin Hosp Pharm 1985;10:223–242.

14   Pedersen-Bjergaard J, Specht L, Larsen SO, Ersbøll J, Struck J, Hansen MM, Hansen HH, Nissen NI: Risk of therapy-related leukaemia and praeleukaemia after Hodgkin's disease: Relation to age, cumulative dose of alkylating agents, and time from chemotherapy. Lancet 1987;ii:83–88.

15   Kaldor JM, Day NE, Petterson F, Clarke EA, Pedersen D, Mehnert W, Bell J, Høst H, Prior P, Karjalainen S, et al: Leukemia following chemotherapy for ovarian cancer. N Engl J Med 1990;332:1–6.

16   Kaldor JM, Day DE, Clarke EA, Van Leeuwen FE, Henry-Amar M, Fiorentino MV, Bell J, Pedersen D, Band P, Assouline D, et al: Leukemia following Hodgkin's disease. N Engl J Med 1990;322:7–13.

17   Pui CH: Myeloid neoplasia in children treated for solid tumours. Lancet 1990;336:417–421.

18   Tarbell NJ, Gelber RD, Weinstein HJ, Mauch P: Sex differences in risk of second malignant tumours after Hodgkin's disease in childhood. Lancet 1993;341:1428–1432.

19   Tucker MA, Meadows AT, Boice JD Jr, Stovall M, Oberlin O, Stone BJ, Birch J, Voûte PA, Hoover, RN, Fraumeni JF Jr: Leukemia after therapy with alkylating agents for childhood cancer. J Natl Cancer Inst 1987;78:459–464.

20   Kyle RA, Gertz MA: Second malignancies after chemotherapy; in Perry MC (ed): The Chemotherapy Source BOOK. Baltimore, Williams & Wilkins, 1992, pp 689–702.

21   Kamel OW, van de Rijn M, Weiss LM, Del Zoppo GJ, Hench PK, Robbins BA, Montgomery PG, Warnke RA, Dorfman RF: Brief report: Reversible lymphomas associated with Epstein-Barr virus occurring during methotrexate therapy for rheumatoid arthritis and dermatomyositis. N Engl J Med 1993;328:1317–1321.

22   Boyle J, MacKie RM, Briggs JD, Junor BJ, Aitchison TC: Cancer, warts, and sunshine in renal transplant patients: A case-control study. Lancet 1984;i:702–705.

23   Krikorian JG, Burke JS, Rosenberg SA, Kaplan HS: Occurrence of non-Hodgkin's lymphoma after therapy for Hodgkin's disease. N Engl J Med 1979;300:452–458.

24   Whitlock JA, Greer JP, Lukas JN: Epipodophyllotoxin-related leukemia. Cancer 1991;68: 600–604.

25   Bokemeyer C, Schmoll HJ, Polidowa H: Sekundäre Leukämien nach Etoposid-haltiger Chemotherapie. Dtsch Med Wochenschr 1994;119:707–713.

26 Nichols CR, Breeden ES, Loehrer PJ, Williams SD, Einhorn LH: Secondary leukemia associated with a conventional dose of etoposide. J Natl Cancer Inst 1993;85:36–40.

27 De Gramont A, Louvet C, Krulik M, Sadja N, Donadio D, Laporte JP, Brissaud P, Smith M, Delâge JM, Drolet Y, et al: Preleukemic changes in cases of non-lymphocytic leukemia secondary to cytotoxic therapy: Analysis of 105 cases. Cancer 1986;58:630–634.

28 Hawkins MM, Wilson LM, Stovall MA, Marsden HB, Potok MH, Kingston JE, Chessells JM: Epipodophyllotoxins, alkylating agents, and radiation and risk of secondary leukemia after childhood cancer. Br Med J 1992;304:951–958.

29 Pedersen-Bjergaard J, Philip P, Larsen So, Jensen G, Byrsting K: Chromosome aberrations and prognostic factors in therapy related myelodysplasia and acute non-lymphocytic leukemia. Blood 1990;76:1083–1091.

30 Le Beau MM, Albain KS, Larson RA, Vardiman JW, Davis EM, Blough RR, Golomb HM, Rowley JD: Clinical and cytogenetic correlations in 63 patients with therapy-related myelodysplastic syndromes and acute non-lymphocytic leukemia: Further evidence for characteristic abnormalities of chromosomes no. 5 and 7. J Clin Oncol 1986;4:325–345.

31 Kaldor JM, Day NE, Band P, Choi NW, Clarke EA, Coleman MP, Hakama M, Koch M, Langmark F, Neal FE, et al: Second malignancies following testicular cancer, ovarian cancer and Hodgkin's disease: An international collaborative study among cancer registries. Int J Cancer 1987;39:571–585.

32 Coltman CA, Dixon DO: Second malignancies complicating Hodgkin's disease: A Southwest Oncology Group 10-year follow-up. Cancer Treat Rep 1982;66:1023–1033.

33 Nelson DF, Cooper S, Weston MG, Rubin P: Second malignant neoplasms in patients treated for Hodgkin's disease with radiotherapy or radiotherapy and chemotherapy. Cancer 1981;48:2386–2393.

34 Pedersen-Bjergaard J, Larsen SO: Incidence of acute myeloproliferative syndrome up to 10 years after treatment of Hodgkin's disease. N Engl J Med 1982;307:965–971.

35 Swerdlow AJ, Douglas AJ, Hudson GV, Hudson BV, Bennett MH, MacLennan KA: Risk of second primary cancers after Hodgkin's disease by type of treatment: Analysis of 2864 patients in the British National Lymphoma Investigation. Br Med J 1992;304:1137–1143.

36 Greene MH, Boice JD Jr, Greer BE, Blessing JA, Dembo AJ: Acute nonlymphocytic leukemia after therapy with alkylating agents for ovarian cancer. N Engl J Med 1982;307:1416–1421.

37 Prosnitz LR: Leukemia after treatment of ovarian cancer or Hodgkin's disease. N Engl J Med 1990;322:1819–1820.

38 Coltman CA, Dahlberg S: Leukemia after treatment of ovarian cancer or Hodgkin's disease. N Engl J Med 1990;322:1820.

39 McLean A, Newell D, Baker G: The metabolism of chlorambucil. Biochem Pharmacol 1976;25:2331–2335.

40 McLean A, Newell D, Baker G, Connors T: The metabolism of chlorambucil. Biochem Pharmacol 1980;29:2039–2047.

41 Bank BB, Kanganis D, Liebes LF, Silber R: Chlorambucil pharmacokinetics and DNA binding in chronic lymphocytic leukemia lymphocytes. Cancer Res 1989;49:554–559.

42 Sunters A, Springer CJ, Bagshawe KD, Souhami RL, Hartley JA: The cytotoxicity, DNA crosslinking ability and DNA sequence selectivity of the aniline mustards Melphalan, Chlorambucil and 4-(Bis(2-chloroethyl)amino)benzoic acid. Biochem Pharmacol 1992;44:59–64.

43 Harrap KR, Gascoigne EW: The interaction of bifunctional alkylating agents with the DNA of tumour cells. Eur J Cancer 1976;12:53–59.

44   Riches PG, Harrap KR: Some effects of chlorambucil on the chromatin of Yoshida ascites sarcoma cells. Cancer Res 1973;33:389–393.

45   Detke S, Stein JL, Stein GS: Influence of chlorambucil, a bifunctional alkylating agent on DNA replication and histone gene expression in HeLa S3 cells. Cancer Res 1980;40:967–974.

46   Begleiter A, Lee K, Israels LG, Mowat MR, Johnston JB: Chlorambucil induced apoptosis in chronic lymphocytic leukemia (CLL) and its relationship to clinical efficacy. Leukemia 1994;8(suppl 1):103–106.

47   Hill BT, Harrap KR: The uptake and utilization of chlorambucil by lymphocytes from patients with chronic lymphocytic leukemia. Br J Cancer 1972;26:439–443.

48   Palmer RG, Doré CJ, Denman AM: Chlorambucil-induced chromosome damage to human lymphocytes is dose-dependent and cumulative. Lancet 1984;i:246–249.

49   Haddow A, Timmis GM: Myleran in chronic myeloid leukemia chemical constitution and biological action. Lancet 1953;1:207–208.

50   Brookes P, Lawley PD: The alkylation of guanosine and guanylic acid. J Chem Soc 1961;3923–3928.

51   Tong WP, Ludlum DB: Crosslinking of DNA by Busulfan. Formation of diguanyl derivates. Biochim Biophys Acta 1980;608:174–181.

52   Bishop JB, Wassom JS: Toxicological review of busulfan (Myleran). Mutat Res 1986; 168:15–45.

53   Alexander P, Stacey KA: Comparison of the changes produced by ionising radiations and by the alkylating agents. Ann N Y Acad Sci 1958;68:1225–1231.

54   Roberts JJ, Warwick GP: Metabolism of myleran (1.4-dimethansulphonyloxybutane). Nature 1959;183:1509–1510.

55   Wheeler GP: Alkylating agents; in Holland JF, Frei E (eds): Cancer Medicine. Philadelphia, PA, Lea & Febinger, 1982, pp 824–843.

56   Wilkinson JF, Turner RL: Chemotherapy of chronic myeloid leukemia with special reference to Myleran; in Tocantins LM (ed): Progress in haematology. New York, NY, Grune & Stratton, 1959, vol 2, p 225.

57   Buggia GP, Locatelli F, Regazzi MB, Zecca M: Busulfan. Ann Pharmacother 1994;28:1055–1062.

58   Meschan I, Hines WB, Scharyj M: Bronchopulmonary dysplasia – What is it? South Med J 1973;66:417–426.

59   Koss LG, Melamed MR, Mayer K: The effect of busulfan on human epithelia. Am Clin J Pathol 1965;44:385–397.

60   Leake E, Smith WG, Woodliff HJ: Diffuse interstitial pulmonary fibrosis after busulfan therapy. Lancet 1963;2:432–434.

61   Juch E, Lauterbach A: Dysplastische Veränderungen am Epithel der Cervix uteri durch Busulfan (Myleran). Geburtshilfe Frauenheilkd 1982;42:43–44.

62   Aksoy M, Erdem S, Bakioglu I, Dincol G: Endometrial cancer due to Busulfan therapy. J Cancer Res Clin Oncol 1984;108:362–363.

63   Nelson BM, Andrews GA: Breast cancer and cytologic dysplasia in many organs after busulfan. Am J Clin Pathol 1964;42:37–44.

64   Feingold ML, Koss LG: The effect of long term administration of busulfan. Arch Intern Med 1969;124:66–71.

65   Landaw SA: Acute leukemia in polycythemia vera. Semin Hematol 1986;23:156–165.

66   Dittmar K: Acute myeloblastic leukemia with polycythemia vera, treated with busulfan and phlebotomy. N Y State J Med 1979;75:758–761.

67   Stott H, Fox W, Girling DJ, Stephens RJ, Galton DA: Acute leukaemia after busulphan. Br Med J 1977;2:1513–1517.

68   Wood PJ, Sansom JM, Newell K, Tannock IF, Stratford IJ: Reduction of tumour intracellular pH and enhancement of melphalan cytotoxicity by the ionophore nigericin. Int J Cancer 1995;60:264–268.

69   Ross WE, Ewig RA, Kohn KW: Differences between melphalan and nitrogen mustard in the formation and removal of DNA cross-links. Cancer Res 1978;38:1502–1506.

70   Brox LW, Gowans B, Belch A: L-Phenylalanin mustard (melphalan) uptake and cross-linking in the RPMI 6410 human lymphoblastoid cell line. Cancer Res 1980;40:1169–1172.

71   Osborne MR, Lawley PD: Alkylation of DNA by melphalan with special reference to adenine derivates and adenine-guanine cross-linking. Chem Biol Interact 1993;89:49–60.

72   Brookes P, Lawley PD: The reaction of mono- and bifunctional alkylating agents with nucleic acids. Biochem J 1961;80:496–503.

73   Stacher A, Lutz D: Antineoplastische Chemotherapie; in Kuemmerle H-P, Hitzenberger G, Spitzy KH (Hrsg): Klinische Pharmakologie. Grundlagen, Methoden, Pharmakotherapie. Lehr- und Handbuch für Klinik und Praxis; 4. Aufl, vol III, pp 1–22. München, Ecomed, 1988.

74   Fernberg JO, Lewensohn R, Skog S: Cell cycle arrest and DNA damage after melphalan treatment of the human myeloma cell line RPMI 8226. Eur J Haematol 1991;47:161–167.

75   Demur C, Chiron M, Saivin S, Attal M, Dastugue N, Bousquet C, Galinier JL, Colombies P, Laurent G: Effect of melphalan against self-renewal capacity of leukemic progenitors in acute myeloblastic leumekia. Leukemia 1992;6:204–208.

76   De Kraker J: Massive bladder haemorrhage. Br Med J 1986;292:628.

77   Schmoll H-J, Höffken K, Possinger K (Hrsg): Kompendium Internistische Onkologie, Teil 1. Heidelberg, Springer, 1996, p 467.

78   Fleer R, Brendel M: Toxicity, interstrand cross-links and DNA fragmentation induced by 'activated' cyclophosphamide in yeast. Chem Biol Interact 1981;37:123–140.

79   Fleer R, Brendel M: Toxicity, interstrand cross-links and DNA fragmentation induced by 'activated' cyclophosphamide in yeast: Comparative studies on 4-hydroperoxy-cyclophosphamide, its monofunctional analogon, acrolein, phosphoramide mustard, and nor-nitrogen mustard. Chem Biol Interact 1982;39:1–15.

80   IARC monographs on the evaluation of the carcinogenic risk of chemicals to human. Some antineoplastic and immunosuppressive agents. International Agency for Research on Cancer, 1981, vol 26.

81   Wall RL, Clausen KP: Carcinoma of the urinary bladder in patients receiving cyclophosphamide. N Engl J Med 1975;293:221–223.

82   Plotz PH, Klippel JH, Decker JL, Grauman D, Wolff B, Brown BC, Rutt G: Bladder complications in patients receiving cyclophosphamide for systemic lupus erythematosus or rheumatoid arthritis. Ann Intern Med 1979;91:221–223.

83   Pedersen-Bjergaard J, Ersbøll J, Hansen VL, Sørensen BL, Christoffersen K, Hou-Jensen K, Nissen NI, Knudsen JB, Hansen MM: Carcinoma of the urinary bladder after treatment with cyclophosphamide for non-Hodgkin's lymphoma. N Engl J Med 1988;318:1028–1032.

84   Travis LB, Curtis RE, Boice JD Jr, Fraumeni JF Jr: Bladder cancer after chemotherapy for non-Hodgkin's lymphoma. N Engl J Med 1989;321:544–545.

85   Connors TA, Cox PJ, Farmer PB, Foster AB, Jarman M: Some studies of the active intermediates formed in the microsomal metabolism of cyclophosphamide and isophosphamide. Biochem Pharmacol 1974;23:115–129.

86 Peter G, Hohorst H-J: Synthesis and preliminary antitumor evaluation of 4-(SR)-sulfido-cyclophosphamides. Cancer Chemother Pharmacol 1979;3:181–188.

87 Weber GF, Waxman DJ: Activation of the anti-cancer drug ifosphamide by rat liver microsomal P450 enzymes. Biochem Pharmacol 1993;45:1685–1694.

88 American Hospital Formulary Services; in McEvoy et al (eds): AHFS Drug Information. Bethesda, MD, American Society of Hospital Pharmacists, 1991, p 490.

89 Green D, Tew KD, Hisamatsu T, Schein PS: Correlation of nitrosourea murine bone marrow toxicity with deoxyribonucleic acid alkylation and chromatin binding sites. Biochem Pharmacol 1982;31:1671–1679.

90 Shimada S, Kawashima M, Watanabe S, Yamada K, Mizoguchi M, Hori Y, Kukita A: Cell kinetic studies of the effect of various kinds of chemotherapeutic agents on a human melanoma cell line (SEKI, II). J Dermatol 1982;9:271–278.

91 Fujiwara T, Nakasone S, Matsumoto K, Ohnishi R, Tabuchi K, Nishimoto A: [Effect of ACNU, a water-soluble nitrosourea, on cell cycle of cultured glioma cells—flow cytometric analysis.] Gan To Kagaku Ryoho 1983;10:2055–2061.

92 Kanawaza H, Miyamoto T: [Effect of ACNU, a water-soluble nitrosourea derivative, on survival and cell progression of cultured HeLa S3 cells.]. Gan To Kagaku Ryoho 1983;10:2007–2015.

93 Wheeler GP, Chumley S: Alkylating activity of l,3-bis(2-chloroethyl)-l-nitrosourea and selected compounds. J Med Chem 1967;10:259–265.

94 Barranco SC, Humphrey RM: The effects of l,3-bis(2-chloroethyl)-l-nitrosourea on survival and cell progression in Chinese hamster cells. Cancer Res 1971;31:191–195.

95 Bhuyan BK, Scheidt LG, Frase TJ: Cell cycle phase specificity of antitumor agents. Cancer Res 1972;32:398–407.

96 Tobey RA, Crissman HA: Comparative effects of three nitrosourea derivates on mammalian cell cycle progression. Cancer Res 1975;35:460–470.

97 Kohn KW, Erickson LC, Laurent G, et al: DNA cross linking and the origin of sensitivity to chloroethylnitrosoureas; in Prestayko AW, Crooke ST, Baker LH, et al (eds): Nitrosoureas: Current Status and New Developments. New York, NY, Academic Press, 1981, pp 69–83.

98 Wheeler GP, Alexander JA: Duration of inhibition of synthesis of DNA in tumors and host tissues after single doses of nitrosoureas. Cancer Res 1974;34:1957–1964.

99 Wheeler GP, Alexander JA: Duration of inhibition of synthesis of DNA in tumors and host tissues after single doses of nitrosoureas. Cancer Res 1976;36:1470–1474.

100 Kann HE Jr: Carbamoylating activity of nitrosoureas; in Prestayko AW, Crooke ST, Baker LH, et al (eds): Nitrosoureas: Current Status and New Developments. New York, NY, Academic Press, 1981, pp 95–105.

101 Erickson LC, Laurent G, Sharkey N, Kohn KW: DNA crosslinking and monoadduct repair in nitrosourea-treated human tumour cells. Nature 1980;288:727–729.

102 Ludlum DB, Kramer BS, Wang J, Fenselau C: Reaction of l,3,bis(2-chloroethyl)-l-nitrosourea with synthetic polynucleotides. Biochemistry 1975;14:5480–5485.

103 Zackheim HS, Feldmann RJ, Lindsay C, Maibach HI: Reaction of l,3-bis(2-chloroethyl)-1-nitrosourea (BCNU, carmustine) in mycosis fungoids. Br J Dermatol 1977;97:65–67.

104 Mellett LB: Physicochemical considerations and pharmacokinetic behavior in delivery of drugs to the central nervous system. Cancer Treat Rep 1977;61:527–531.

105 Reed DJ, May HE: Alkylation and carbamoylation intermediates from the carcinostatic 1-(2-chloroethyl)-3-cyclohexyl-l-nitrosourea (CCNU). Life Sci 1975;16:1263–1270.

106 Wheeler GP, Johnston TP, Bowdon BJ, McCaleb GS, Hill DL, Montgomery JA: Comparison of the properties of metabolites of CCNU. Biochem Pharmacol 1977;26:2331–2336.

107 Wheeler GP, Alexander JA: Duration of inhibition of synthesis of DNA in tumours and host tissues after single doses of nitrosoureas. Cancer Res 1974;34:1957–1964.

108 Wheeler GP, Bowden BJ: Effects of l,3-bis(2-chloroethyl)-l-nitrosourea and related compounds upon the synthesis of DNA by cell free systems. Cancer Res 1975;35:460–470.

109 Ewig RAG, Kohn KW: DNA-protein cross-linking and DNA interstrand cross-linking by haloethylnitrosoureas in L1210 cells. Cancer Res 1978;38:3197–3203.

110 Erickson LC, Bradley MO, Ducore JM, Ewig RA, Kohn KW: DNA crosslinking and cytotoxicity in normal and transformed human cells treated with antitumour nitrosoureas. Proc Natl Acad Sci USA 1980;77:467–471.

111 Boice JD, Greene MH, Killen JY Jr, Ellenberg SS, Fraumeni JF Jr, Keehn RJ, McFadden E, Chen TT, Stablein D: Leukemia after adjuvant chemotherapy with semustine (methyl-CCNU) – evidence of a dose-response effect. N Engl J Med 1986;314:119–120.

112 Devereux S, Selassie TG, Vaughan Hudson G, Vaughan Hudson B, Linch DC: Leukaemia complicating treatment for Hodgkin's disease: The experience of the British National Lymphoma Investigation. Br Med J 1990;301:1077–1080.

113 Ozegowski W, Krebs D: IMET 3393, g-(l-Methyl-5-bis-(ß-chloräthyl)-amino-benzimidazolyl-(2))-buttersäure-hydrochlorid, ein neues Zytostatikum aus der Reihe der Benzimidazol-Loste. Zentralbl Pharm 1971;110:1013–1019.

114 Wemer W: Experimental characterization of bendamustin. J Cancer Res Clin Oncol 1990; 116:467(abstr A4124.02).

115 Hartmann M, Zimmer C: Investigation of cross-link formation in DNA by the alkylating cytostatica IMET 3106, 3393, 3943. Biochim Biophys Acta 1972;287:386–389.

116 Heinecke H, Glittner J: Zur mutagenen Wirkung des N-Lost-Derivates IMET 3393. Zentralbl Pharm 1971;110:1079–1086.

117 Güttner J, Bruns G, Jungstand W: Onkogene Wirkung von g-(l-Methyl-5-bis-(ß-chloräthyl)-amino-benzimidazolyl-(2))-buttersäure-hydrochlorid bei der Maus. Arch Geschwulstforsch 1974;43:16–21.

118 Feit PW, Rastrup-Andersen N, Matagne R: Studies in epoxide formation from (2S, 3S)-Threitol-l,4-Bismethane-sulfonate. The preparation and biological activity of (2S, 3S)-l,2-Epoxy-3.4-butanediol-4-methanesulfonate. J Med Chem 1970;13:1173–1175.

119 Feit PW: Treosulfan, eine Spezialform aus der Gruppe der Alkylantien; in Bastert G, et al (Hrsg): Treosulfan i.v. Mehr Lebensqualitat in der Therapie des Ovarialkarzinoms. Zuckschwerdt, München; Akt Onkol 1988;45:9–18.

120 Egorin MJ, Akman SR, Gutierrez PL: Plasma pharmacokinetics and tissue distribution of ThioTEPA in mice. Cancer Treat Rep 1984;68:1265–1268.

121 Cohen BE, Egorin MJ, Kohlhepp EA, Aisner J, Gutierrez PL: Human plasma pharmacokinetics and urinary excretion of thiotepa and its metabolites. Cancer Treat Rep 1986; 70:859–864.

122 Cohen BE, Egorin MJ, Nayar MSB, Gutierrez PL: Effect of pH and temperature on the stability and decomposition of N,N',N'-Triethylenethiophosphoramide in urine and buffer. Cancer Res 1984;44:4312–4316.

123 Teicher BA, Lee JB, Antman K, Frei E: Evidence for metabolic activation of ThioTEPA. Proc AACR 1988;29:487.

124 Hartley JA: Report on molecular pharmacology of treosulfan. Medac, 1996.

125 Feit PW: Treosulfan: 'Prodrug' für Epoxid-Verbindungen und analytische Bestimmungen im Serum und Urin des Hundes. Symposien Hannover, Karlsruhe, März l982.

126 Matagne R: Induction of chromosomal aberrations and mutations with isomeric forms of L-threitol-l,4-bismethanesulfonate in plant materials. Mutat Res 1969;7:241–247.

127 Zeiger E, Pagano DA: Mutagenicity of the human carcinogen treosulphan in Salmonella. Environ Mol Mutagen 1989;13:343–346.

128 Kelly M, Hartwell J: The biological effects and chemical composition of podophyllin. A review. J Natl Cancer Inst 1954;14:967–1010.

129 Keller-Justin C, Kuhn M, Von Wartburg A: Synthesis and antimitotic activity of glycosidic lignan derivates related to podophyllotoxin. J Med Chem 1971;14:936–940.

130 Misra NC, Roberts DW: Inhibition by 4'-demethyl-epipodophyllotoxin 9-(4,6-O-2-thenyli-dene-beta-D-glucopyranoside) of human lymphoblast cultures in G2 phase of the cell cycle. Cancer Res 1975;35:99–105.

131 Ross WE, Towe T, Glisson BS, Yalowich J, Liu L: Role of topoisomerase II in mediating epipodophyllotoxin-induced DNA cleavage. Cancer Res 1984;44:5857–5860.

132 Glisson BS, Ross WE: DNA topoisomerase II: A primer on the enzyme and its unique role as a multidrug target in cancer chemotherapy. Pharmacol Ther 1987;32:89–106.

133 Krishan A, Paikg K, Frei E: Cytofluorometric studies on the action of podophyllotoxin and epipodophyllotoxins (VM-26 and VP-16–213) on the cell cycle traverse of human lym-phoblasts. J Cell Biol 1975;66:521–530.

134 Smith PJ, Anderson CO, Watson JV: Predominant role for DNA damage in etoposide-induced cytotoxicity and cell cycle perturbation in human SV40-transformed fibroblasts. Cancer Res 1986;46:5641–5645.

135 Chatterjee S, Trivedi D, Petzold SJ, Berger NA: Mechanism of epipodophyllotoxin-induced cell death in poly(adenosine diphosphate-ribose) synthesis-deficient V7 Chinese hamster cell lines. Cancer Res 1990;50:2713–2718.

136 Pedersen-Bjergaard J, Daugaard G, Hansen SW, Philip P, Larsen SO, Rørth M: Increased risk of myelodysplasia and leukaemia after etoposide, cisplatin and bleomycin for germ-cell tumors. Lancet 1991;338:359–363.

137 Pui CH, Behm FG, Raimondi SC, Dodge RK, George SL, Rivera GK, Mirro J Jr, Kalwinsky DK, Dahl GV, Murphy SB: Secondary acute myeloid leukemia in children treated for acute lymphoid leukemia. N Engl J Med 1989;321:136–142.

138 Meadows AT, Robison LL, Neglia JP, Sather H, Hammond D: Potential long-term toxic effects in children treated for acute lymphoblastic leukemia. N Engl J Med 1989; 321:1830–1831.

139 Pui CH, Ribeiro RC, Hancock ML, Rivera GK, Evans WE, Raimondi SC, Head DR, Behm FG, Mahmoud MH, Sandlund JT et al: Acute myeloid leukemia in children treated with epipodophyllotoxins for acute lymphoblastic leukemia. N Engl J Med 1991;325:1682–1687.

140 Ratain MJ, Kaminer LS, Bitran JD, Larson RA, Le Beau MM, Skosey C, Purl S, Hoffman PC, Wade J, Vardiman JW, et al: Acute nonlymphocytic leukemia following etoposide and cisplatin combination chemotherapy for advanced non-small-cell carcinoma of the lung. Blood 1987;70:1412–1417.

141 DeVore R, Whitlock J, Hainsworth JD, Johnson DH: Therapy-related acute nonlymphocytic leukemia with monocytic features and rearrangement of chromosome 11q. Ann Intern Med 1989;110:740–742.

142 Winick NJ, McKenna RW, Shuster JJ, Schneider NR, Borowitz MJ, Bowman WP, Jacaruso D, Kamen BA, Buchanan GR: Secondary acute myeloid leukemia in children with acute lym-phoblastic leukemia treated with etoposide. J Clin Oncol 1993;11:209–217.

143 Kelly M, Hartwell JL: The biological effects and chemical composition of podophyllin. A review. J Natl Cancer Inst 1954;14:967–1010.

144 Kelly M, Hartwell JL: Podophyllum. A review. J Natl Cancer Inst 1954;14:647.

145 Kaplan IW: Condylomata acuminata. New Orleans M & SJ. 1942;94:338–390.

146 Lonn U, Lonn S, Nylen U, Winblad G: Altered formation of DNA in human cells treated with inhibitors of DNA topoisomerase II (etoposide and teniposide). Cancer Res 1989;49:6202–6207.

147 Qiu J, Catapano CV, Fernandes DJ: Formation of topoisomerase II alpha complexes with nascent DNA is related to VM-26-induced cytotoxicity. Biochemistry 1996;35:16354–16360.

148 Chen GL, Yang L, Rowe TC, Halligan BD, Tewey KM, Liu LF: Nonintercalative antitumor drugs interfere with the breakage-reunion reaction of mammalian DNA topoisomerase II. J Biol Chem 1984;259:13560–13566.

149 Kreissmann SG, Gelber RD, Sallan SE, Leavitt P, Cohen HJ: Secondary acute myeloic leukemia (AML) in children treated for acute lymphoblastic leukemia (ALL) (meeting abstract). Proc Am Soc Clin Oncol 1990;9:219.

150 Preusser P, Achterrath W, Niederle N, Seeber S: Cisplatin. Arzneimitteltherapie 1985;3:50–65.

151 Roberts JJ: Cisplatin; in Pinedo HM (ed): Cancer Chemotherapy 1983. The EORTC Cancer Chemotherapy Annual. Amsterdam, Excerpta Medica, 1983, vol 5, pp 107–119.

152 Achterrath W, Wilke H, Kroll-v. Haeseler E: Carboplat, Zytostatikum für die Mono- und Polychemotherapie maligner Neoplasien. Neu-Isenburg, Bristol-Arzneimittel, 1988.

153 Rosenberg B: Anticancer activity of cis-dichloro-diammine-platinum (II) and some relevant chemistry. Cancer Treat Rep 1979;63:1433–1438.

154 Lippert B: Aktuelle Cis-Platin-Derivate; in Seeber S, Osteka R, Sack R, Schoneberger H (Hrsg): Das Resistenzproblem bei der Chemo- und Radiotherapie maligner Tumoren. Basel, Karger, 1984, pp 36–47.

155 Drewinko B, Patchen M, Yang LY, Barlogie B: Differential killing efficacy of twenty antitumor drugs on proliferating and non-proliferating human tumor cells. Cancer Res 1981;41:2328–2333.

156 Ducore JM, Erickson LC, Zwelling LA, Laurent G, Kohn KW: Comparative studies of DNA-cross-linking and cytotoxicity in Burkitt's lymphoma cell lines treated with cis-diamine-dichloro-platinum(II) and L-phenylalanine mustard. Cancer Res 1982;42:897–902.

157 Rozencweig M, von Hoff DD, Abele R, Mugia FM: Cisplatin; in Pinedo HM (ed): Cancer Chemotherapy 1979. The EORTC Cancer Chemotherapy Annual. Amsterdam, Excerpta Medica, 1979, vol 1, pp 107–125.

158 Snowden JA, Laidlaw ST, Champion AE, Reilly JT: Acute promyelocytic leukaemia after treatment for seminoma with carboplatin. Lancet 1994;344:1361.

159 Travis LB, Holowaty EJ, Bergfeldt K, Lynch CF, Kohler BA, Wiklund T, Curtis RE, Hall P, Andersson M, Pukkala E, Sturgeon J, Stovall M: Risk of leukemia after platinum-based chemotherapy for ovarian cancer. N Engl J Med 1999;34:351–357.

Dr. W. Haussmann, Kliniken Landkreis Sigmaringen GmbH, Hohenzollernstraße 40,
D–72488 Sigmaringen (Germany)
Tel. +49 7571 100 22 33

Rüther U, Nunnensiek C, Schmoll H-J (eds): Secondary Neoplasias following Chemotherapy, Radiotherapy, and Immunosuppression. Contrib Oncol. Basel, Karger, 2000, vol 55, pp 62–93

Mechanisms of Action of Immuno-suppressants and Immunoinductors

W. Haussmann

Kliniken Landkreis Sigmaringen GmbH, Sigmaringen, Deutschland

In many countries, laws governing transplantation are being set down in writing for the first time, while in others, existing ones are undergoing amendment. This, plus the increasing number of transplantation centers, has led to more organ transplantations the world over.

The first successful human renal transplantation was conducted in 1954. Taking place between identical twins, it was syngenic, so that their genetic compatibility made immunosuppression unnecessary. Since that time, much progress has been made, thanks in part to the use of various immunosuppressants [1]. Consequently, kidney, heart and liver transplantations are routine procedures today, and the number of lung and combined transplantations is also growing.

Most organ transplantations are still allogenic ones of parenchymatous solid organs; that is, between genetically different individuals. Due to their inherent histoincompatibility, however, such operations are hampered by four basic problems: (1) the risk of *acute or chronic rejection* of the transplant [2, 3]; (2) the risk of *infection* in conjunction with transplantation and during the subsequent phase of immunosuppression; (3) medicinal *side effects,* and (4) the risk of posttransplantation *tumorigenesis* resulting from obligatory life-long medication. The expensive treatment and high morbidity rates associated with these problems make them a major issue in modern health care and health-care economics.

Immunosuppression inhibits the immune system's response to transplanted foreign tissue. Here, we differentiate between inhibition of an established immune reaction and the blockade of one which has just begun or is expected to. Defining the scope of immunosuppression is the question of whether only one clone is selectively inhibited, or if all are targeted.

This chapter will not discuss: physical methods of immunosuppression, such as irradiation; immunobiologic methods, such as using cytotoxic antisera against immunocytes, or cytokines that interfere in regulation mechanisms, such as interferon-γ (IFN-γ). Instead, this chapter deals with clearly defined chemical substances and substance groups that inhibit, suppress or eliminate an immune reaction threatening the transplant.

Mechanisms of Immunologic Rejection Reactions

In the acute rejection process, the immune system of the genetically different recipient recognizes surface proteins of the major histocompatibility complex (MHC) of the transplant as foreign. The high concentration of foreign MHC peptides helps trigger immune system mechanisms that lead to tissue destruction and scarring, thus progressively worsening transplant function or even causing its loss [4–7]. However, the risk of immunologic rejection can be reduced considerably by using the HLA (human leukocyte antigen) system to carefully match donor and recipient [8].

Primarily T cells are responsible for cell-mediated immunity. Their activators include antigen-presenting cells (superantigens) – such as monocytes, macrophages, B cells and dendritic cells. The T lymphocytes are subsequently differentiated and proliferated in effector cells. T-killer cells may also directly recognize the foreign MHC structure of the allogenic transplant, and be activated by it. These processes enable the vital differentiation of antigen structures into 'self' and 'foreign'. Consequently, the allograft's concentration of foreign MHC peptide structures will also classify it as foreign (host-versus-graft reaction).

T-helper cells (CD4+) recognize the foreign antigen primarily in conjunction with (MHC)HLA class II (HLA)DR molecules, and cytotoxic T cells (CD8+) in conjunction with HLA class I molecules. If a T cell is activated, it produces interleukin (IL)-2 and IL-6, which leads to differentiation and proliferation of further T cells [9]. IL-2 , however, also activates macrophages and B cells, and the latter differentiate into antibody-producing plasma cells. Antigen-activated and IL-2-stimulated T cells secrete additional cytokines, such as IL-4, IL-5 and IL-6, which lead to clonal expansion of B cells. As when stimulated by IL-2, these B cells differentiate into antibody-producing plasma cells of high specificity.

Transplantation antigens (histocompatibility antigens) are glycoproteins of the cell membrane that play a dominant role in the rejection process. It is the preformed antibodies in recipient serum which are responsible for hyperacute rejections (those occurring within a few minutes to a few hours after transplantation). The T-cell-mediated immunomechanisms described above, however, are responsible for acute (7–21 days) and chronic (3 or more months) rejections. Today, hyperacute rejections can be nearly eliminated by cross-matching HLA-specific antibodies.

Humoral or antibody-mediated immunity, in which antibodies are produced against foreign surface structures, is in the scope of functions of B cells. This mechanism is probably at the root of both acute and chronic rejection. Via various cy-tokines/lymphokines, communication takes place between T- and B-cell-mediated immunity, while reactions are regulated by cytokines.

Acute-rejection mechanisms are better understood than those of chronic rejection. But regardless of the kind of transplant, the same pathophysiologic mechanism appears to be at work: Tissue damage leads to the proliferation of endothelial and smooth-muscle cells, and hence concentric narrowing of microvessels and vessels serving the transplant.

Without therapy to suppress the immune attack on the transplant, every graft would be rejected. This is why medicative immunosuppression starting shortly before or during transplantation is necessary for the rest of the patient's life. Without the immunosuppressants described in the following and the latest advances in immune system mechanisms, modern transplantation medicine would not be possible.

At the same time, we need to redefine transplanted organs. For example, 'passenger leukocytes' from the donor organ have been found in some recipients decades after transplantation. Also reported are patients who, despite years of immunosuppressive therapy, did not reject their donor organs when therapy was stopped. These kinds of transplants can no longer be classified as foreign organs, for they have united with the recipient organism [10, 11].

The mechanisms of immunosuppressants, immunomodulators and immunoinductors available to today's transplantation medicine are discussed in this chapter. Since transplantation of an allogenic organ makes the recipient's lymphocyte count skyrocket – usually in the first postoperative phase – in response to the 'invasion' by foreign MHC peptides, antiproliferative substances such as azathioprine and glucocorticoids are usually administered. Methotrexate and thalidomide, also discussed in this chapter, are not approved for immunosuppression after solid-organ transplantation, but are included because of the experience gained from their use in transplantation medicine.

Chemically Defined Substances

Azathioprine, first synthesized in 1959, is a nitroimidazole derivative of 6-mercaptopurine. An antimetabolite, it nonspecifically inhibits the lymphocytic cell cycle by integrating into DNA and RNA, thereby exerting a cytostatic effect, with inhibition of cellular and humoral immune resistance. Azathioprine inhibits the recipient organism's antigen reaction – the proliferation of immunocompetent cells – to the foreign graft [12, 13].

Azathioprine is also called active or activated 6-mercaptopurine, into which it is metabolized in vivo. It probably does not have any effect itself, but is rather a prodrug. The actual effective metabolite, thioinosinic acid (mercaptopurine ribonu-

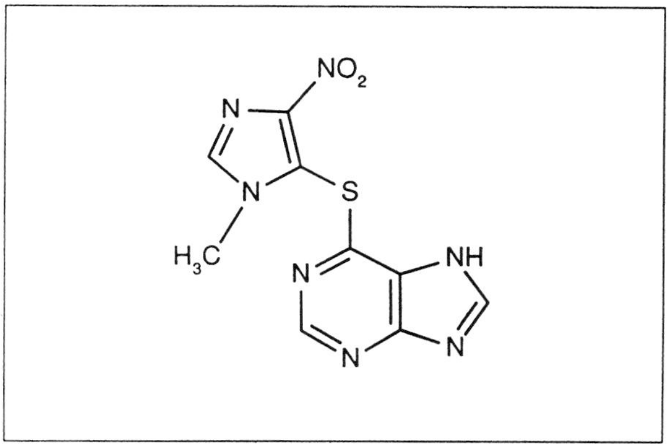

Fig. 1. Azathioprine.

cleotide), is formed intracellularly only. In vivo, the first step in purine synthesis is inhibited by inhibition of glutamine-5-phosphoribosyl-pyrophosphate dehydroge-nase, as are inosine monophosphate dehydrogenase (IMPDH) and adenylosuccinate synthetase, which catalyzes conversion of inosinic acid into guanosine monophos-phate and adenosine monophosphate, respectively.

Azathioprine may cause bone marrow depression and even leukopenia by di-rectly integrating ribosylated mercaptopurine into DNA and by generally inhibiting cells of various organ systems. Also reported are dose-related leukopenia and throm-bocytopenia, gastrointestinal disturbances, hepatotoxicity and an increased tumor risk. This makes careful blood level monitoring essential with azathioprine therapy. Unlike glucocorticoids, azathioprine cannot suppress initial gene activation (activa-tion of the accessory cells of the IL-1 gene). However, by integrating into DNA or RNA, it can very effectively prevent gene replication and T-cell proliferation. Hence, azathioprine targets a distal area of the T-cell activation cascade. It has also been proven to inhibit K cells, a lymphocyte subpopulation that can lyse target cells via antibody-dependent cytotoxicity.

In addition, azathioprine suppresses the number of migratory mononuclear and granulocytic cells, as well as the proliferation of promyelocytes in bone marrow. As a consequence, the number of circulating monocytes able to differentiate into macrophages drops. This accounts in part for the increased susceptibility to infec-tion and tumors with azathioprine. The substance also has a general antiphlogistic effect and, by inhibiting proline hydroxylase and sulfate incorporation into acidic mucopolysaccharides, inhibits connective tissue biosynthesis.

Glucocorticoids/Corticosteroids (Such as Prednisone, Dexamethasone and Methylprednisolone)

Corticosteroids are used in today's basic immunosuppressive therapy and to treat rejection reactions (in the latter case, using short-term high doses, called

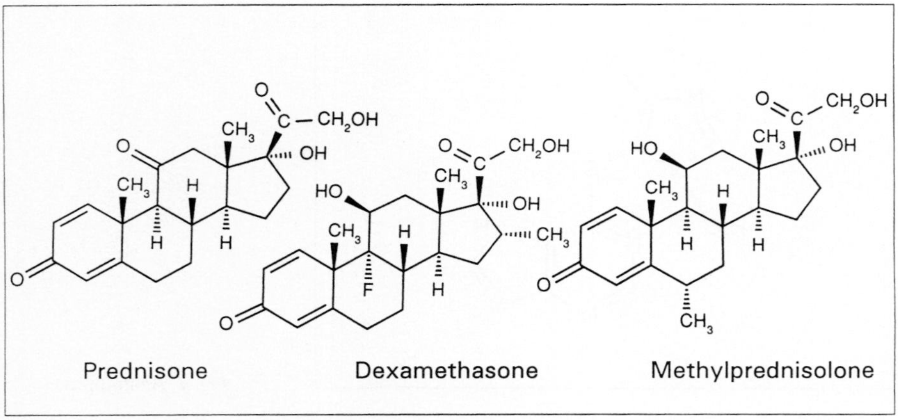

Fig. 2. Prednisone, dexamethasone, methylprednisolone.

'pulsed doses'). To minimize the risk of unwanted side effects and to increase immunosuppression, glucocorticoids are usually administered with cyclosporine or azathioprine or both. When combined with cyclosporine, less glucocorticoid is given than when combined with azathioprine. Combinations are chosen depending on the individual's risk of rejection and the risk of toxicity that could result from kidney and/or liver dysfunction.

Whether intra- or postoperatively administered, corticosteroids act as immunosuppressants by nonspecifically inhibiting the cell cycle (as do azathioprine and methotrexate), and by inhibiting the anti-inflammatory activity of macrophages and other phagocytes [14]. We also know that glucocorticoids trigger programmed cell death (apoptosis) of lymphocytes [15].

In cytoplasma of target cells (accessory cells), glucocorticoids bind to a special intracellular glucocorticoid receptor. When the steroid binds to the C-terminal end of the receptor, translocation of the ligand into the nucleus is induced. Binding of the steroid receptor complex (acting as a transcription factor) to specific DNA sequences in the nucleus inhibits the expression of a number of genes in lymphoid cells. This inhibits activation and transcription of postsynaptic genes of lymphoid cells through the stimulation of monocytes and macrophages. The T-cell activation cascade is then 'proximally' blocked. Subsequently, activation of accessory, antigen-presenting cells is inhibited by the blocked transcription of IL-1 and IL-6 genes. With higher doses, glucocorticoids also inhibit the release of tumor necrosis factor-α (TNF-α).

Only recently was it discovered that transcription factor NF-κB, a dimer of p50 and p60 subunits, probably plays the key role in glucocorticoid-dependent gene regulation [16, 17].

In cytosol of nonactivated cells, NF-κB is suppressed by repressor molecules of the I-κ1B family, such as I-κBα. I-κBα is broken down as soon as TNF-α binds to its receptor. Transcription factor NF-κB then migrates into the nucleus and activates various genes. Synthesis of repressor I-κBα is then stimulated, which suppresses stimulation of TNF-α. Glucocorticoids stop this activation by activating gene transcription of the I-κB repressor and complexing transcription factor NF-κB, which was released by the TNF-α stimulus. This is why it cannot enter the nucleus. Various glucocorticoids have also been found to bind directly to NF-κB. In addition to these effects exerted directly by the steroid receptor complex as a transcription factor, there are also indirect mechanisms. For example, glucocorticoids inhibit transcription factor AP-1 from activating its target genes [18], suppress proliferation of T cells, and reduce the expression of IL-2 and the IL-2 receptor. An indirect IL-2 blockade is explained by the fact that the release of IL-2 depends on an IL-1-triggered release of IL-6.

Glucocorticoids have not only an immunospecific effect, but also a wide range of nonspecific immunosuppressive and antiphlogistic capabilities. For example, they suppress the migration of monocytes to inflammatory foci.

This complete blockade of the inflammatory system during pulsed-dose therapy for acute rejection reactions is a disadvantage of steroid therapy, as is the modification of other glucocorticoid regulatory centers ('permissive effect'). This total blockade causes a number of side effects, such as slower wound healing, aseptic bone necrosis, hyperglycemia, edema, and hypertension.

Methotrexate (MTX)

Another substance used to treat acute rejection reactions is the folate antagonist MTX, a drug well established in oncologic practice. Although the only folate antagonist on the market, it is not approved for use as an immunosuppressant for solid-organ transplantation, since its toxicity, as detailed below, is very high, and sufficient alternative drugs are available. MTX is therefore purely an alternative medication.

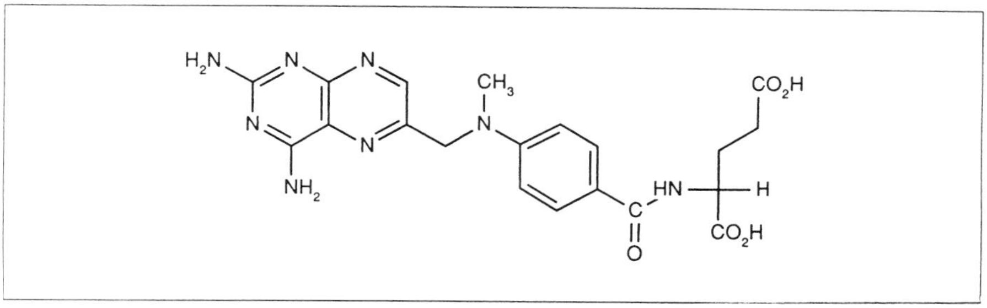

Fig. 3. Methotrexate.

Numerous studies have been published on using MTX to prevent graft-versus-host reaction after allogenic bone marrow transplantation [19–23].

A slight structural alteration of folic acid into MTX results in much higher affinity to dihydrofolate reductase than folic acid itself has. The resulting inhibition of the transfer of one-carbon fragments (hydroxymethyl groups, formyl groups) disrupts nucleic acid synthesis and thus cell division.

MTX therefore has a relatively unspecific effect, since it influences all rapidly proliferating cells, and not only activated T and B cells that are subject to proliferation. This accounts for its high toxicity and limited use as an immunosuppressant in transplantation therapy. To protect the organism's cells from destruction, folinic acid must be given soon after MTX as an antidote.

Thalidomide

Thalidomide (2-(2,6-dioxo-piperidin-3-yl)-iso-indole-1,3-dione) was developed by Grünenthal Co. and put on the market in 1956. In the 1960s, it was prescribed to pregnant women as a sedative, but caused a large number of birth defects. Since 1970, it has been used as an immunosuppressant/antiphlogistic for leprosy patients (erythema nodosum leprosum), and to treat various autoimmune disorders [24–28].

Thalidomide's value in solid-organ transplantation is unclear, since there are not enough studies involving humans. Only inhibition of a graft-versus-host reaction after allogenic bone marrow transplantation has been demonstrated in animal and human experiments, although dosage has not yet been optimized [29–32]. Thalidomide appears indicated when a graft-versus-host reaction does not respond to cyclosporine or glucocorticoids. The efficacy of various thalidomide derivatives, such as 3-aza- and 4-aza-thalidomide, in treating graft-versus-host reactions has also been studied.

Experiments have shown that both of thalidomide's enantiomers inhibit release of TNF-α by monocytes; synthesis of IFN-γ, and, probably via inhibition of en-

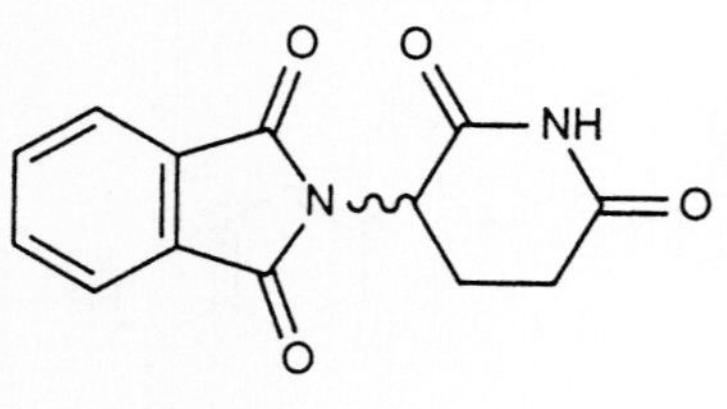

Fig. 4. Thalidomide.

dothelial cell proliferation, angiogenesis [33]. Elevated TNF-α levels have been measured in the course of graft-versus-host reactions. Toxicity of natural killer cells cannot be inhibited by thalidomide [34].

Racemic separation or purification and application of pure enantiomers does not appear useful, since racemization takes places in vivo again [35].

The substances described below, such as cyclosporine, tacrolimus, sirolimus, gusperimus, mycophenolate mofetil, mizoribine and brequinar, incorporate a relatively new mechanism by which intracellular signal processes and various enzyme systems in T cells are inhibited.

Cyclosporine

Cyclosporine is a low-molecular-weight cyclical peptide made up of 11 amino acids, and was originally isolated from *Tricoderma polysporum*. It is also produced by *Tolypocladium inflatum* Gams (Fungi imperfecti), from which it was isolated for the first time [36]. The substance was discovered on the Hardangervidda Plateau in Norway. Its complex stereochemical structure plays a key role in its immunosuppressive activity, so that a semisynthetic preparation has not yet been developed. When use of cyclosporine in international clinical transplantation medicine began in 1983, it helped provide the breakthrough in treating refractive organ failure. Today, it is considered the most effective basic immunosuppressive medication to prevent rejection reactions or crises after organ and bone marrow transplantations, and for treating graft-versus-host reactions.

Immunosuppression consisting of cyclosporine, corticosteroids and azathioprine has since become standard therapy for routine transplantations. Because it targets the distal end of T-cell activation, however, cyclosporine is of limited value in treating acute manifest rejection episodes.

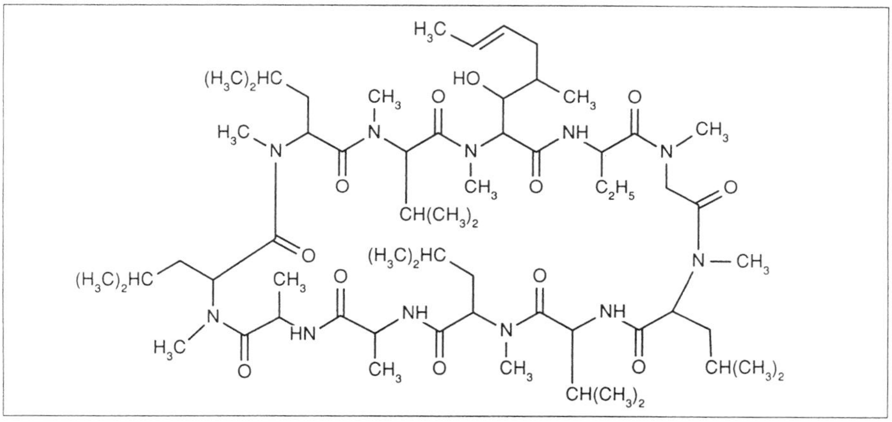

Fig. 5. Cyclosporine.

Cyclosporine acts immunosuppressively in vivo by binding to a cytosolic protein, 'cyclophilin', and inhibiting its peptidyl-prolyl isomerase (PPI) activity [37]. Because of the catalysis of *cis/trans*-rearrangement of peptidyl-prolyl bonds, cyclophilins are also called rotamases. While cyclosporine surface receptors have been described, it is more likely that the substance's lipophilia permits it to simply diffuse through the membrane into cytoplasm.

Cyclophilins, a family of cyclosporine-binding proteins of high affinity, are today called 'immunophilins', and have been found in calf thymus, plants, yeasts and bacteria [38]. Because they are widespread and highly conserved, they are assumed to have an essential function. Four different cyclophilins (Cyp A, Cyp B, Cyp C and S-Cyp) have been described in various tissues. This tissue specificity probably explains cyclosporine's nearly exclusive effect on T cells.

By binding to cyclophilin, cyclosporine interferes with intracellular calcium-dependent signal pathways essential for T-cell activation. The latest findings indicate that the cyclosporine-cyclophilin complex interacts with other regulatory proteins, such as with the calcium-binding protein calmodulin and with the serine-threonine phosphatase, calcineurin (phosphatase 2B) [39]. This pentameric unit probably controls the key regulators of gene transcription in the target cell. Uninhibited calcineurin dephosphorylates the cytosolic subunit of nuclear factor NF-ATc in activated T cells. If this dephosphorylated subunit does enter the nucleus, the combination of NF-ATc with its nuclear subunit NF-ATn there activates transcription of the IL-2 gene.

Cyclosporine, in other words, inhibits the physiologic activity of PPI such that it is no longer able to bind epitopes containing proline, nor generate isomeric rearrangement or exposition of DNA binding sites with which the genes for IL-2, IL-3, IL-4 and IFN-γ are calcium-dependently activated. The c-myc gene is also inhibited [40, 41]. T cells, on the other hand, do not lose their ability to produce other cytokines, such as granulocyte/macrophage colony-stimulating factor (GM-CSF). More recent studies, however, show that at immunosuppressive concentrations, cyclosporine occupies only 1–2% of the attachment sites on cyclophilin. The resulting inhibition of PPI activity can thus be only minimal, so that this mechanism cannot be solely responsible for cyclosporine's effects in the cell, although it may explain an increase in the scope of function.

The immunosuppressive effect of cyclosporine is therefore based primarily on inhibition of the T-cell population of lymphocytes. Like tacrolimus, cyclosporine inhibits the calcium- and calmodulin-dependent protein phosphatase calcineurin [42]. By inhibiting this calcineurin phosphatase, production of various cytokines involved in rejection reactions is suppressed [43].

Depending on concentration, cyclosporine inhibits the release of IL-2 by T-helper cells, thereby delaying proliferation of further T cells – whose proliferation is aided by the autocrine and paracrine effects of IL-2 – and indirectly blocks the

T-cell-dependent release of IL-1 by macrophages [44, 45]. The most important mechanism, suppression of IL-2 synthesis in activated T cells, is effected via suppression of the 'transcription' of IL-2-encoding mRNA. The resulting deficiency of (IL-1 and) IL-2 makes potentially reactive T cells unable to mature into cytotoxic T cells [46]. This is the reason behind cyclosporine's selective effect on immunocompetent T cells, and why allograft rejection and the graft-versus-host reaction are prevented. Cyclosporine cannot, however, completely stop activation of the IL-2 receptor gene nor, consequently, IL-2 receptor expression on superantigen-stimulated T cells.

Suppressing IL-2 production not only inhibits clonal expansion of antigen-stimulated T cells, but also prevents activation of antigen-nonspecific natural killer cells and B cells. Nor can T cells secrete IFN-γ, which would activate macrophages.

Cyclosporine also inhibits induction of HLA class II determinants, which need macrophages to present superantigen structures. This is probably caused by T cells inhibiting production of IFN-γ and IL-4.

As is discussed in the section on the mechanism of tacrolimus, cytokine transforming growth factor-β (TGF-β) is physiologically involved in wound healing and cicatrization, and promotes proliferation and differentiation of, for example, smooth-muscle cells. It may also trigger fibrosis and glomerulosclerosis. In vitro and in vivo, cyclosporine stimulates TGF-β production and the expression of receptors for TGF-β [47]. Measuring TGF-β levels in patients after kidney transplantation shows that they are significantly higher in the cyclosporine group than in the tacrolimus group. High levels of TGF-β, however, also inhibit IL-2-stimulated T-cell proliferation and generation of cytotoxic T cells, which explains cyclosporine's antiproliferative effect selectively targeting T cells.

In higher concentrations, though, cyclosporine directly affects not only T cells. There are indications that it inhibits production of TNF-α. This may take place independently of any effect on TNF-α-mRNA levels. It also inhibits connective tissue cells, including bone, cartilage and synovial cells, all of which can produce a number of cytokines.

To ensure adequate absorption when administered orally, cyclosporine should be dissolved in cocoa, orange or grapefruit juice. Bioavailability is improved when cyclosporine is given in capsules, or, with more recent galenics, in Sandimmun optoral®, a liposomal micro-emulsion. Patient blood levels should be checked morning and evening directly before drug administration.

It is also of interest that in late 1997, cyclosporine was approved for basic therapy for severe rheumatoid arthritis on account of its influence on T cells.

Tacrolimus

In 1995, tacrolimus (Prograf®) was approved in Germany, in combination with corticosteroids, for liver transplant rejection prophylaxis; for the treatment of mani-

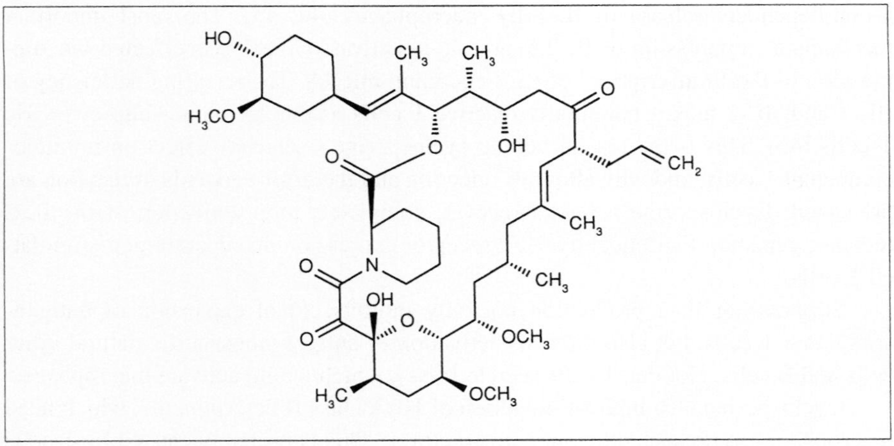

Fig. 6. Tacrolimus.

fest steroid-refractory liver transplant rejection, and as a second-line attempt to treat manifest kidney transplant rejection if no alternative is available [48–50]. Tacrolimus can be administered orally and parenterally.

Also known as Fujimycin or FK-506, tacrolimus, like sirolimus, is a macrolide lactone similar to the macrolide antibiotics, and is obtained from culture medium of *Streptomyces tsukubaensis*. It was named after its place of discovery, Mount Tsukuba, Japan.

Tacrolimus inhibits the production of cytotoxic T cells, which are the main cause of transplant rejection [51–54]. It also suppresses the production of cytokines/lymphokines such as IL-1B, IL-2, IL-3, IL-4, IL-6, IL-7, IL-8, GM-CSF and IFN-γ, as well as the expression of IL-2 receptor. IL-8, as a proinflammatory cytokine, triggers leukocyte migration at the start of an acute rejection reaction.

As a consequence, T-cell activation, and B-cell proliferation dependent on T-helper cells, are suppressed. Tacrolimus' immunosuppressive potential is somewhat higher than that of cyclosporine, but its side effects are comparable [55, 56].

The inhibition of T-cell activation occurs very early in the cell cycle: between the G_0 and G_1 phases. This inhibition of T cells, in turn, indirectly inhibits B-cell activation. Moreover, B-cell activation is also directly inhibited via a blockade of TNF-α gene transcription by an anti-Ig antibody.

Tacrolimus acts as an immunosuppressant only when bound to intracellular receptors termed FK-506-binding proteins (FK-BP-12, or macrophilin) [57]. Just like cyclosporine-binding cyclophilins, these proteins are called immunophilins, and in terms of genetic evolution are very highly conserved [58]. This binding to cytosolic proteins probably also accounts for the intracellular uptake of tacrolimus.

By binding to FK-BPs, tacrolimus interferes with intracellular calcium-dependent signal pathways essential for T-cell activation. Like cyclosporine, tacrolimus inhibits the calcium- and calmodulin-dependent protein phosphatase, calcineurin [59, 60].

Tacrolimus also inhibits matrix synthesis induced by cytokine TGF-β [61]. As a result, there is less graft fibrosis, since higher concentrations of TGF-β promote its formation. TGF-β is physiologically involved in wound healing and cicatrization, and promotes proliferation and differentiation of, for example, smooth-muscle cells. It is known to trigger fibrosis and glomerulosclerosis in animals. In swine, TGF-β gene transfection in endothelial cells can induce arteriosclerosis.

In post-lung-transplantation patients, elevated TGF-β levels have been found in conjunction with increased rates of lung fibrosis. Because TGF-β genes vary from person to person, the extent of TGF-β production varies.

With tacrolimus, there are fewer steroid-resistant rejection reactions; perhaps because tacrolimus inhibits the TGF-β-induced blockade of steroid-induced apoptosis (programmed cell death) of activated T cells [62, 63].

Due to (a) wide fluctuations in bioavailability from individual to individual; (b) a strong bond to erythrocytes and to plasma proteins (plasma protein bond of over 98.8%); (c) the significant impact of food ingested on absorption (average oral bioavailability is about 20%), and (d) a number of drug interactions, a blood trough level must be used to adjust dosage appropriately. Trough level and the area under curve (AUC) correlate closely.

In the early post-renal transplantation phase, the tacrolimus trough level should be measured 2–3 times weekly, and should be 10–20 ng/ml [64]. After 3 months, a trough level of 5–10 ng/ml is sufficient, and 1 year after transplantation, 5 ng/ml. After dosage adaptation, the new steady state is not reached until after about 3 days.

Sirolimus

Sirolimus (rapamycin) is a macrolide lactone and thus structurally closely related to tacrolimus. In the United States, this substance was clinically tested by Wyeth-Ayerst under the abbreviated designation AY-22989. Sirolimus is isolated from *Streptomyces hygroscopicus* (actinomycetes, Easter Islands), and has antibiotic, antimycotic and immunosuppressive properties [65, 66].

Blocking the cytokine-mediated effect on the cell cycle inhibits T- and B-cell response, which explains sirolimus' immunosuppressive effect [67]. Even so, the immunosuppressive effect of sirolimus differs from those of tacrolimus and cyclosporine [68, 69]. Like tacrolimus, sirolimus binds to FK-BP and inhibits its rotamase activity. Unlike cyclosporine, however, sirolimus does not bind to cyclophilins [70–72]. Furthermore, unlike tacrolimus and cyclosporine, sirolimus does not affect expression of cytokine genes, but does inhibit the antigen- and IL-2-stimulated proliferation of T cells [73, 74].

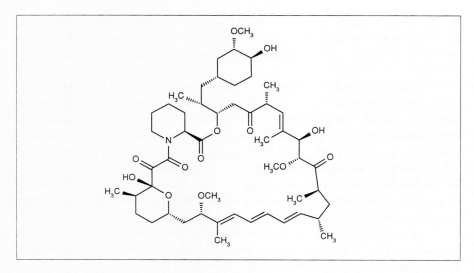

Fig. 7. Sirolimus.

Unlike tacrolimus, sirolimus directly inhibits B cells by inhibiting both their calcium-dependent proliferation (as do tacrolimus and cyclosporine) and their calcium- and T-cell-independent proliferation [75]. It is also reported that sirolimus inhibits natural killer cells and antibody-dependent cytotoxicity, and it blocks growth factor-induced proliferation of fibroblasts, endothelial cells, hepatocytes and muscle cells, i.e., the proliferation of nonimmunocompetent cells as well.

The target structures of the sirolimus FK-BP complex have been identified in mammalian cells as proteins (RAFT1/FRAP) evincing phosphatidylinositol-3-OH-kinase activity [76]. These target structures, termed TOR (Targets of RAPA), were first isolated in yeasts [77, 78]. Phosphatidylinositol-3-OH-kinases are activated by growth factor receptors, among other things, and help regulate growth and differentiation.

Exactly how sirolimus inhibits T-cell proliferation is unknown, because phosphatidylinositol-3-OH-kinases are not inhibited by sirolimus itself. It is known, however, that when a sirolimus FK-BP complex is present, p70S6 kinase is not activated. Phosphorylation of ribosomes is then disrupted, and thus the cell cycle as well [79–81].

Gusperimus/15-Deoxyspergualin

Gusperimus (15-DSG) as an immunosuppressant is undergoing clinical tests, but is already available on the Japanese market. In 1981, the parent substance, spergualin, was isolated from *Bacillus laterosporus*. Because it was found to be one of

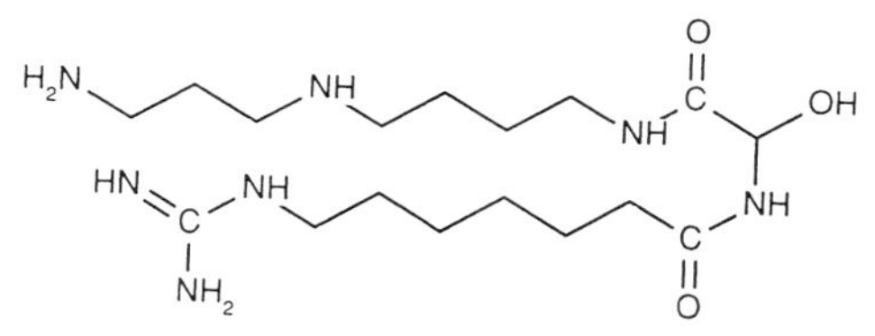

Fig. 8. Gusperimus/15-Deoxyspergualin.

the most active antitumoral substances known, its over 400 chemically modified derivatives have been researched intensively. Today, gusperimus is no longer derived from spergualin, but is a completely synthetic racemate [82].

Compared to cyclosporine, tacrolimus or sirolimus, gusperimus has a totally new mechanism of effect which could enhance immunosuppressive therapy [83, 84]. Gusperimus interferes in intracellular signal transduction by binding to cytosolic heat-shock protein hsp70, a protein which facilitates protein transport within the cell [85]. This may explain why transcription factor NF-κB can no longer be transported into the nucleus. This then inhibits the production of the κ light chain in antibodies, which in turn inhibits T-cell-dependent and T-cell-independent antibody production [86, 87].

Nonimmunosuppressive analogues of gusperimus do not bind to hsp70, which explains the link between gusperimus' binding to hsp70 and its immunosuppressive potency.

Gusperimus has not been found to inhibit proliferation of stimulated T and B cells, but it does inhibit T cells' differentiating into cytotoxic T cells. It also reduces IL-2 receptor expression on both CD4 and CD8 cells. However, IL-1 and IL-2 production is suppressed only very slightly, if at all.

Gusperimus has been shown to inhibit IFN-γ-induced maturation of B cells [88, 89]. It also exerts a potentiated immunosuppressive effect when administered together with tacrolimus, cyclosporine or mycophenolate mofetil to prevent the rejection of allogenic grafts.

Mycophenolate Mofetil (MPM)

Mycophenolic acid (MPA) is a product of fermentation of various species of fungus of the Penicillium genus, and was first tested as an antibiotic and antitumoral medication [90–92]. In 1996, MPM was approved in Europe as an immunosuppressant.

MPA or MPM (RS-61443) has proved successful in preventing acute and chronic rejection reactions of kidney transplants. Its use has recently begun in heart

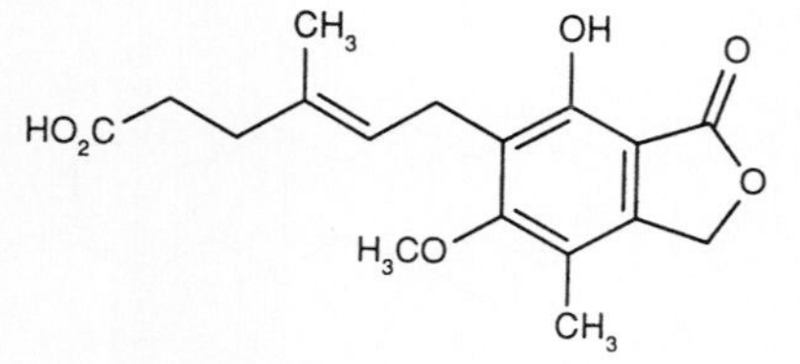

Fig. 9. Mycophenolic acid.

transplantation as well. In 1998, the FDA approved the use of CellCept®, in combination with other immunosuppressants, to prevent organ rejection in post-heart transplant patients. In Germany, in combination with cyclosporine and corticosteroids, CellCept® has been approved as a prophylactic for acute allogenic kidney transplant rejection.

When orally administered, MPM is quickly and almost completely absorbed and is fully converted into the active metabolite, MPA. MPA is itself a highly effective, selective, noncompetitive, reversible inhibitor of IMP (inosine monophosphate) dehydrogenase (IMPDH), the key enzyme of de novo purine synthesis, and thus inhibits guanosine monophosphate (GMP) synthesis without being integrated into DNA. If key enzyme IMPDH is inhibited, GMP is degraded, which normally phosphorylates into GTP (guanosine triphosphate) and is converted into dGTP. Via DNA polymerase, dGTP is then integrated into DNA [93, 94a, b].

Breakdown of GMP, and hence that of GTP and dGTP as well, leads to a deficiency of guanosine nucleotides. This deficiency inhibits two other speed-regulating key enzymes for lymphocytic DNA synthesis, namely phosphoribosyl-pyrophosphate (PRPP)-synthetase and ribonucleotide reductase. This additionally inhibits proliferation of lymphocytes [95].

After conversion into the actual drug, MPA, immunosuppression is effected by inhibiting de novo purine synthesis (de novo synthesis of guanosine nucleotides) and by consequently suppressing T- and B-cell responses. The resulting inhibition of B-cell proliferation suppresses production of antibodies. MPA has a stronger cytostatic impact on lymphocytes than on other cells. This is because lymphocytes are primarily dependent on de novo synthesis and cannot, like other cell types, reconstruct themselves out of other structures.

MPA also inhibits glycosylation of lymphocytic glycoproteins, especially the transfer of mannose and fucose sugars. Some of these glycoproteins are involved in the adhesion of leukocytes to endothelial and target cells [96].

In vitro studies show that MPM inhibits DNA synthesis of mitogen-activated lymphocytes, but not that of neutrophils, fibroblasts, or endothelial cells. It has also been demonstrated that neither MPA nor MPM inhibits the production of IL-1β by mitogen-activated human lymphocytes. This indicates that the early signal transduction systems of T cells are not influenced. It has also been shown that MPM inhibits superantigen-induced, but not mitogen-induced, cytokine production [97]. Various models, moreover, show that MPA almost completely stops antibody formation of polyclonal activated human B cells [98].

In vivo studies on rats, hamsters, dogs and primates have confirmed the vast majority of findings of the in vitro studies. The prevention of graft-versus-host reaction has also been demonstrated in rats which had undergone intestinal and bone marrow transplantation. In studies on preventing rejection reactions, the incidence of malignoma (only lymphoproliferative diseases) was higher in the MPM group than in the placebo or azathioprine groups.

Since a large-scale study has confirmed MPM's benefits for heart transplantation patients as well, it should soon gain approval for additional uses.

Mizoribine (Bredinin)

Like azathioprine and MPM, mizoribine is an antiproliferative. It was discovered in a screening program to develop new antibiotics, and was first isolated from *Eupenicillium brefeldianum* fungus by Toyo Jozo Co. of Japan in 1974. Mizoribine has an imidazole nucleoside structure, and is used in Japan as an immunosuppressant [99], for which use it has not yet been approved in Europe. It may eventually grow in importance also outside of Japan, being at least as immunosuppressive as azathioprine, but with lower myelo- and hepatotoxicity [100].

Like MPM, mizoribine inhibits IMPDH and GMP synthetase, and thus de novo purine synthesis as well [101]. Mizoribine is a prodrug; the actual competitive inhibitor of IMPDH and GMP synthetase is mizoribine-5-monophosphate. The active metabolite itself is not incorporated in DNA or RNA, but is dephosphorylated intracellularly via a 5'-nucleotidase and flushed out of the cell when the extracellular concentration drops.

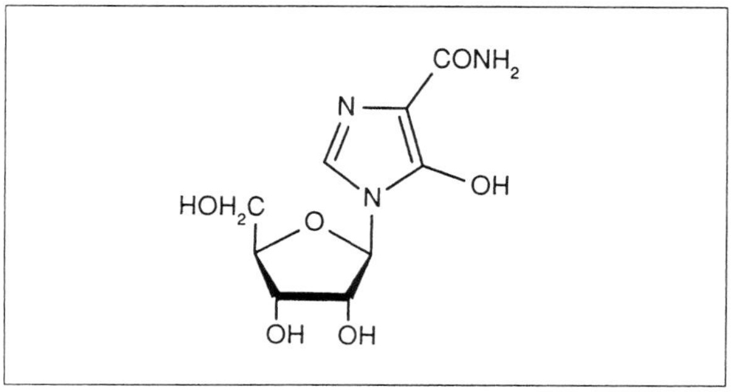

Fig. 10. Mizoribine (Bredinin).

Mizoribine has no effect on IL-2 synthesis, nor on its expression [102, 103], but when combined with cyclosporine or tacrolimus, enhances inhibition of T-cell proliferation.

Various animal trials have shown that mizoribine can suppress acute graft-versus-host reactions and the generation of memory-B and T-helper cells.

Brequinar (Brequinar Sodium, DUP-785)

Brequinar sodium has not yet been approved in Europe for use as an immunosuppressant. Completely synthetic, it is derived from 4-quinolinecarboxylic acid. Brequinar was developed in the United States by DuPont-Merck as part of a program to synthesize new antitumoral substances [104].

Like MPM, azathioprine and mizoribine, brequinar acts antiproliferatively [105]. It takes a fully new approach to immunosuppression in that it inhibits pyrimidine synthesis by inhibiting dehydroorotate dehydrogenase (DHO-DH), subsequently blocking production of orotate (as a precursor of uridine monophosphate). Its mechanism is based on a reversible, noncompetitive inhibition of the DHO-DH enzyme, which is involved in de novo pyrimidine synthesis. This reduces the pyrimidine pool in activated T and B cells, especially of UTP, CTP, dTTP and dCTP [106, 107].

Studies have shown that brequinar suppresses the proliferation of activated lymphocytes more strongly than that of certain tumor cell lines. This is because T and B cells require large amounts of pyrimidine bases to proliferate [108]. The antiproliferative effect can be antagonized by administering uridine.

In 1991, the first report was published of brequinar preventing graft rejection in humans, although great fluctuations in sensitivity from individual to individual were reported. It was found that in vivo, brequinar suppresses both T-cell-dependent and T-cell-independent antibody production, as well as generation of cytotoxic T cells. Combination with cyclosporine improved transplant rejection prevention [109, 110],

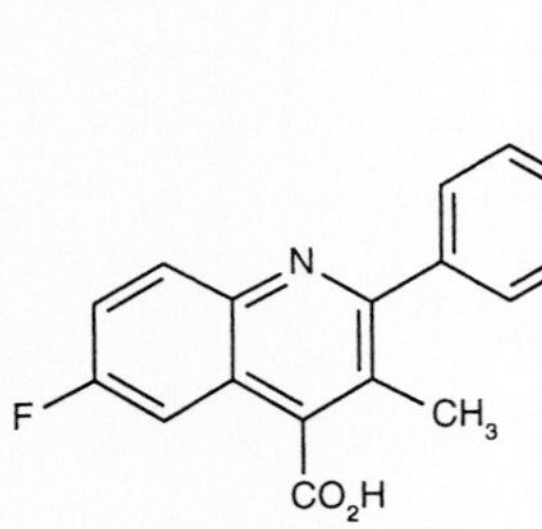

Fig. 11. Brequinar.

and it was reported that brequinar inhibits IL-2 production, IL-2 gene transcription, and the expression of IL-2 receptor. Adding cytidine, moreover, was found to potentiate brequinar's immunosuppressive effect, so that brequinar is also assumed to inhibit cytidine deaminase in pyrimidine synthesis.

Leflunomide (HWA 486, LFM)

Leflunomide was developed by HMR in Germany, and is one of the newest substances under study for its immunosuppressive possibilities. Leflunomide's precursor substances were originally developed in the search for new herbicides, and only later was their anti-inflammatory potential recognized. Leflunomide is a fully synthetic, organic isoxazol derivative which is metabolized into its active form, A77 1726, in intestinal mucosa and perhaps in the liver. Because it has negative pharmacokinetics – in particular, a half-life that lasts several days in humans – HMR is working on a successor substance.

Animal experiments studying leflunomide's effect on autoimmune disorders showed that it inhibits T-cell-dependent antibody production and that it antagonizes the cytokinic effect of immune cells. In vitro, it was demonstrated that the active metabolite, A77 1726, inhibits both T- and B-cell proliferation, although its effect was stronger on B cells [111–113].

While leflunomide does not appear to affect the production of immunocytokines, its antagonism of the biologic effects of IL-3, IL-4, G-CSF, GM-CSF and TNF-α has been described.

One of its main effects in vivo appears to be its inhibition of tyrosine kinase, which accounts for the inhibition of tyrosine phosphorylation of IL-2-stimulated T cells [114]. It has also been demonstrated that leflunomide inhibits pyrimidine synthesis in vivo, a finding supported by the fact that administering uridine, cytidine or pyrimidine nucleotides antagonizes the antiproliferative effect [115].

Genetic engineering has created substances with which T-cell surface structures can be specifically masked and the cascade of immune reactions thereby suppressed. Some of these substances are discussed below.

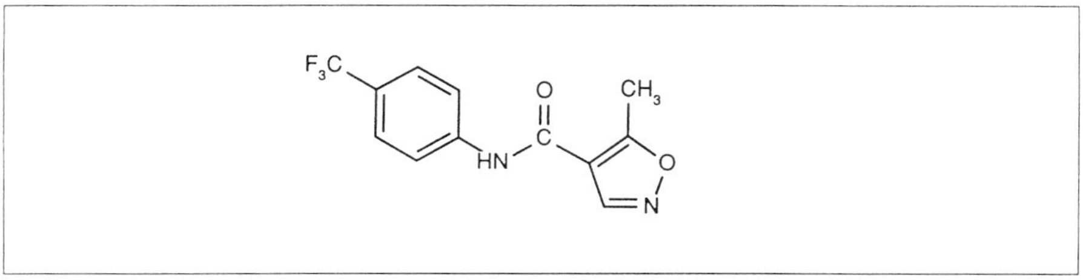

Fig. 12. Leflunomide.

Monoclonal Antibodies

Muronomab CD3

Even though polyclonal immunoglobulin fractions targeted against T-cell surfaces had proven effective, monoclonal antibodies were also developed [116, 117] to circumvent the drawbacks of polyclonal antibodies. For example, polyclonal antibodies must be administered in large doses, vary in makeup from batch to batch, and contain certain antibodies that do not target immunocompetent cells, but which do cause many side effects.

Hence, various monoclonal antibodies (OKT1, OKT3, OKT4, OKT6, OKT8, OKT11) were developed against specific surface structures of T cells that target various CD classes [118]. One of these is orthoclone® OKT3, a monoclonal humanized antibody of murine origin targeted against the T3 antigen; i.e., against the CD3 molecule (CD = cluster of differentiation) of the T-cell receptor complex [119, 120]. The CD3 structure is found on all mature peripheral T cells, and is part of the T-cell antigen recognition complex of the T-cell receptor, whereby the CD3 structure is noncovalently bound to the T-cell receptor complex, and helps facilitate its expression [121].

Orthoclone's antibodies against T3 antigens are class IgG_{2a} immunoglobulins [122]. Because the hybridoma technique is used that Köhler and Milstein developed in 1975, they are manufactured identically, and react specifically only to peripheral T cells and mature thymocytes.

By specifically blocking T3 antigens, orthoclone prevents T cells with T-cell receptors from binding to superantigens (antigen structures of the graft) which, for example, are presented by phagocyting macrophages or dendritic cells. This inhibits production of immunocomplexes and the correlating activation of transmembranous signals [123].

Because extracellular CD3 proteins are not polymorphous, antibody muronomab CD3 recognizes these structures regardless of the individual in which they are found. With muronomab CD3 treatment, T cells are eliminated from peripheral circulation and phagocytically opsonized in the liver and spleen. As therapy continues, the number of T cells rises again, but because fewer T-cell receptors are expressed, immunosuppression occurs.

Additional mechanisms reported are cell clearance of alloreactive T cells via sequestration or lysis due to uptake into the reticuloendothelial system (primarily of the liver and spleen), as well as modulation or induction of receptor shedding. This deactivates the inductor/effector phase of alloreactive T-cell activation. Binding to the CD3 unit also disrupts T-cell function where receptor modulation is deficient. Once OKT3 is bound, class I and class II MHC antigens inhibit T-cell proliferation. It is also assumed that sessile T cells in the graft are blocked [124, 125].

Muronomab CD3's binding to the T-cell receptor temporarily activates the T cell, causing a rise in serum concentrations of TNF-α, IFN-γ, IL-2 and other interleukins (in the cytokine release syndrome) [126]. This accounts for muronomab's side effects such as fever and chills. Also reported is complement activation and macrophage migration into the lungs with subsequent lung edema. In about 6% of the patients, neutralizing idiotypical antibodies are produced, and are accompanied by an increasing number of circulating CD3+ cells, which limits the efficacy of a second course of therapy [127, 128].

In Germany, orthoclone has been approved for treating acute (especially gluco-corticoid-resistant) rejection of allogenic kidney, heart and liver transplants. Previously, OKT3 was also in induction and rejection therapy after heart transplantation. In 1998, the FDA approved its use in combination with other immunosuppressants to prevent heart transplant rejection. The side effects of OKT3 are nearly the same as those of polyclonal antibodies ALG and ATG. In addition, an increased frequency of malignoma has been observed under OKT.

Monoclonal Antibody BMA 031

Murine monoclonal antibody BMA 031, an IgG2b immunoglobulin, is targeted at structures of the T-cell receptor and indicated for acute rejection reactions and crises. It is presently undergoing phase II and III tests involving transplantation of solid organs. The mechanism of BMA 031 resembles that of muronomab CD3, but BMA 031 does not modulate the T-cell receptor/CD3 complex. BMA 031 is targeted at the α and β chains of T-cell receptors on T lymphocytes, and thus blocks intracellular signal transmission during T-cell activation.

Monoclonal Antibody WT31

Murine monoclonal antibody WT31 is still in the preclinical development phase. It is an IgG1 fraction, which, like BMA 031 and T10B9, is targeted against structures of the T-cell receptor.

Monoclonal Antibody T10B9

T10B9 is a murine antibody of the IgMk class. Like BMA 031, antibody T10B9 is presently in phase II and III tests involving transplantation of solid organs.

Monoclonal Antibody Anti-TAC (IgG2a)

Murine monoclonal IL-2 antibody anti-TAC (IgG2a) has been tested in various clinical trials. This antibody binds to the α chain of IL-2 receptors, which inhibits T-cell activation and facilitates cell destruction. Antibodies targeted at IL-2 recognize only T cells that are positive for IL-2 receptors; i.e., only activated T cells, because these receptors are expressed almost solely on these cells, and only rarely on activated B cells [129].

Monoclonal Antibody 33B3.1

Monoclonal antibody 33B3.1 is an IgG2b fraction in the class of anti-IL-2 antibodies. Animal trials have proved its prophylactic efficacy in solid-organ transplantation, although about 14 days after therapy had commenced, IgG and IgM antibodies against 33B3.1 were detected, which led to a loss of effect [130].

Basiliximab

Murine monoclonal antibodies used on humans quickly cause production of neutralized antibodies, which limits the success of therapy and may result in dose escalation. To counteract this effect, chimeric or humanized antibodies were developed. These are monoclonal antibodies that contain the variable region of the mouse and the constant regions of the human. Basiliximab is this kind of chimeric antibody.

As a CD25 antibody, basiliximab has high affinity for binding to CD25 protein, one of the three transmembranous protein chains that make up the IL-2 receptor. Large amounts of this IL-2 receptor develop on antigenically activated T cells. By binding to these CD25 receptors, IL-2 stimulates the T cells to rapidly proliferate, so that the organism is stimulated to reject the foreign transplant [131]. By blocking these receptors with basiliximab, this process can be halted [132].

In a randomized European-Canadian double-blind study, 380 patients received a cadaverous kidney with at least HLA class I or class II incompatibility. They were administered either a placebo or were given 20 mg of basiliximab 2 h before, and on the fourth day after, transplantation [133]. 40 mg of basiliximab inhibit CD25 formation and thus the effect of IL-2 for 4–6 weeks. All 380 patients also received cyclosporine and glucocorticoids concomitantly. Biopsy after 6 months proved that 33% of the patients in the basiliximab group had had an acute rejection reaction, and 44% in the placebo group. Frequency of acute rejection was thus significantly reduced by one third. Basiliximab was as well tolerated as placebo, and no evidence of cytokine release syndrome was observed.

Daclizumab/Dacliximab

Daclizumab/dacliximab, which will be marketed under the trademarked name of Zenapax®, is a new, humanized monoclonal antibody that has been clinically tested on nearly 500 patients. It has been approved for use in the United States and Switzerland, and is expected to gain approval in Germany soon. The humanized monoclonal antibody daclizumab was discovered by Protein Design Labs of Mountain View, Calif., and developed to marketability by Hoffmann-La Roche.

This genetically engineered antibody (IgG_1-immunoglobulin) binds specifically to the α chain (the TAC or T-cell-activating antigen) of the IL-2 receptor [134–136]. It is therefore also known as humanized anti-TAC. This bond prevents the actual ligand, IL-2, from triggering the clonal replication of superantigen-stimulated T cells by binding to the IL-2 receptor. These stimulated T cells express the α chain of the IL-2 receptor. The β and γ chains of the IL-2 receptor, which are also expressed on nonactivated T cells, form, together with the α subunit, an IL-2 receptor complex of high affinity.

In placebo-controlled studies, 1 mg/kg b.w. of daclizumab was given intravenously, over 15 min, prior to kidney transplantation and every 2 weeks thereafter for a total of five doses. This dosage significantly reduced the frequency of acute rejection reactions [137–140].

Unlike other immunosuppressants, which paralyze the entire immune system and increase the patient's risk of infection, daclizumab inhibits only those T cells activated by the allogenic transplant.

Antithymocytic or Antilymphocytic Globulins

Induction Therapy with Antithymocytic or Antilymphocytic Globulins
To supplement standard prophylaxis and therapy using immunosuppressants, induction therapy using polyclonal antithymocyte or antilymphocyte globulins has been introduced over the past few years [141].

Polyclonal immunoglobulins are generated by injecting animals (horses, rabbits, rats, and so on) with human lymphatic cells, such as lymphoblasts of the B-cell line or peripheral lympho- or thymolymphocytes. The resulting immunosera are harvested, and the immunoglobulin-γ fractions purified. Even so, the result is a fairly heterogenic mix of polyclonal antibodies, and only a few of them evince affinity to lymphatic tissue [142]. Some of the immunoglobulins bind to B cells, T cells or macrophages, but the majority binds in a relatively general manner [143].

It is very difficult to standardize polyclonal immunoglobulin fractions, since the composition of antibodies fluctuates so widely. This also accounts for the variability of effects and side effects. Nonspecific antibodies can cause thrombocytopenia, granulocytopenia, serum sickness with fever and shaking chills, and glomerulonephritis [144, 145]. In combination with other immunosuppressants there is a higher risk of 'oversuppression', which may account for the increased frequency of cytomegaloviral infections.

Administration of these kinds of immunoglobulin fractions has been found to further reduce the incidence of acute rejections in the early phase of postoperative immunosuppression [146]. One advantage of immunoinductor therapy is that it prevents more serious rejection reactions in the early postoperative phase than does glucocorticoid therapy. This permits patients with renal insufficiency to be saturated more slowly with cyclosporine [147].

There may be reactions to its foreign protein structure, with intermittent fever, shaking chills, and even anaphylaxis, so that therapy must usually be limited to

10–14 days. This reaction can be lessened with prophylactic administration of paracetamol, antihistamines and methylprednisolone.

The mechanisms of action of polyclonal immunoglobulins comprise complement-induced lysis of lymphocytes, as well as lymphocyte clearance due to uptake by the reticuloendothelial system. Also reported are the expansion of suppressor subpopulations and the masking of T-cell antigens, which can inhibit lymphocytic function. Moreover, the binding of specific antibodies to the lymphocytes temporarily brings about a manifest lymphopenia, and it is this reduction in circulating T cells which is at the root of the primary immunosuppressive effect. But when therapy has stopped and the number of circulating T cells increases again, proliferation continues to be inhibited and suppressor subpopulations expand, as described above, which is why immunosuppression continues after the end of therapy.

Horse Anti-Human Lymphocyte Immunoglobulin

Lymphoglobulin Mérieux contains an anti-T-cell immunoserum / polyclonal horse antithymocyte globulin, with an IgG_2 content of 14–26 mg/ml. It has been approved in Germany for prophylactic and therapeutic use in rejection crises after organ transplantation, as well as for aplastic anemia. Prior to beginning therapy, which is in combination with glucocorticoids, a test for hypersensitivity to equine protein is recommended, and administration of an antihistamine.

Rabbit Anti-Human Lymphocyte Immunoglobulin

Thymoglobulin® is a product of the further development of horse polyclonal antilymphocyte immunoglobulins, and contains immunoglobulin G (polyclonal) from the serum of immunized rabbits (rabbit ATG). It has been approved as a prophylactic for rejection reactions after transplantation of the kidney, heart or liver, for rejection crises after kidney transplantation, and for treating aplastic anemia when other therapies have failed [148–151].

Antibodies specifically active against surface structures of T cells have been identified in Thymoglobulin Mérieux®, and include anti-CD2, anti-CD4, anti-CD8, anti-CD18, anti-HLA-DR, and small amounts of anti-CD3 antibodies [152].

Like Thymoglobulin Mérieux®, ATG Fresenius S® contains polyclonal immunoglobulin G from the serum of immunized rabbits (rabbit ATG).

Fusion Proteins

Proteins created by fusing cytokines and toxins enable a completely new approach towards suppressing or destroying activated T cells, as described below.

CTLA4-Ig Fusion Protein

A solid-organ transplantation generally activates T cells because antigen-presenting cells, such as macrophages, present superantigen structures of the graft. But before the T-cell population can be fully activated against the foreign antigen, the T-cell receptor must recognize these presented superantigens, and additional surface proteins of the T cell, such as CTLA4, must find their counterpart on the antigen-presenting cell.

The possible use of these interactive mechanisms for immunosuppressive therapy has thus far been tested only in animal experiments on CTLA4-Ig fusion proteins. This chimera was developed out of the CTLA4 surface molecule of the T cell and the heavy chain of the IgG_1. It prevents communication between the T cell and the MHC molecules on the surface of the antigen-presenting cell. One of the results of this barrier to molecular communication is an adaptive immunity to, or acceptance of, the foreign organ. This acceptance is called T-cell anergy.

IL-2 Toxin

Studies are underway on using fusion proteins gained from IL-2 and diphtheria toxin to destroy activated T cells. These fusion proteins bind selectively to IL-2-positive (and thus activated) T cells, and destroy them with their toxin. The IL-2 component of the fusion protein guarantees the highly affine binding to the IL-2 receptor and subsequent uptake into the cell, in which the diphtheria toxin is then activated. Animal experiments have demonstrated the efficacy of this fusion protein, and of fusion proteins combining IL-4 and diphtheria toxin, or IL-2 and Pseudomonas exotoxin. Clinical trials, however, have yet to be conducted.

Outlook: Transplantations without Immunosuppression!

After receiving a solid-organ graft, the recipient must take immunosuppressants for the rest of his/her life, and is therefore very susceptible for all kinds of infection. This drawback makes the goal of organ transplantation without any form of immunosuppression that much more important.

The Medical Center of the University of Pennsylvania has taken a major step in this direction. In animal studies, the institute has found that the activation of immunocompetent T cells, and thus the attack on transplanted tissue, is triggered only when two signals have been given. The first signal comes from the MHC (major histocompatibility complex), and the second from protein CTLA4-Ig.

While a blockade of MHC might be possible, it would probably have undesirable side effects. Instead, the animal experiment at the Medical Center entailed placing the organ to be transplanted in a cooled solution containing adenoviruses loaded with CTLA4-Ig genes. The adenoviruses acted as vectors along which the CTLA4-Ig genes entered the graft cells. The organ thus treated actually did express the CLTA4-Ig protein desired. What is more, even though its MHC signaled to the recipient's T cells that the transplant was foreign, the T cells did not attack because the second signal, the costimulatory signal, was missing.

Despite this success, it may be some time before this experiment will be conducted on humans, since adenoviruses are usually just agents of the common cold. It would in any case first have to be ascertained that no other genes could be 'smuggled in' by the adenoviruses to cause illness or genetic disorders. Additionally, the CTLA4-Ig proteins expressed by the organ thus treated would have to be stable enough to be passed on reliably by every mitosis. But if these experiments some day evince the same long-term success in humans, the transplantation of solid organs will be possible without hazardous, extremely expensive life-long immunosuppression.

References

1   Meire JP: Successful homotransplantation of human kidneys between identical twins. JAMA 1956;160:277–282.
2   Janeway CA, Travers P: Immunologie. Heidelberg, Spektrum Akademischer Verlag, 1995.
3   Ferguson R: Acute rejection episodes – Best predictor of long-term primary cadaveric renal transplant survival. Clin Transplant 1994;8:328–331.
4   Tilney NL, Kupiec-Weglinski JW: The immunobiology of acute allograft rejection; in Brent L, Sells RA (eds): Organ Transplantation: Current Clinical Immunological Concepts. London, Bailliere Tindall, 1989, pp 19–38.
5   Zanker B, Walz G, Wieder KJ, Strom TB: Evidence that glucocorticosteroids block expression of the human interleukin-6 gene by accessory cells. Transplantation 1990;49:183–185.
6   Tilney NL, Strom TB, Macpershon SG, Carpenter CB: Surface properties and functional characteristics of infiltrating cells harvested from acutely rejecting cardiac allografts in inbred rats. Transplantation 1975;20:323–330.
7   Bainbridge DR, Gowland G: Studies on transplantation immunity. The nature of the response to allogenic Cr-labelled lymphoid cells and its relationship to homograft immunity. Cell Immunol 1971;2:115–127.
8   Beatty PG, Mickelson EM, Petersdorf EW: Histocompatibility 1991. Transfusion 1991;31:847–856.
9   Beato M: Gene regulation by steroid hormones. Cell 1989;56:335–344.
10 Starzl TE, Demetris AJ: Transplantation milestones: Viewed with one- and two-way paradigms of tolerance. JAMA 1995;273:876–879.
11 Rao AS, Starzl TE, Demetris AJ, Trucco M: The two-way paradigm of transplantation immunology. Clin Immunol Immunopathol 1996;80:41–46.
12 Folb PI: Elective pharmacological inhibition of lymphocyte stimulation. Lancet 1971;ii:221–222.
13 Elion GB: Summary of investigations with 6-((1-methyl-4-nitro-5-imidazolyl)thio)purine. Cancer 1961;14:93–98.
14 Marx J: How the glucocorticoids suppress immunity. Science 1995;270:232–233.
15 Wyllie AH: Glucocorticoid-induced thymocyte apoptosis is associated with endogenous endonuclease activation. Nature 1980;284:555–556.

16 Scheinman RI, Cogswell PC, Lofquist AK, Baldwin AS Jr: Role of transcriptional activation of IκBα in mediation of immunosuppression by glucocorticoids. Science 1995;270:283–286.

17 Auphan N, DiDonato JA, Rosette C, Helmberg A: Immunosuppression by glucocorticoids: Inhibition of NF-κB activity through induction of IκB synthesis. Science 1995;270:286–289.

18 Kerppola TK, Luk D, Curran T: Fos is a preferential target of glucocorticoid receptor inhibition of AP-1 activity in vitro. Mol Cell Biol 1993;13:3782–3791.

19 Olsen SL, O'Connell JB, Bristow MR, Renlund DG: Methotrexate as an adjunct in the treatment of persistent mild cardiac allograft rejection. Transplantation 1990;50:773–775.

20 Michael B, Francos GC, Burke JF, Gaughan WI: Methotrexate is effective in preventing acute and potentially chronic renal allograft rejection. Transplant Proc 1994;26:3046–3047.

21 Zhao SC, Banerjee D, Mineishi S, Bertino JR: Mice bearing a transplanted carcinoma tolerate curative doses of methotrexate after transplantation with a retroviral construct containing a mutated dihydrofolate reductase cDNA. Proc Am Assoc Cancer Res 1996;37:343.

22 Przepiorka D, Ippoliti C, Khouri I, Anderlini P, Le Bherz D, van Besien K, Ueno N, Mehra R, Giralt S, Gajewski J, Fritsche H, Cleary K, Claxton D, Champlin R, Andersson B, Koerbling M: Microdose methotrexate vs. methylprednisolone in combination with tacrolimus for prevention of acute graft-vs.-host disease after allogenic blood stem cell transplantation. Blood 1996;88:418A.

23 Yu C, Seidel K, Fitzsimmons WE, Sale G, Storb R: Glucocorticoids fail to enhance the effect of FK-506 and methotrexate in prevention of graft-versus-host disease after DLA-nonidentical, unrelated marrow transplantation. Bone Marrow Transplant 1997;20:137–141.

24 Ochonisky S, Verroust J, Bastuji-Garin S, Gherardi R, Revuz J: Thalidomide neuropathy incidence and clinicoelectrophysiologic findings in 42 patients. Arch Dermatol 1994;130:66–69.

25 McBride WG: Thalidomide and congenital abnormalities. Lancet 1961;ii:1358.

26 Keller H, cited in Wenzel D, Wenzel KH (eds): Der Contergan-Prozess. Berlin, Wissenschaft und Forschung, 1968, vol 2, pp 56–70.

27 Sheskin J: Thalidomide in the treatment of lepra reactions. Clin Pharmacol Ther 1965;6: 303–306.

28 Sheskin J: The treatment of lepra reaction in lepromatous leprosy. Int J Dermatol 1980;19: 318–322.

29 Vogelsang GB, Farmer ER, Hess AD, Altamonte V, Beschorner WE, Jabs DA, Corio RL, Levin LS, Colvin OM, Wingard JR, Santos GW: Thalidomide for the treatment of chronic graft-versus-host disease. N Engl J Med 1992;326:1055–1058.

30 Cole CH, Rogers PCJ, Pritchard S, Phillips G, Chan KW: Thalidomide in the management of chronic graft-versus-host disease in children following bone marrow transplantation. Am Marrow Transplant 1994;14:937–942.

31 Parker PM, Chao N, Nademanee A: Thalidomide as salvage therapy for chronic graft-versus-host disease. Blood 1995;86:3604–3609.

32 Duval M, Rohrlich P, Thomas E, Fenneteau O, Nafa S, Schlegel N, Jacqz-Aigrain E, Vilmer E: Three cases of neutropenia and thrombopenia attributable to thalidomide in the treatment of GVHD. Bone Marrow Transplant 1995;15:147.

33 Sampaio EP, Sarno EN, Galilly R, Cohn ZA, Kaplan G: Thalidomide selectively inhibits tumor necrosis factor alpha production by stimulated human monocytes. J Exp Med 1991;173:699–703.

34 Wnendt S, Finkam M, Winter W, Raabe G, Ossig J, Zwingenberger K: Enantiospecific inhibition of TNF-α release by thalidomide and thalidomide analogues. Chirality 1996;8: 390–396.

35 Hague D, Smith RL: Enigmatic properties of (+/–)-thalidomide. An example of a stable racemic compound. Br J Clin Pharmacol 1988;26:623.

36 Rüegger A, Kuhn M, Lichti H, Loosli HR: Cyclosporin A, a peptide metabolite from *Trichoderma polysporum,* with a remarkable immunosuppressive activity. Helv Chim Acta 1976;59:1075–1092.

37 Handschuhmacher RE, Harding MW, Rice J, Drugge RH: Cyclophilin: A specific cytosolic binding protein for cyclosporin A. Science 1984;236:544–547.

38 Wiederrecht G, Etzkorn F: The immunophilins. Perspect Drug Disc Design 1994;2:57–84.

39 Clipstone NA, Crabtree GR: Calcineurin is a key signaling enzyme in T-lymphocyte activation and the target of the immunosuppressive drugs cyclosporin A and FK-506. J Biol Chem 1993;696:20–30.

40 Bram RJ, Hung DT, Martin PK, Schreiber SL: Identification of the immunophilins capable of mediating inhibition of signal transduction by cyclosporin A and FK-506: Roles of calcineurin and cellular location. Mol Cell Biol 1993;13:4760–4769.

41 Herold KC, Lancki DW, Moldwin RL, Fitch TW: Immunosuppressive effects of cyclosporin A on cloned T cells. J Immunol 1986;136:1315–1321.

42 Siekierka JJ, Hung SH, Poe M, Lin CS: A cytosolic binding protein for the immunosuppressant FK-506 has peptidyl-prolyl isomerase activity but is distinct from cyclophilin. Nature 1989;341:755–757.

43 Harding MW, Galat A, Uehling DE, Schreiber SL: A receptor for the immunosuppressant FK-506 is a *cis-trans* peptidyl-prolyl isomerase. Nature 1989;341:758–760.

44 Elliot JF, Lin Y, Mizel SB, Bleackley RC: Induction of interleukin 2 messenger RNA inhibited by cyclosporin A. Science 1984;226:439–441.

45 Kronke M, Leonard WJ, Depper JM, Arya SK: Cyclosporin A inhibits T cell growth factor gene expression at the level of mRNA transcription. Proc Natl Acad Sci USA 1984;81:5214–5218.

46 Hess AD, Tutschka PJ: Effect of cyclosporin A on human lymphocyte responses in vitro. J Immunol 1988;124:2601–2608.

47 Schwaninger M, Blume R, Oetjen E, Knepel W: The immunosuppressive drugs cyclosporin A and FK-506 inhibit calcineurin phosphatase activity and gene transcription mediated through the cAMP-responsive element in a nonimmune cell line. Naunyn Schmiedebergs Arch Pharmacol 1993;348:541–545.

48 Peters DH, Fitton A, Plasker GL: Tacrolimus. A review of pharmacology and therapeutic potential in hepatic and renal transplantation. Drugs 1993;46:746–794.

49 Przepiorka D, Ippoliti C: Tacrolimus and minidose methotrexate for prevention of acute graft-versus-host disease after matched unrelated donor marrow transplantation. Blood 1996;88:4383–4389.

50 Uberti JP, Silver SM, Adams PT, Jacobson P, Scalzo A, Ratanatharathorn V: Tacrolimus and methotrexate for the prophylaxis of acute graft-versus-host disease in allogenic bone marrow transplantation in patients with hematologic malignancies. Bone Marrow Transplantation 1997;19:1233–1238.

51 Dumont FJ, Staruch MJ, Koprak SL: Distinct mechanism of suppression of murine T cell activation by the related macrolides FK-506 and rapamycin. J Immunol 1990;144:251–258.

52 Bierer BE, Mattila PS, Standaert RF: Two distinct signal transmission pathways in T lymphocytes are inhibited by complexes formed between an immunophilin and either FK-506 or rapamycin. Proc Natl Acad Sci USA 1990;87:9231–9235.

53 Venkataramanan R, Warty VS: Pharmacokinetics and monitoring of FK-506 (tacrolimus); in

Thomson A, Starzl TS (eds): Immunosuppressive Drugs: Developments in Anti-Rejection Therapy. London, Arnold, 1994, pp 84–94.

54 Thomson A, Woo J, Zeevi A: The influence of FK-506 on lymphocyte responses in vitro and in vivo; in Thomson A, Starzl TS (eds): Immunosuppressive Drugs: Developments in Anti-Rejection Therapy. London, Arnold, 1994, pp 96–111.

55 Sigal NH, Dumont FJ: Cyclosporin A, FK-506 and rapamycin: Pharmacologic probes of lymphocyte signal transduction. Annu Rev Immunol 1992;10:519–560.

56 Schreiber SL, Crabtree GL: The mechanism of action of cyclosporin A and FK-506. Immunol Today 1992;13:136–142.

57 Dawson TM: Immunosuppressant, FK-506, enhances phosphorylation of nitric oxide synthase and protects against glutamate neurotoxicity. Proc Natl Acad Sci USA 1993;90: 9808–9812.

58 Cohen P, Cohen PTW: Protein phosphatases come of age. J Biol Chem 1989;264: 21435–21438.

59 Cardenas ME, Hemenway C, Muir RS: Immunophilins interact with calcineurin in the absence of exogenous immunosuppressive ligands. EMBO J 1994;13:5944–5957.

60 Flanagan WM, Corthesy B, Bram RJ: Nuclear association of a T cell transcription factor blocked by FK-506 and cyclosporine A. Nature 1991;352:803–807.

61 Demirci G, Pichlmayr R, Nashan B: TGF-β_1 expression in comparison to cyclosporine levels in chronic rejection of human liver allografts. XVIth Int Congr Transplant Soc, Barcelona, 1996, abstr 318.

62 Green DR, Bissonnette RP, Glyn JM: Activation-induced apoptosis in lymphoid cells. Semin Immunol 1992;4:379–388.

63 Staruch MJ, Sigal NH, Dumont FJ: Differential effects of the immunosuppressive macrolides FK-506 and rapamycin on activation-induced T cell apoptosis. Int J Immunopharmacol 1991;13:677–685.

64 Pichlmayr R, Bismuth H, Calne R: Three-Year data from the European Multicentre Tacrolimus Liver Study. XVIth Int Congr Transplant Soc, Barcelona 1996, abstr 307.

65 Vezina C, Kudelki A, Sehgal SN: Rapamycin, a new antifungal antibiotic. Taxonomy of the producing streptomycete and isolation of the active principle. J Antibiot 1975;28:721–726.

66 Vezina C, Kudelki A, Sehgal SN: Rapamycin, a new antifungal antibiotic. J Antibiot 1975;28: 721–732.

67 Kahan BD: Sirolimus: A new agent for clinical renal transplantation. Transplant Proc 1997; 29:48–50.

68 Sehgal SN, Baker H, Vezina C: Rapamycin, a new antifungal antibiotic. Fermentation, isolation and characterization. J Antibiot 1975;28:727–732.

69 Sehgal SN, Molnar-Kimber K, Ocain T, Weichman BM: Rapamycin: A novel immunosuppressive macrolide. Med Res Rev 1994;14:1–22.

70 Sidorowicz A, Baker H, Vezina C: Rapamycin, a new antifungal antibiotic: In vitro and in vivo studies. 15th Intersci Conf Antimicrob Agents Chemother, 1975, abstr 26.

71 Fretz H, Albers M, Galat A, Standaert R: Rapamycin and FK-506 binding proteins (immunophilins). J Am Chem Soc 1991;113:1409.

72 Wood MA, Bierer BE: Rapamycin: Biological and therapeutic effects, binding by immunophilins and molecular targets of action. Perspect Drug Disc Design 1994;2:163–184.

73 Kelly PA, Gruber SA, Behbod F, Kahan BD: Sirolimus, a new, potent immunosuppressive agent. Pharmacotherapy 1997;17:1148–1156.

74 Bierer BE, Mattila PS, Standaert RF: Two distinct signal transmission pathways in T lym-

phocytes are inhibited by complexes formed between an immunophilin and either FK-506 or rapamycin. Proc Natl Acad Sci USA 1990;87:9231–9235.

75 Molnar-Kimber KL, Rhoads A, Warner L: Evidence that the anti-tumor and immunosuppressive effects of rapamycin are mediated via similar mechanisms. Cold Spring Harbor Symp 1994;141.

76 Sabers CJ, Martin MM, Brunn GJ, Williams JM: Isolation of a protein target of the FK-BP12-rapamycin complex in mammalian cells. J Biol Chem 1995;270:815–822.

77 Kunz J, Henriquez R, Schneider U, Deuter-Reinhard M: Target of rapamycin in yeast, TOR2, is an essential phosphatidylinositol kinase homolog required for G1 progression. Cell 1993;73:585–596.

78 Cafferkey R, Young PR, McLaughlin MM, Bergsma DJ: Dominant missense mutations in a novel yeast protein related to mammalian phosphatidylinositol 3-kinase and VPS34 abrogate rapamycin cytotoxicity. Mol Cell Biol 1993;13:6012–6023.

79 Chen Y, Chen H, Rhoad M, Warner L: A putative sirolimus effector protein. Biochem Biophys Res Commun 1994;203:1–10.

80 Sabatini D, Erdjument-Bromage H, Lui M, Tempst P, Snyder SH: RAFT1: A mammalian protein that binds to FK-BP12 in a rapamycin-dependent fashion and is homologous to yeast TORs. Cell 1994;78:35–43.

81 Brown E, Albers MW, Shin TB, Ichikawa K, Kieth CT, Lane WS, Schreiber SL: A mammalian protein targeted by G1-arresting rapamycin receptor complex. Nature 1994;369:756–758.

82 Maeda K, Umeda Y, Saino T: Synthesis and background chemistry of 15-deoxyspergualin. Ann NY Acad Sci 1993;685:123–135.

83 Kaufman D, Jones J, Matas AJ: New immunosuppressive agents: FK-506, rapamycin, RS-61443, 15-deoxyspergualin. J Transplant Coord 1992;2:20–27.

84 Yuh D, Morris RE: The immunopharmacology of immunosuppression by 15-deoxyspergualin. Transplantation 1993;55:578–591.

85 Nadler SG, Eversole ACB, Tepper MA, Cleaveland JS: Elucidating the mechanism of action of the immunosuppressant 15-deoxyspergualin. Ther Drug Monit 1995;17:700–703.

86 Tepper M: Deoxyspergualin. Mechanism of action studies of a novel immunosuppressive agent. Ann NY Acad Sci 1993;696:123–132.

87 Ramos EL, Nadler SG, Grasela DM, Kelley SL: Deoxyspergualin: Mechanism of action and pharmacokinetics. Transplant Proc 1996;28:873–875.

88 Alegre ML, Sattar H, Herold KC, Smith J, Tepper MA, Bluestone JA: Prevention of the humoral response induced by an anti-CD3 monoclonal antibody by deoxyspergualin in a murine model. Transplantation 1994;57:1785–1794.

89 Kerr P, Nikolic-Patterson DJ, Lan HY, Tesch G, Rainone S, Atkins RC: Deoxyspergualin suppresses local macrophage proliferation in rat renal allograft rejection. Transplantation 1994;58:596–601.

90 Carter S, Franklin TJ, Jones DF, Leonard BJ, Mills SD, Turner RW, Turner WB: Mycophenolic acid: An anticancer compound with unusual properties. Nature 1969;223:848–851.

91 Suzuki S, Kimura T, Ando K, Sawada T, Tamura G: Antitumor activity of mycophenolic acid. J Antibiot 1969;22:197–302.

92 Mitsui A, Suzuki S: Immunosuppressive effects of mycophenolic acid. J Antibiot 1969;22:358–363.

93 Allison A, Eugui EM, Sollinger HW: Mycophenolate mofetil: Mechanism of action and effects in transplantation. Transplant Rev 1993;7:129–139.

94a Allison A, Eugui EM: Immunosuppressive and other effects of mycophenolic acid and an ester prodrug, mycophenolate mofetil. Immunol Rev 1993;136:5–28.

94b Morris R, Hoyt EG, Eugui EM, Allison A: Mycophenolic acid morpholinoethylester is a new immunosuppressant that prevents and halts heart allograft rejection by selective inhibition of T- and B-cell purine biosynthesis. Transplant Proc 1990;22:1659–1662.

95 Laurent AF, Dumont S, Poindron P, Muller CD: Mycophenolic acid suppresses protein N-linked glycosylation in human monocytes and their adhesion to endothelial cells and some substrates. Exp Hematol 1996;24:59–67.

96 Nagy S, Andersson JP, Andersson UG: Effect of mycophenolate mofetil on cytokine production: Inhibition of superantigen-induced cytokines. Immunopharmacology 1993;26:11–20.

97 Figueroa J, Fuad SA, Kunjummen-Platt J, Bacj FH: Suppression of synthesis of natural antibodies by mycophenolate mofetil. Transplantation 1993;55:1371–1374.

98 Mizuno K, Masatoshi T, Takada M, Hayashi M, Atsumi K, Asano K, Matsuda T: Studies on bredinin: Isolation, characterization and biological properties. J Antibiot 1974;27:775–782.

99 Morris RE: Mechanisms of action of new immunosuppressive drugs. Ther Drug Monit 1995;17:564–569.

100 Gruber S, Erdman GR, Burke BA: Mizoribine pharmacokinetics and pharmacodynamics in a canine renal allograft model of local immunosuppression. Transplantation 1992;53:12–19.

101 Dayton J, Turka LA: Mizoribine; in Kupiec-Weglinski J, Austin RG (eds): New Immunosuppressive Modalities and Anti-Rejection Approaches in Organ Transplantation. Trappe, PA, Landes, 1994.

102 Amemiya H, Itoh H: Mizoribine (Bredinin): Mode of action and effects on graft rejection; in Thomson A, Starzl TE (eds): Immunosuppressive Drugs: Developments in Anti-Rejection Therapy. London, Arnold, 1994.

103 Makowka L, Sher L, Cramer DV: The development of brequinar as an immunosuppressive drug for transplantation. Immunol Rev 1993;136:51–70.

104 Cramer D, Chapman FA, Makowka L: The use of brequinar sodium for transplantation. Ann NY Acad Sci 1993;696:216–226.

105 Makowka L, Cramer DV: Brequinar sodium: Mode of action and effects on graft rejection; in Thomson A, Starzl TE (eds): Immunosuppressive Drugs: Developments in Anti-Rejection Therapy. London, Arnold, 1994.

106 Murphy M: Brequinar sodium is a highly potent antimetabolite immunosuppressant that suppresses heart allograft rejection. Med Sci Res 1991;19:835–836.

107 Forrest T, Ware RE, Howard T, Jaffee BD, Denning SM: Novel mechanisms of brequinar sodium immunosuppression on T cell activation. Transplantation 1994;58:920–926.

108 Cramer DV, Makowka I: Brequinar sodium; in Przepiorka D (ed): New Immunosuppressive Drugs. Glenview, IL, Physicians and Scientists Publishing, 1994.

109 Kakowka L, Cramer DV: Brequinar sodium: A new immunosuppressive drug for transplantation. Transplant Proc 1993;25:1–83.

110 Bartlett RR, Campion G, Musikic P, Schleyerbach R, Zielinski T, Schorlemmer HU: Leflunomide: A novel immunomodulating drug; in Lewis AJ, Furst DE (eds): Nonsteroidal Anti-Inflammatory Drugs. New York, Dekker, 1994, pp 349–366.

111 Chong ASF, Xiao F, Xu X, Williams JW: In vivo and in vitro immunosuppression with leflunomide; in Przepiorka D (ed): New Immunosuppressive Drugs. Glenviews, IL, Physicians and Scientists Publishing, 1994, pp 163–177.

112 Xiao F, Chong ASF, Bartlett R, Williams JW: Leflunomide: A promising immunosuppressant in transplantation; in Thomson A, Starzl TE (eds): Immunosuppressive Drugs: Developments in Anti-Rejection Therapy. London, Arnold, 1994.

113 Nikcevich D, Finnegan A, Chong ASF, Williams JW, Bremer EG: Inhibition of interleukin-2 stimulated tyrosine kinase activity by leflunomide. Agent Action (in press).

114 Zelinski T, Zeitter D, Mullner S, Bartlett RR: Leflunomide, a reversible inhibitor of pyrimidine biosynthesis? Agent Action (in press).

115 Cosimi AB: Anti-T-cell monoclonal antibodies in transplantation therapy. 1983;15: 1889–1892.

116 Cosimi AB, Colvin RB, Burton RC, Goldstein G: Use of monoclonal antibodies to T-cell subsets for immunologic monitoring and treatment in recipients of renal allografts. N Engl J Med 1981;305:308–313.

117 Von Willebrand E: OKT4/8 ratio in the blood and in the graft during episodes of human renal allograft rejection. Cell Immunol 1983;77:196–201.

118 Walz G: Aktuelle Aspekte der Transplantationsimmunologie: Möglichkeiten einer selektiven Immunsuppression. Z Transplantationsmed 1990;2:36–43.

119 Reinherz EL, Meuer S, Fitzgerald KA: Antigen recognition by human T lymphocytes is linked to surface expression of the T3 molecular complex. Cell 1982;30:735–743.

120 Van Wauwe JP, De Mey JR, Goosens JG: A monoclonal anti-human T lymphocyte antibody with potent mitogenic properties. J Immunol 1980;124:2708–2713.

121 Kung PC, Goldstein G, Reinherz EL, Schlossman SF: Monoclonal antibodies defining distinctive human T cell surface antigens. Science 1979;206:347–349.

122 Norman DJ: Mechanism of action and overview of OKT3. Ther Drug Monit 1995;17: 615–620.

123 Chatenoud L, Baudrihaye MF, Kreis H: Human in vivo antigenic modulation induced by the anti-T cell OKT3 monoclonal antibody. Eur J Immunol 1982;12:979–982.

124 Giorgi JV, Cosimi AB, Colvin RB: Monitoring immunosuppression following renal transplantation. Diagn Immunol 1983;1:174–178.

125 Norman DJ, Shield CF, Barry JM, Henell KR: Therapeutic use of OKT3 monoclonal antibody for acute renal allograft rejection. Nephron 1987;46:41.

126 Cosimi AB, Burton RC, Colvin RB: Treatment of acute renal allograft rejection with OKT3 monoclonal antibody. Transplantation 1981;32:535–539.

127 Cosimi AB, Colvin RB, Burton RC: Use of monoclonal antibodies to T cell subsets for immunologic monitoring and treatment in recipients of renal allografts. N Engl J Med 1981;305: 308–314.

128 Tsudo M, Kozak RW, Goldman CK, Waldmann TA: Demonstration of a non-TAC peptide that binds IL-2. A potential participant in a multichain IL-2 receptor complex. Proc Natl Acad Sci USA 1986;83:9694–9698.

129 Soulillou JP, Cantarovich D, Le Mauff B: Randomized controlled trial of a monoclonal antibody against the interleukin-2 receptor (33B3.1) as compared with rabbit antithymocyte globulin for prophylaxis against rejection of renal allograft. N Engl J Med 1990;322:1175–1182.

130 Taniguchi T, Minami Y: The IL-2/IL-2 receptor system: A current overview. Cell 1993;73:5–8.

131 Kupiec-Weglinski JW, Diamantstein T, Tilney NL, Strom TB: Therapy with monoclonal antibody to interleukin-2 receptor spares suppressor T cells and prevents or reverses acute allograft rejection in rats. Proc Natl Acad Sci USA 1986;83:2624–2627.

132 Nashan B: Randomised trial of basiliximab versus placebo for control of acute cellular rejection in renal allograft recipients. Lancet 1997;350:1193–1198.

133 Queen C, Schneider WP, Selick HE: A humanized antibody that binds to the interleukin-2 receptor. Proc Natl Acad Sci USA 1989;86:10029–10033.

134 Hakimi J, Chizzonite R, Luke DR: Reduced immunogeneticity and improved pharmacokinetics of humanized anti-TAC in cynomolgus monkeys. J Immunol 1991;147:1352–1359.

135   Vincenti F, Lantz M, Birnbaum J: A phase I trial of humanized anti-interleukin-2 receptor antibody in renal transplant recipients. Transplantation 1997;63:33–38.

136   Kirkman RL, Shapiro ME, Carpenter CB: A randomized prospective trial of anti-TAC monoclonal antibody in human renal transplantation. Transplantation 1991;51:107–113.

137   Van Gelder T, Zietse R, Mulder AH: A double-blind, placebo-controlled study of monoclonal anti-interleukin-2 receptor antibody administration to prevent acute rejection after kidney transplantation. Transplantation 1995;60:248–252.

138   Brown PS Jr, Parenteau GL, Dirbas FM: Anti-TAC-H, a humanized antibody to the interleukin-2 receptor, prolongs primate cardiac allograft survival. Proc Natl Acad Sci USA 1991;88:2663–2667.

139   Anasetti C, Hansen JA, Waldmann TA: Treatment of acute graft-versus-host disease with humanized anti-TAC: An antibody that binds to the interleukin-2 receptor. Blood 1994;84:1320–1327.

140   Shield CF, Cosimi AB, Rubin RM: Use of antithymocyte globulin for reversal of acute allograft rejection. Transplantation 1979;28:461–464.

141   Bonnefoy-Berard N, Vincent C, Revillard JP: Antibodies against functional leukocyte surface molecules in polyclonal antilymphocyte and antithymocyte globulins. Transplantation 1991;51:669–673.

142   Skamene E, Russell PS: A quantitative study of the binding of ALS to various cell types. Clin Exp Immunol 1971;8:195–204.

143   Vernier I, Giraud P, Eche JP, Durand D, Suc JM: Hematological side effects of antilymphocyte globulins: Prevalence and impact on therapeutical protocol. Transplant Proc 1985;6:2765–2766.

144   Noordally R, Berland Y, Robert A, Olmer M: Side effects of rabbit and horse anti-lymphocyte serum. Transplant Clin Immunol 1985;32:255.

145   Thomas F, Thomas J, Flora R: Effect of antilymphocyte-globulin potency on survival of cadaver renal transplants. Lancet 1977;ii:672–674.

146   Matas AJ, Tellis VA, Quinn T, Glicklich D, Soberman R, Weiss R, Karwa G, Veith FJ: ALG treatment of steroid-resistant rejection in patients receiving cyclosporine. Transplantation 1986;41:579–583.

147   Storb R, Gluckman E, Thomas ED: Treatment of established human graft-versus-host disease by antilymphocyte globulin. Blood 1974;44:57–63.

148   Young N, Speck B: Antithymocyte and antilymphocyte globulin: Clinical trials and mechanisms of action. Aplastic anaemia: Stem Cell Biology and Advances; in Young NS, Levine AS, Humphries RK (eds): Treatment. New York, Liss, 1984.

149   Monaco AP, Campion JP, Kapnick SJ: Clinical use of antilymphocyte globulin. Transplant Proc 1977;9:1007–1018.

150   Gray JG, Monaco AP, Wood ML, Russell PS: Studies on heterologous anti-lymphocyte serum in mice: In vitro and in vivo properties. J Immunol 1966;96:217–221.

151   Leimenstoll G, Zerrenthien N, Niedermayer W, Steinmann J: An antithymocyte globulin of rabbit origin inhibits the antigen-induced activation of alloreactive T cells by blocking CD2. Transplant Proc 1991;23:982–984.

Dr. W. Haussmann, Kliniken Landkreis Sigmaringen GmbH, Hohenzollernstraße 40,
D–72488 Sigmaringen (Germany), Tel. +49 7571 100 22 33

Rüther U, Nunnensiek C, Schmoll H-J (eds): Secondary Neoplasias following Chemotherapy, Radiotherapy, and Immunosuppression. Contrib Oncol. Basel, Karger, 2000, vol 55, pp 94–116

Immune Surveillance and Tumor Recognition

Sören T. Eichhorst, Bernd Elser

Forschungsschwerpunkt Tumorimmunologie, Abteilung Immungenetik, Deutsches Krebsforschungszentrum, Heidelberg, Deutschland

Introduction: Tumorigenesis and Antitumor Immune Response

Tumors evolve out of uncontrolled clonal mitosis. They are the product of an autonomous and aggressive increase in autologous tissue, a process in which atypical cells are always involved. Tumorigenesis, especially of a malignant neoplasm, generally entails several individual steps. Illustrative of this process is the hepatocellular carcinoma induced by aflatoxins. Here, tumorigenesis begins when grains and cereals are stored incorrectly. The excess moisture in them promotes the growth of *Aspergillus flavus,* a mold which produces aflatoxins. Once ingested, this precarcinogen is converted hepatically, by the cytochrome-dependent P450 system, into a carcinogen. The new carcinogen binds to hepatocytic DNA, damaging the genetic makeup of the affected cells. This probably activates proto-oncogenes, while additional factors such as hepatides (especially B) further tumor progress. Yet even if the prerequisites for tumor growth to start are met, the body's immune response mechanisms must fail before this, or any other, tumor can grow. It is this immune response and its deficiency, which are the subjects of this chapter.

There are two main kinds of mechanisms that inhibit tumor growth: (1) genetic, or tumor suppressor genes, and (2) immunologic mechanisms. The latter (immunologic antitumor response) is based on specific and nonspecific mechanisms which are discussed in detail below within the context of neoplasms.

Let us first look at the genetic mechanisms, in particular at tumor suppressor genes. In the last two decades, a sequential model for the tumorigenesis of colon carcinoma has been developed, and shows that its pathogenesis involves genetic mutations, including the activation of oncogenes and the deactivation of tumor suppressor genes. This model thus illustrates that an antitumor immune response mechanism is switched off [1]. In the chain of events, previously normal colon epithelium loses tumor suppressor gene APC on chromosome 5q, so that epithelium proliferates faster. Subsequent DNA hypomethylation reactivates genes that are normally deactivated, and enables early adenomas to develop. Activation of oncogenes (e.g., K-RAS on chromosome 12p) then leads to what is termed an intermediate adenoma. The loss of two additional tumor suppressor genes, DCC (on chromosome 18q) and p53 (on chromosome 17p), facilitates the genesis of late adenomas and, eventually, of colon carcinomas. A similar sequential tumorigenesis has been established for some melanomas.

Whether a tumor can actually develop and metastasize depends on specific and nonspecific immunomechanisms of antitumor response. Here, tumor immunology has greatly profited from the concept of immune surveillance, which postulates that all tissue is constantly monitored by T cells. If a T cell recognizes an altered cell as nonself, or as threatening to the entire organism, this altered cell will be eliminated by various mechanisms. The primary method is to trigger apoptosis in target cells. Natural killer (NK) cells also patrol throughout the body, but do not recognize their target cells as specifically as do T cells, since the NK cell lacks a T-cell receptor.

These are the mechanisms that can be disrupted by many influences, especially immunosuppression necessitated by transplantation or resulting from chemo- or radiotherapy. Deactivation of just one of the two antitumor immune response defense mechanisms has grave consequences.

The concept of immune escape, in which tumor cells evade detection by immunosurveillance, has been elaborated in the last few years. According to this model, tumor cells can 'turn the tables' on the attacking lymphocyte with the latter's own weapons (see below). The fact that this system can also be modulated by chemotherapy may be a clue to the genesis of secondary neoplasms.

Basically, the immune system reacts to tumors the way it does to 'usual' antigens. This is why we need to know how the immune system recognizes antigens before we can understand tumor immunology and the influence of primary and secondary neoplasms on immune response.

Overview of the Immune System

Introduction
In the immune system, differentiation is made between innate, versus acquired or adaptive, immune mechanisms. Innate mechanisms are present in all individuals at birth and react quickly but nonspecifically. This immune response does not improve despite repeated contact with the offending antigen.

The acquired, or adaptive, immune system reacts more slowly but more specifically, and repeated contact with the same antigen improves immune response significantly. The acquired immune system is derived from bone-marrow stem cells, and consists of T and B cells. This immune system is stimulated to respond or react when accessory cells take up and process antigens and present them to T cells via special cell-surface molecules. If an antigen is recognized as such, certain mediators and cytokines are released that activate T and B cells and induce their proliferation. The immune response then culminates in a cellular and humoral effector phase. Although the innate and the adaptive immune systems differ in their mechanisms of antigen recognition, their similar effector mechanisms eliminate antigen in a like manner.

Innate immunologic mechanisms have humoral elements, such as the complement system, as well as cell-bound elements like phagocytes and lymphocytes with limited receptor diversity. Of special importance are the phagocytes. They help eliminate bacteria, dead cells and other waste products, and can utilize special molecules to present antigens, after phagocytosis, on their surface. Phagocytes can also transmit messenger substances via cytokines. They thus influence the adaptive immune system. Of the lymphocytes, the NK cells deserve special mention: without previous sensitization, they can kill affected cells after interacting with cell-surface molecules or surface-bound antibodies.

To understand the course of an immune system reaction, we must first know what triggers one. At the heart of this process is the antigen, a substance which the living organism recognizes as foreign and at which it can target a specific immune response. Antigen recognition by the immune system is highly sensitive: the mutation or deletion of just one amino acid in a protein can suffice to mark the altered protein as foreign.

In the adaptive immune system, antigen recognition is the catalyst for specific immune response. Playing a key role here are B and T lymphocytes distinguished by two kinds of highly variable receptor molecules on their cell surfaces. B cells are characterized by the synthesis and secretion of immunoglobulins or antibodies, making this a humoral immune response. B cells not only synthesize immunoglobulins, but also present them as antigen receptors on their cell surfaces.

Thymus-dependent lymphocytes, or T cells, feature CD3 antigen and the T-cell receptor. They are the mediators of cell-mediated immune response. Mature T cells express either CD4+ (T-helper) cells or CD8+ (T-suppressor and T-killer) cells in a mutually exclusive manner.

The central function of antigen recognition is carried out by two kinds of highly variable receptor molecules: antigen-specific receptors of T cells, and the immunoglobulins of B cells. These are detailed in the following.

Recognition of Antigens

Antigen Recognition by B Cells

The antigen receptor of the B cell is a membrane-bound antibody, the antigen-specific product of B cells. Antibodies have two functions: (1) they bind the antigens that provoked the immune response, and (2) recruit other molecules and cells to eliminate the antigen.

Since nearly any substance can trigger antibody production, the antigen-binding region must be highly variable to specifically recognize the wide variety of antibodies. Therefore, for each section of the variable region, there are several genes available, from which one is selected for antibody synthesis [2, 3]. With this mechanism of somatic recombination, a limited number of genes can be combined in an almost unlimited number of ways [4, 5]. Point mutation and alterations at the sites of individual segment linkage additionally enhance antibody diversity [6, 7].

These mechanisms facilitate the production of highly specific antibodies against antigens that differ from the organism's own proteins by just one amino acid. This is important for antitumor immune response, since tumors often evince somatic mutations of autologous proteins. Such substitutions of single amino acids can produce an antigen that gives the tumor its own fingerprint [8].

To trigger effective antibody synthesis and secretion, B cells need the help of T-helper cells. Activated T-helper cells produce not only cytokines, which influence proliferation and antibody synthesis, but also provide a co-signal, the CD40 ligand, which binds to the CD40 molecule on the B-cell surface. Without this co-signal facilitated by CD40/CD40 ligand, only weak, ineffective humoral immune responses are generated [9]. In such cases, the antigen may not be eliminated, but tolerated instead.

When B cells develop, some evolve with immunoglobulins rearranged against autoantigens. These are either eliminated, or stimulated to again rearrange their genes so that only immunoglobulins develop that do not react to autoantigens. This prevents the production of autoreactive antibodies as early as during B-cell development [10]. If this control mechanism fails, additional monitoring is available with antigen recognition and B-cell activation.

Naive B cells activated by antigen and the necessary co-stimulus will proliferate, produce antibodies, and become resistant to CD95-induced apoptosis [11]. In contrast, B cells in permanent contact with autologous antigens become desensitized to them and can no longer be activated. These anergic, autoreactive B cells are therefore not resistant to apoptosis, so that CD95 can induce their cellular death [12–14].

This is particularly important for antitumor immune response. Since tumors evolve out of the body's own tissue and thus possess autologous antigens, B cells that can produce antibodies against these antigens are rare. In addition, constant contact with these autoantigens desensitizes these B cells and makes them especially susceptible to apoptosis. Nor can support from T-helper cells – which is required for effective antibody synthesis – be expected, for such help would necessitate the T cell recognizing the antigen, and such recognition of autoantigens is already blocked during T-cell maturation. This is why humoral resistance to tumors is difficult.

Antibody attacks on tumors may also be hindered by tumor inaccessibility if the tumor does not have satisfactory vascularization for circulating antibodies to reach it, their target. Moreover, secreted or circulating soluble tumor antigens can prevent the antibodies from binding to the antigen on tumor cells and marking them. In this case, antibody-dependent effector mechanisms cannot take effect [15].

Even so, efforts to treat tumors with monoclonal antibodies are bearing fruit. In particular, lymphomas, which are easier to access, appear to respond well to therapy with antibodies against surface proteins – with response rates of more than 75% in some cases [16]. Antibody therapy is also very promising as an adjuvant for colorectal carcinoma and mammary carcinoma, as discussed below.

Once an antigen has been marked with antibodies, there are various mechanisms for its elimination. For example, IgG and IgM immunoglobulins can activate classic-pathway complements and trigger destruction of the cells affected. Also, phagocyting cells have receptors which recognize the constant region of the immunoglobulins and which destroy antibody-marked materials and cells (antibody-dependent cellular cytotoxicity). However, these mechanisms for eliminating antigens can function only if an antibody has recognized and bound itself to the antigen.

However, not only secreted immunoglobulins play a role here, but also those presented on the B cell's surface. If an antigen binds to an antibody on the cell surface, the complex created by the two will be taken up. Once inside, B-cell activation and antigen processing are stimulated.

The section on antigen presentation discusses in detail the role of the B cell as an antigen-presenting cell (APC) in antitumor immune response.

Antigen Recognition by T Cells

The function of T cells depends on their ability to recognize antigens on the surface of body cells. Body cells, in turn, make use of two classes of glycoproteins, the major histocompatibility complex molecules (or MHC molecules), to present antigens on their surfaces. The first class, MHC-I molecules, transports intracellular peptides to the cell surface, where the MHC-I peptide complexes are recognized by CD8+ T cells, which are also termed cytotoxic or killer cells. After recognizing the antigen, these cytotoxic or killer cells can kill the presenting cell. MHC-II molecules are expressed only by the APCs. They enable the CD4+ T-helper cells to trigger an immune response [17].

The receptors of T cells recognize an antigen only if the antigen is bound to an MHC molecule and presented as an MHC-peptide complex. This phenomenon is termed MHC restriction of the T-cell response.

The T-cell antigen receptor consists of two polypeptide chains which, like immunoglobulins, are constructed of one variable and one constant region each. In order to recognize a wide variety of antigens, a vast range of T-cell receptors is generated by somatic recombination of the gene segments, as is the case for B cells. On the T-cell surface, the T-cell receptor is associated with CD3 complexes, without which there is no signal transduction into the cell interior. Serving the T-cell receptor-CD3 complex as co-receptors are CD4 or CD8 molecules. They enhance the T cell's sensitivity for MHC-peptide complexes.

To prevent T-cell antigen receptors from recognizing autoantigens and to consequently stop T cells from attacking the body's own cells, all T lymphocytes undergo a twofold selection process during their development in the thymus. Although these mechanisms are not yet fully understood, there is, in any case, first positive selection, during which only those T cells are allowed to proliferate which recognize MHC molecules. This ensures that mature T cells also interact with the proteins that body cells use for antigen presentation. After this, those T cells that recognize complexes of autoantigens and MHC molecules are eliminated by negative selection. This results in autotolerance, or nonresponse by the immune system to autologous antigens. While this dual mode of selection is essential for auto-tolerance and prevention of autoimmunity, negative selection creates functional gaps in the antigen receptor reservoir of the T cells.

It is this auto-tolerance which weakens T-cell response to tumors, since tumors develop from autologous tissue and thus have autoantigens. Since the autoreactive T cells have been eliminated by negative selection, antitumor immune response must depend on the tumor producing antigens that distinguish it from the body's own cells; that is, tumor-specific antigens. These will be discussed in detail later in this chapter.

Cytotoxic T cells in particular work directly to eliminate antigens, as will be demonstrated later. When cytotoxic CD8 cells recognize antigen presented on MHC-I molecules, they deploy a variety of mechanisms to eliminate the APC. To do so, they polarize opposite the cell to be killed, and this polarization enables the cytotoxic cell to recognize, select and kill individual cells within cell aggregates and tissues.

To this end, stored cytokines may be released, of which perforin and granzymes are the most important. Perforin facilitates granzyme absorption through the membrane of the cell to be killed. Granzymes are proteases that help induce apoptosis (programmed cell death): Via direct cleavage, granzymes activate Casp-8, for example, and thereby trigger apoptosis.

In addition, through the expression of CD95 ligands, cytotoxic cells can induce apoptosis in cells with the appropriate CD95 receptor on their surface. Activated cytotoxic T cells secrete, moreover, substances that modulate immune response.

Now that antigen recognition by T- and B-cell receptors has been described, we shall consider how MHC-I and MHC-II molecules present antigens so that they are recognizable as such.

Antigen Presentation

MHC-I molecules are expressed on almost all nucleic cells of the body, albeit in various densities. The mass of constitutive MHC-I expressed affects T-cell activation: If the cell surface evinces only a few MHC molecules, the cytotoxic T cell has difficulty recognizing the MHC-I peptide complex and cannot kill the cell as easily. A loss of MHC molecules, particularly in the case of a tumor, can enable the tumor to escape recognition and immunosurveillance. Then, T cells will not be activated nor will cytotoxic T cells attack the tumor.

The binding of peptides to MHC molecules involves several intracellular steps. During their synthesis, proteins designated for the cell surface are translocated from cytosol into endoplasmic reticulum. Since intracellular proteins are constantly being degraded and replaced by newly synthesized ones, protein fragments (peptides) are produced. These peptides are transported by TAP (transporters associated with antigen processing) molecules into endoplasmic reticulum, where they are inspected by MHC molecules. If the peptide is found to be firmly bound to the MHC molecule, the entire MHC-I-peptide complex is transported to the cell surface. TAP molecules therefore mediate the loading of MHC-I molecules, making them essential for the efficient processing and presentation of antigens.

With tumors, antigen recognition by TAP molecules and MHC can be disrupted in a number of ways. For example, the genetic instability and mutation of tumors can disrupt or destroy TAP transport so that antigens cannot be processed nor subsequently bound to MHC molecules. The frequency of such TAP dysfunctions varies significantly according to tumor type, ranging from 14% for primary colorectal carcinomas to 49% for cervical carcinomas which are positive for human papillomavirus 16 [18]. Metastases from breast cancers and malignant melanomas are reported to have a higher incidence of loss of TAP molecules than do primary tumors [19]. However, it is still unclear whether this is a specific event in tumor progression or a general epiphenomenon stemming from the greater genetic instability of metastases. This type of disruption of antigen presentation considerably lessens the T-cell's ability to recognize tumors.

As noted above, the tumor can also avoid detection by the immune system when MHC-I molecules are deficient or missing. In fact, the complete loss of these surface antigens is a common phenomenon arising with 9–52% of tumors [19]. There may also be loss of individual MHC-I molecules – particularly devastating if they are tumor-specific antigen presenters. This may take place under the pressure of selection of a T-cell response targeted at a tumor antigen [20]. Causing such upheavals in MHC expression are point mutations, partial deletions of MHC genes, and chromosomal breakage.

Because of their MHC restriction, T cells can assume their surveillance function only if antigens are presented bound to MHC molecules. Without the correlating MHC molecules or the correlating antigen processing by TAP molecules, the tumor cannot be detected by the immune system.

MHC-II molecules are expressed primarily on B lymphocytes, macrophages and other APCs, such as dendritic cells. Common to all of these cells is the ability to phagocytize and/or to absorb antigen-antibody complexes, which is why they present extracellular antigens in particular. Like class I MHC molecules, class II MHC molecules are synthesized in endoplasmic reticulum, but are transported by vesicles to cytoplasm, where they come into contact with antigens.

Acidic proteases degrade phagocytosed extracellular antigens into peptides in intracellular vesicles. When vesicles with degraded extracellular antigens fusion with vesicles containing MHC-II molecules synthesized in the endoplasmic reticulum, peptides can then bind to MHC-II molecules, and the MHC-II-peptide complex will be transported to the cell surface.

Antigen presentation by specialized cells using MHC-II molecules is one of the most effective mechanisms for triggering a response from the adaptive immune system.

Stimulating an Immune Response
An immune response is invoked in peripheral lymphatic organs where specialized APCs present antigens to T cells circulating in the blood and lymph systems. Macrophages, dendritic cells and B cells are particularly efficient APCs. When antigens are present in tissue, APCs must first exit the circulatory system and enter tissue.

This leukocytic extravasation involves several steps – rolling, sticking, diapedesis and transmigration – which are initiated and propelled by inflammatory mediators: First, the leukocytes simply roll along the vascular endothelium because at this stage, the leukocyte-endothelium bond is reversible. A permanent bond is achieved only when chemokines such as interleukin(IL)-8 express additional adhesion molecules on the endothelium, e.g., ICAM-1 (intercellular adhesion molecule-1). In the next step, the leukocyte squeezes through the space between the endothelial cells. It must then dissolve the basal membrane with proteolytic enzymes in order to enter the tissue. Once there, the leukocyte follows the concentration gradient of the chemokines to reach the foci of inflammation, where it finds foreign bodies and antigens. The leukocyte can then present these and trigger an adaptive immune response.

It is in tumors in particular where this multistage process of leukocytic extravasation is disrupted, because a tumor's mutated constitution causes it to produce an insufficient number of adhesion molecules and an altered basal membrane. Also postulated is a disruption in the regulation of adhesion-molecule synthesis. In addition, the tumor-induced vascular system may be abnormal in many other areas as well, making it difficult for the immune system to reach the tumor.

But if leukocytes have managed to reach the tissue, come into contact with the antigen and recognized it as such, then antigen presentation can take place.

The type of antigen presentation determines the activation of T and B cells. Of key importance are antigen concentration, affinity to the antigen receptor, chronology of the antigen presentation, and co-stimulation.

Surprisingly, high concentrations of antigen do not necessarily induce a strong immune response. In fact, if antigenicity is low, they may instead induce anergy, as is the case for autoantigens. On the other hand, antigen with a high affinity for its receptor is much more likely to induce an immune response. If antigens are directly presented together with the correlating co-stimulation, they will trigger T- and B-cell activation and proliferation. In contrast, chronic stimulation, such as by autoantigens, induces a reduction in antigen receptors and occasionally death of the correlating cell.

For an antigen to trigger activation and proliferation of T cells, two signals are required: First, through the interaction between the T-cell receptor and the MHC-peptide complex of the APC, and in cooperation with the CD4 or CD8 molecule, the T cell is signaled that antigen has been recognized. Then, to activate T cells, a second co-stimulating signal is needed, which is given when B7 molecules of the APC bind to CD28 protein of the T cell. When activated by additional signals such as TNF (tumor necrosis factor) or complement, APCs express B7.1 (CD80) or B7.2 (CD86).

The fact that an APC must evince *both* an antigen *and* a co-stimulating signal to trigger an immune response, prevents the body's own tissue from being destroyed. If the co-stimulating signal is missing, the T cell will not be activated, but rather its anergy, so that the T cell can no longer be activated.

Tumors, however, are characterized by the very fact that they do not correctly present any tumor antigens they may have. Their lack of a correlating co-stimulating signal in particular makes their detection by immunosurveillance impossible.

A murine tumor model demonstrated that transfer of tumor cells of a B-cell lymphoma and of CD4+ cells that reacted specifically to a tumor antigen of the B-cell lymphoma rendered the CD4+ T cells tolerant of the tumor. Although T cells were present which specifically recognized the tumor antigen, antitumor immune response was not initiated. Instead, the tumor induced immune-system anergy [21].

What is more, the *type* of co-stimulation appears to influence antitumor immune response, because signals emitted by B7.1 and B7.2 evince both overlapping and mutually independent functions. Depending on tumor type, tumor expression of B7.1 and/or B7.2 leads to progression or regression. In other words, the *kind* of co-stimulation helps determine whether the immune system will repel or tolerate a tumor [22–24].

Co-stimulation by B7.1/B7.2 is closely associated with the behavior of CD4 cells: the subgroups of CD4+ cells employ cytokines to influence the immune system's reaction to a tumor. For example, type 2 T-helper cells and IL-4 promote tumor growth [22–24].

While macrophages and dendritic cells primarily present large phagocytosed antigens via MHC-II molecules, B cells primarily present soluble antigens bound to immunoglobulins on the B-cell surface. Even so, nearly any normal body cell can use MHC-I molecules to present intracellular antigens and their correlating co-stimulation, and can thus activate T cells.

Since most tumors possess MHC-I but not MHC-II molecules, T-cytotoxic cells are important for tumor recognition and defense. However, research is showing that T-helper cells are also involved in tumor growth control. In particular, when there is no inflammatory reaction, T-cytotoxic cell reactivity depends that much more on T-helper cells. This is because APCs, such as dendritic cells, must first be activated by antigen-specific T-helper cells before they can trigger immune response from T-cytotoxic cells [25]. Here, T cells must use co-signals such as CD40/CD40 ligand to trigger an interaction in order to stimulate APCs to activate cytotoxic cells [26].

This role of T-helper cells is underscored by the fact that mice lacking CD8+ cells evince dysfunctional antitumor immune response, while mice lacking CD4+ cells are able to eliminate the tumor. This shows that the antitumor immune response observed in these studies depends on T-helper-cell-mediated effects [27].

An additional central function of co-stimulation by B7/CD28 is to stimulate synthesis and secretion of cytokines and correlating surface receptors. These are prerequisites for the proliferation and differentiation of T and B cells. Without co-stimulation, the adaptive immune system cannot be induced to respond effectively to antigens.

Let us now turn to the questions of what characterizes a tumor, and what makes a tumor grow from the point of view of the immune system.

Tumor Antigens

During tumorigenesis, normal body cells are transformed and become genomically unstable. Once tumor cells, they express antigens which they either did not previously possess in this form (neoantigens) or which they possessed only during their fetal age (oncofetal antigens) [28].

Oncofetal antigens are often found in human tumors, and sometimes serve as tumor markers. These include α-fetoprotein, which is produced by hepatocarcinoma and yolk-sac tumor; carcinoembryonic antigen, produced by gastrointestinal tumors, and a few others.

Since the body already produces oncofetal antigens during the fetal period, the immune system considers them to be autologous. They are thus not specific for the tumor, but only associated with it. And, since the tumor usually under- or overexpresses oncofetal antigens, any deviation from the norm is usually quantitative, not qualitative. Oncofetal antigens appear not only in tumors, but also with other reactions such as inflammatory or healing processes. This is why immune response to these antigens is suppressed, or else the consequences would be devastating.

However, an immune response can also be triggered against autologous, non-mutated proteins if they are overexpressed by the tumor. An interesting example is tumor suppressor gene p53, which is overexpressed in some tumors. This overexpression of nonmutated protein can be detected by the immune system, enabling cytotoxic T cells to find and destroy the tumor cells [29].

Tumor-specific antigens that appear solely in the tumor and nowhere else in the body give the tumor its specific antigenic 'fingerprint' and are particularly suited to eliciting an antitumor immune response. The alteration of just one amino acid can result in a tumor-specific antigen that can be recognized by immunocells [8].

Here, differentiation is made between tumor antigen mutated from one of the body's own proteins, making the antigen specific for one individual tumor, and tumor antigens occurring in several individual tumors. There are many examples of neoantigens evolving from somatically mutated proteins in the body, such as the point mutation of β-catenin, a signal transduction gene that was found in a malignant melanoma. This point mutation can also be recognized by cytotoxic T cells and is specific for this tumor [30].

In some cases, mutations produce antigens that become the target of an immune response, but the immune response to the tumor is impeded by the mutations themselves. In a squamous-cell carcinoma of the head and neck region, a mutation was found of Casp-8, a protease involved in programmed cell death. This is an example of impedance of an antitumor immune response deploying induction of apoptosis [31] (see below).

Tumor antigens that occur in not just one, but in many kinds of tumors are useful proving grounds for diagnostic and therapeutic methods. A well-known example is the Philadelphia chromosome in chronic myeloid leukemia: translocation of the c-abl gene from chromosome 9 to the proximity of the BCR gene on chromosome 22 produces a fusion gene, which disrupts regulation of tyrosine kinase. This is functionally significant because tyrosine kinases influence many growth and differentiating processes.

A further example of neoantigenic genesis is the MUC-1 (mucin-1) antigen, a reduced glycosylated mucin that develops, through abnormal posttranslational modification, in mammary carcinomas [32]. This mucin molecule, however, can trigger apoptosis in activated T cells, thus inhibiting effective antitumor immune response [see also Tumor Counterattack, 33].

Oncofetal proteins of the MAGE family appear to have a special tumor specificity, being produced only by malignomas and in the testis, an immunologically privileged organ [34]. The genes of the MAGE family are reactivated in the course of general, nonspecific gene activation by DNA methylation – which often occurs as general transcriptional deregulation in tumors [35]. MAGE tumor antigens are a good target for cytotoxic T cells, being relatively specific for the tumor and sufficiently antigenic to induce an immune response. MAGE antigens are produced by various tumors, such as malignant melanomas, small-cell bronchial carcinomas and esophageal carcinomas, although often only some of the tumors express this antigen.

Tumors associated with viral infections sometimes have viral antigens. Since cervical carcinomas are often linked with infection by human papillomaviruses 16 and 18, the tumor produces the E6/E7 oncoproteins of these viruses [36]. To what extent an immune response targets these oncoproteins is still unclear, however, because papillomaviral infection occurs far in advance of tumorigenesis.

For immunotherapeutic strategy, antigens that develop in various tumors and in several individuals, such as those of the MAGE family, are of special interest. Therapies targeting such antigen families may someday enable applications for broad groups of tumors. In juxtaposition are many of the tumor antigens devolving from mutation of the body's own proteins. Because mutation is random, many such antigens are specific for only one individual tumor in one patient. Therapeutic use of this kind of antigen would be limited to just one single tumor.

In summary, the following can be said about tumor antigens: many tumors possess only autoantigens because they have developed out of the body's own cells. Some tumors produce oncofetal antigens, which, however, are not specific for that tumor since they developed in the fetal period and are thus seen as part of the body. Tumor-specific antigens can arise from somatic mutations in the tumor. Here, even slight changes in the protein sequence suffice to trigger an immune reaction. Tumor-specific antigens, while rare, are the antigens best suited for stimulating a response against tumors, since they appear only in the tumor. Unfortunately, some of them inhibit effective antitumor immune response themselves.

In addition to deficient or missing antigenicity, the tumor has other means of escaping detection by the immune system. These mechanisms and concepts are discussed in the sections below.

General Concepts in Tumor Immunology

The principles of tumor immunology can be summarized as follows: (1) Only rarely is the immune system a significant barrier to tumor growth; (2) tumors present more or less specific antigens, and (3) modulation of the immune system (whether positive or negative) can lead to the complete eradication of the tumor (immunotherapy).

Of course, these are only the basic principles; the actual situation is more complex. For example, lymphocytes inhibit the growth of only some tumors. Although some tumors present antigens on their surface that are more or less specifically expressed, the immune system usually accepts these as autoantigens and does not launch a significant attack against them. Moreover, the third principle mentioned above has proven clinically successful in only a few cases, such as for renal cell carcinomas.

It is generally accepted that tumors are nearly always antigenic, but only rarely induce an antitumor immune response. This brings up one of the main topics of research in modern tumor immunology: Why are tumors so rarely immunogenic, and how can immunogenicity be improved? Since most tumor cells are not APCs, perhaps immunogenicity can be increased by loading professional APCs with tumor antigen. Studies are underway to see whether dendritic cells that present tumor antigens are able to trigger an effective antitumor immune response.

But even if immune response to the tumor can be initiated, the tumor has a number of mechanisms to repel the attack. For example, genomic instability, a basic feature of many tumors, could lead to the loss of specific antigenicity. This, in turn, would mean the loss of the immune response if the response were directed at only one individual antigen.

The tumor can also suppress immune response by secreting immunosuppressive cytokines such as TGF-β or IL-10, which inhibits antigen presentation by down-regulating MHC molecules and TAP transporters [37].

The CD95 (APO-1/Fas) system probably plays a special role in many areas of tumorigenesis. Research in the past few years has shown that by expressing CD95 ligands, tumors may create an immunoprivileged zone. In addition, the CD95 system may also bolster resistance to chemotherapy. In any case, the role of the CD95 system is more complex than previously assumed, as is discussed later in this paper.

Finally, factors leading to dysfunctional extravasation of lymphocytes may prevent sufficient antitumor immune response. One example may be a cytokine-modulated expression of adhesion molecules on endothelial cells supplying the tumor: loss of adhesion molecules – which are essential to the sticking-rolling transmigration process – can render the tumor inaccessible for the lymphocytic pool, resulting in dysfunctional antitumor immune response.

Adhesion molecules play an important role in tumor growth: when modulated by certain influences, tumor cells circulating in the bloodstream can assume a pattern of expression of adhesion molecules. This enables them to metastasize into certain organs [38], such as when lymphoma cells metastasize into lymph nodes. This process is regulated by lymphocyte-homing receptors, which are also important for normal lymphocytic circulation [39]. Hence, metastasis may take place passively, or be actively steered. Studies on human endothelium have shown that activation by IL-1, TNF or endotoxin leads to increased adhesion of melanoma cells. This, in turn, points to an interesting coincidence of inflammatory processes and tumors [40]. Medications may also influence the expression of adhesion molecules and contribute to the genesis of tumors and metastases.

Recognition of Tumors by the Immune System

A fundamental concept of tumor surveillance is that tumors express antigens which differ from normal tissue. Unfortunately, surveillance of tumor-specific antigens is often insufficient, although certain tumor-specific antigens have recaptured clinical interest in recent years.

A tumor cell has many ways of producing a neoantigen, such as by losing parts of surface antigens; acquiring antigens not normally present in the tissue; or through mutation of known antigens. What is more, most tumors are heterogenic. Although they evolve out of one cell, new mutations in the course of tumor growth generate phenotypes beneficial for further tumor progression. These are then selected, and the tumor becomes increasingly inhomogeneous. This is why resistance to cytostatic agents often develops after initially successful primary chemotherapy, resulting in a recurring tumor. It is most likely a case of therapy having selected cytostatically resistant tumor cells which then recur.

Only a few therapies based on specific tumor antigens have shown promise, such as 17–1A antibodies used adjuvantly in treating colorectal carcinoma; anti-CD20 antibodies for treating malignant B-cell lymphomas; anti-HER2/neoantibodies for therapy of breast cancer; while recently, monoclonal antibodies have been tested for neuroblastoma in children.

There are some promising immunovaccination therapies, such as MAGE-3 vaccines based on peptide inoculations. Vaccination for the idiotypes of B-cell lymphomas has also shown promise, as have approaches using adoptive T cells.

The Concept of Immune Surveillance

Immune surveillance is based on the premise that tumor cells possess specific antigens and that the body recognizes these antigens as foreign. The immune system, in other words, recognizes the tumor as foreign, and if all goes well, proceeds to eliminate it. Immunosurveillance also stipulates a recirculating lymphocyte pool: lymphocytes continually exit the bloodstream, travel through all body tissues, and immunologically survey them. This principle was formulated for the first time in 1959 [41], and later modified and published by Burnet [42].

The prerequisite here is that the immune system is able to distinguish between the body's own structures and structures foreign to it [43]. Although this model remains very attractive, it has been increasingly questioned in recent years because no one has been able to produce large-scale, truly effective immunotherapies.

One fundamentally new concept of immunosurveillance is not based on self/nonself differentiation by the immune system, but on threatening vs. nonthreatening. This better explains the phenomenon of tumors evading detection by the immune system. Unlike the self/nonself differentiation model, this theory does not presume that tumors per se are dangerous to the immune system. That is why there is no automatic, standard response by T cells to tumor cells. Only when there is additional damage that threatens the immune system can tumors act immunogenically [44].

What led to the model of differentiating between body and foreign tissues? First, it was observed that dizygotic twins linked at the placental level are tolerant of each other's tissue. This led to the conclusion that the immune system learns to differentiate before birth between 'self' and 'foreign'. Accordingly, if allogenic cells were injected prenatally into a fetus, the immune system would automatically recognize these cells as belonging to the body and would tolerate them.

It was therefore assumed that all antigens with which the immune system came into contact *after maturation* would automatically be attacked. Today, this concept is seen as the pathophysiologic basis for many autoimmune diseases. Its mechanics are simple: while lymphocytes are developing, contact with any antigen kills them. If the lymphocytes are mature, however, contact with an antigen activates them to attack the presenting tissue. Yet tumors often repeatedly manage to evade detection by the immune system even though they frequently form new antigens, such as by mutating existing proteins. On the other hand, if the required co-stimulatory signal is already missing, adequate immune response cannot be launched in the first place.

One model that resolves these contradictions is the danger model of immune response. It postulates that proteins foreign to the body that are taken up and presented by any body cell will not trigger an immune reaction. Only when a second (danger) signal is given can the foreign antigen stimulate the immune system. Along these lines, a virus that infects a cell population can remain undetected until cellular damage occurs, causing cellular and viral components to be released and viral peptides to be expressed on APCs, which in turn can trigger a lymphocytic response. Correlating danger signals that could trigger an immune reaction include infections, heat, cold, hypoxia and trauma [45].

What role does the danger model play in tumor immunology? First of all, it may explain why some tumors spontaneously regress or even disappear without specific therapy, as does the neonatal hemangioma in 80–90% of cases. This tumor generally appears 2–4 weeks after birth, grows quickly, but soon begins to shrink. It is usually gone by the age of 10 years, leaving only a scar. Reports have also been published on spontaneously regressing renal cell carcinomas, neuroblastomas, melanomas and choriocarcinomas. There are also reports of metastases regressing after excision of the primary tumor, although these rare cases are probably somewhat overrepresented in the literature.

Hence, according to the self/nonself model, the tumor basically 'hides' from the immune system, which responds to it only if the tumor becomes detectable due to trauma, local infection, and so on. With the danger model, on the other hand, the tumor does not initially present a threat to the immune system. Only if a danger signal is sent are the APCs activated, which is what leads to an immune response. What makes the danger model the more likely explanation is that the immune reaction is maintained only as long as the danger signal is present. By contrast, the self/nonself model postulates continual activation of the lymphocytes – which should lead to tumor elimination once the system has been activated, but which is usually not the case.

Against this backdrop, it is interesting to know that many of the spontaneous regressions have been directly associated with patient infections – a clinical observation that was made as far back as the 18th century. For example, in 1774, a Parisian physician treated a female patient with an inoperable breast tumor by injecting pus into her leg. As the infection in her leg developed, the breast carcinoma regressed. A modified version of this method is used today as well: BCG vaccine is superficially instilled to treat superficial urinary bladder tumors. Randomized studies have proven that this approach is at least partially successful.

The CD95 (APO-1/Fas)/CD95 Ligand System

Introduction

CD95 is a glycosylated surface molecule which spans the cell membrane. It is a type I transmembrane receptor, with its amino-terminal end lying outside of the cell. CD95 was discovered when it was found that in CD95+ tumor cells, apoptosis can be triggered by agonistic antibodies [46]. CD95 belongs to the TNF receptor superfamily, which is characterized by extracellular domains rich in cysteine. Some members of this family are able to induce programmed cell death via activation. In addition to CD95, this subgroup contains TNF receptor I, APO-3, CD40 and CD30, and others. The correlating ligands also make up a family.

After CD95 stimulation, an additional protein, FADD, is attached intracellularly to the cytoplasmic part of CD95. FADD, in turn, recruits FLICE (Casp-8), a member of the caspase family. These are proteases that have cysteine in the active center. When recruited by FADD, casp-8 is autocatalytically activated. This leads either to activation of additional caspases, the sum of whose activations then induces apoptosis, or to the CD95 system triggering apoptosis via the release of cytochrome c from mitochondria [47].

Both CD95 and its associated ligand, CD95L, are present in the immune system and in extralymphatic tissue, and crucial to many physiologic and pathophysiologic processes. For example, the system plays a key role in restricting immune responses by inducing the programmed death of peripheral T cells (AICD) [48]. This apoptosis can proceed: (1) via fratricide, in which a CD95L-carrying T cell induces apoptosis in a neighboring cell (a CD95-receptor-carrying T cell); (2) via paracrine death, in which soluble CD95L binds to the receptor and induces apoptosis, and (3) via autocrinal death, where the receptor and the ligand are expressed on the same cell, causing its apoptotic death.

The CD95 system is present not only in the immune system, but also in both the developing and the mature liver. It is probably involved in tissue homeostasis, since mice deficient in CD95 evince liver hyperplasia and increased renal cellularity. It also plays an important role in acute liver damage of various etiology.

In other organs, CD95 seems to play a less prominent role, although it is a main factor in the formation of immunoprivileged regions. These are sites where expression of the CD95 ligand more or less protects from the impact of an immune response, and include the testicles and the anterior chamber of the eye. The CD95 system thus directly affects tumorigenesis, because many tumors express CD95/CD95L and since the system can be modulated by a wide variety of antitumor therapies.

Tumors and the CD95 System

The CD95 system plays a key role in tumorigenesis because it can fight the immune system with its own weapons [49]. This defense mechanism, called the CD95 counterattack, was recently demonstrated in colon carcinoma, liver tumors and melanomas [50]. Certain tumor cells express CD95L, but are resistant to CD95-induced apoptosis. As a result, T cells attacking such a tumor may be eliminated by CD95-mediated apoptosis. This is why tumor cells that express little or no CD95 are not only resistant to a decisive effector from T cells, but in fact attack them. This can lead to deletion of the tumor-specific T-cell clone, an outcome very conducive for tumor growth.

Numerous studies have demonstrated that most tumors are at least partially resistant to CD95-induced apoptosis. In many cases, the original cell is CD95-positive, but becomes unreceptive to CD95-induced apoptosis during tumorigenesis. This defect does not necessarily stem solely from the loss of expression of CD95, because a number of molecular defects have been identified in the CD95 signal pathway in tumor cells.

In addition to these various defects in the signal pathway of CD95, the increased expression of antiapoptotic proteins, such as Bcl-2, may be involved in resistance to CD95 [51]. Inversely, underexpression of proapoptotic molecules of the Bcl-2 family (bax, for example) can also contribute to the phenotype of CD95 resistance [52], as has been demonstrated for breast cancer. In breast cancer cell lines, transfection by bax restored sensitivity to CD95.

Additionally affecting antitumor response in vivo is the interaction of genetic and immunologic mechanisms. Tumor suppressor genes also influence, to varying degrees, the sensitivity of the CD95 system. For example, p53 status plays a key role in the ability to catalyze apoptosis in certain tumor cells. As was recently demonstrated for hepatoma cell lines, via a transcriptionally regulated mechanism, functional (not mutated) p53 can control CD95-induced apoptosis. p53 binds to an enhancer element located in the first intron of the CD95 gene. p53 can then activate the expression of CD95, and sensitize the cell to apoptosis. If mutation causes p53, the cellular 'watchman', to fail (which happens in about 50% of tumors), tumor cells are less likely to undergo apoptosis. They become resistant to various influences, including attacks by the immune system.

Being relatively resistant to CD95-induced apoptosis, the tumor cell can more easily proceed to the next step, expression of CD95L. Otherwise, the increased expression of the apoptotic ligand would result in fratricide or even autocrinal suicide. In all of the tumors examined, CD95 expression in vivo was either down-regulated or completely missing whenever expression of CD95L was simultaneously increased.

In vivo studies also show that expression of CD95L actually does trigger apoptosis in tumor-infiltrating lymphocytes (TIL). The CD95 system therefore appears to facilitate development of an immunoprivileged site in the tumor.

Is launching an attack, therefore, the tumor's best defense? Perhaps, for studies show that resistance to CD95-induced apoptosis offers the tumor relatively little protection against attacking lymphocytes. These lymphocytes, namely, can deploy alternative effector systems, such as the perforin/granzyme system, and cells resistant solely to CD95 will hardly be resistant to other forms of apoptosis. That is why expression of a molecule able to fend off lymphocytes and NK cells attacking the tumor is bound to be a great advantage for the neoplasm. Not surprisingly, experimental data indicate that CD95L-expressing tumors metastasize more quickly than CD95L-negative ones [53].

An immunoprivileged zone can have additional far-reaching consequences. For example, studies of the anterior chamber of the eye found that contact with an antigen within an immunoprivileged zone can lead to systemic tolerance of that antigen. The mechanism behind this tolerance is still unclear, but it probably involves cytokines such as IL-10 and TGF-β. In addition to protecting the tumor from infiltrative lymphocytes, the development of such a zone by expression of CD95L may facilitate systemic tolerance of tumor antigens. This, in turn, would promote further tumor growth and metastasis.

Production of soluble CD95L may also have systemic consequences. Soluble CD95L is primarily produced by metalloproteases cleaving cell-surface CD95L. Increased concentrations of this soluble ligand in serum may trigger systemic apoptosis. It has recently been demonstrated that soluble CD95L is much less effective than the cell-surface version. In cells highly sensitized to CD95-triggered apoptosis, however, the soluble ligand also catalyzes apoptosis. The exact role of this mechanism in systemic immunosuppression is therefore still unclear.

Chemotherapy and Apoptosis
Researchers have known for many years that most chemotherapeutic drugs invoke apoptosis. Only recently, however, have experiments demonstrated the role of

the CD95 system in tumor cell apoptosis. Here, via CD95, cytotoxic substances trigger an autocrinal or paracrinal apoptotic mechanism [54]. For example, it has been shown that bleomycin triggers induction of both CD95 and CD95L on hepatoma cells (HepG2). The subsequent increase in apoptotic activity can then be inhibited by suppressing the CD95 system [55].

Inhibiting the effector mechanisms of cell death also inhibits the effect of chemotherapy: for instance, suppression of caspases in tumor cells makes them resistant to chemotherapy. In addition, some chemotherapeutic drugs apparently activate the caspase cascade directly. Betulinic acid, for example, circumvents the CD95/CD95L system to directly activate casp-8, as has been proven by proteolytic cleavage of the molecule [56].

In tumors with chemotherapeutically enhanced expression of CD95 and CD95L, the system can help eliminate tumors. However, if (1) only one component is increased – in the worst case, only CD95L – or if (2) tumor cells resistant to CD95-induced apoptosis are selected, then therapy may encounter another obstacle: the CD95L+ clone – which would basically be the sole component of the tumor – would render the tumor an immunoprivileged zone. That mode of selection would bolster this tumor's resistance to chemotherapy, and probably make it more aggressive than the original tumor as well. This greater aggressiveness, as noted above, would stem from the tumor's relative protection from the immune system and greater potential for metastasis.

CD95L is not the only catalyst of chemotherapeutically induced apoptosis, although it is probably the most important. Other apoptosis-inducing ligands, such as TNF-α or TRAIL, are also influenced by therapy with cytostatic agents. The TRAIL system in particular is a promising therapeutic approach since it is highly tumor-selective [57].

In sum, systems that trigger apoptosis in tumor cells – especially CD95 – play a key role in resistance to chemotherapy. The functionality of these systems is thus significant for tumor therapy where temporary T-cell resistance is sought without sacrificing tumor cell sensitivity, and is involved in the latent development of secondary neoplasms [58].

The effects discussed above occur in addition to those directly generated by the substances administered. For example, the cytostatic effect of most chemotherapeutic regimens administered today directly suppresses the immune system. Since this immunosuppression brings immunosurveillance to a standstill, it obviously promotes tumor growth. What is more, these substances may themselves stimulate tumor growth directly, although this has not been irrefutably proven.

Cyclosporine, for example, is an immunosuppressant commonly administered after organ transplantation and for autoimmune disorders. Its immunosuppressive effect has long been thought to stimulate tumor growth in vivo, casting a negative light on this substance. Aggravating the situation is that the latest data indicate that cyclosporine is probably not *indirectly* carcinogenic (via its immunosuppressive effect). Instead, it appears to *directly* promote tumorigenesis in vitro and in vivo, probably by boosting production of TGF-β, which influences tumor cells directly through its receptors. Given the heightened risk of developing malignancy after administration of cyclosporine, a shift in paradigms is appropriate. However, these most recent data do not have any impact on the risk that was already present and taken into account when the decision was made to administer cyclosporine [59].

References

1   Stanbridge EJ: The reemergence of tumor suppression. Cancer Cells 1989;1:31–33.
2   Cook GP, Tomlinson IM: The human immunoglobulin V-H repertoire. Immunol Today 1995;16:237–242.
3   Schatz DG: V(D)J recombination – Molecular biology and regulation. Annu Rev Immunol 1992;10:359–383.
4   Tonegawa S: Somatic generation of immune diversity. Scand J Immunol 1993;38:305–317.
5   Wagner SD, Neuberger MS: Somatic hypermutation of immunoglobulin genes. Annu Rev Immunol 1996;14:441–457.
6   Fanning LJ, Connor AM, Wu GE: Development of the immunoglobulin repertoire. Clin Immunol Immunopathol 1996;79:1–14.
7   DeFranco AL, Blum JH, Stevens TL, Law DA, Chan VW, Foy SP, Datta SK, Matsuuchi L: Structure and function of the B-cell antigen receptor. Chem Immunol 1994;59:156–172.
8   Monach PA, Meredith SC, Siegel CT, Schreiber H: A unique tumor antigen produced by a single amino acid substitution. Immunity 1995;2:45–49.
9   Korthauer U, Graf D, Mages HW, Briere F, Padayachee M, Malcolm S, Ugazio AG, Notarangelo LD, Levinsky RJ, Kroczek RA: Defective expression of T-cell CD40 ligand causes X-linked immunodeficiency with hyper-Ig. Nature 1993;361:539–543.
10 Nussenzweig MC: Immune receptor editing: Revise and select. Cell 1998;95:875–878.
11 Rothstein TL, Wang JK, Panka DJ, Foote LC, Wang Z, Stanger B, Cui H, Ju ST, Marshak-Rothstein A: Protection against Fas-dependent Th1-mediated apoptosis by antigen receptor engagement in B cells. Nature 1995;374:163–165.
12 Rathmell JC, Cooke MP, Ho WY, Grein J, Townsend SE, Davis MM, Goodnow CC: CD95 (Fas)-dependent elimination of self-reactive B cells upon interaction with CD4+ T cells. Nature 1995;376:181–184.
13 Cooke MP, Heath AW, Shokat KM, Zeng Y, Finkelman FD, Linsley PS, Howard M, Goodnow CC: Immunoglobulin signal transduction guides the specificity of B cell – T cell interactions and is blocked in tolerant self-reactive B cells. J Exp Med 1994;179:425–439.
14 Ho WY, Cooke MP, Goodnow CC, Davis MM: Resting and anergic B cells are defective in CD28-dependent costimulation of naive CD4+ T cells. J Exp Med 1994;179:1539–1549.
15 Kaklamanis L, Leek R, Koukourakis M, Gatter KC, Harris AL: Loss of transporter of antigen processing 1 transport protein and major histocompatibility complex class I molecules in metastatic versus primary breast cancer. Cancer Res 1995;55:5191–5194.
16 Kaminski MS, Zasadny KR, Francis IR, Fenner MC, Ross CW, Milik AW, Estes J, Tuck M, Regan D, Fisher S, Glenn SD, Wahl RL: Iodine-131-anti-B1 radioimmunotherapy for B-cell lymphoma. J Clin Oncol 1996;14:1974–1981.

17   Ager A: Immune receptor supplement. Immunol Today 1996;5:17.

18   Seliger B, Maeurer MJ, Ferrone S: TAP off – tumors on. Immunol Today 1997;6:292–299.

19   Garrido F, Ruiz-Cabello F, Cabrera T, Perez-Villar JJ, Lopez-Botet M, Duggan-Keen M, Stern PL: Implications for immunosurveillance of altered HLA class I phenotypes in human tumors. Immunol Today 1997;2:89–95.

20   Ikeda H, Lethe B, Lehmann F, van Baren N, Baurain JF, de Smet C, Chambost H, Vitale M, Moretta A, Boon T, Coulie PG: Characterization of an antigen that is recognized on a melanoma showing partial HLA loss by CTL expressing an NK inhibitory receptor. Immunity 1997;6:199–208.

21   Staveley-O'Carroll K, Sotomayor E, Montgomery J, Borrello I, Hwang L, Fein S, Pardoll D, Levitsky H: Induction of antigen-specific T cell anergy: An early event in the course of tumor progression. Proc Natl Acad Sci USA 1998;95:1178–1183.

22   Stremmel C, Greenfield EA, Howard E, Freeman GJ, Kuchroo VK: B 7.2 expressed on EL4 lymphoma suppresses antitumor immunity by an IL-4 dependent mechanism. J Exp Med 1999;189:919.

23   Matulonis U, Dosiou C, Freeman G, Lamont C, Mauch P, Nadler LM, Griffin JD: B 7.1 is superior to B 7.2 costimulation in the induction and maintenance of T-cell-mediated antileukemia immunity. Further evidence that B7.1 and B7.2 are functionally distinct. J Immunol 1996;156:1126–1131.

24   Yang G, Hellstrom KE, Hellstrom I, Chen L: Antitumor immunity elicited by tumor cells transfected with B7.2, a second ligand for CD28/CTLA 4 costimulatory molecules. J Immunol 1995;154:2794–2800.

25   Ridge JP, Di Rosa F, Matzinger P: A conditioned dendritic cell can be a temporal bridge between a CD4+ T-helper and a T-killer cell. Nature 1998;393:474–478.

26   Bennett SR, Carbone FR, Karamalis F, Flavell RA, Miller JF, Heath WR: Help for cytotoxic T cell responses is mediated by CD40 signaling. Nature 1998;393:478–480.

27   Hung K, Hayashi R, Lafond-Walker A, Lowenstein C, Pardoll D, Levitsky H: The central role of CD4+ T cells in antitumor immune response. J Exp Med 1998;188:2357–2368.

28   Van den Eynde BJ, van der Bruggen P: T cell defined tumor antigens. Curr Opin Immunol 1997;9:684–693.

29   Vierboom MP, Nijman HW, Offringa R, van der Voort EI, van Hall T, van den Broek L, Fleuren GJ, Kenemans P, Kast WM, Melief CJ: Tumor eradication by wild-type p53-specific cytotoxic T lymphocytes. J Exp Med 1997;186:695–704.

30   Robbins PF, El-Gamil M, Li YF, Kawakami Y, Loftus D, Appella E, Rosenberg SA: A mutated ß-catenin gene encodes a melanoma-specific antigen recognized by tumor infiltrating lymphocytes. J Exp Med 1996;183:1185–1192.

31   Mandruzzato S, Brasseur F, Andry G, Boon T, van der Bruggen P: A CASP-8 mutation recognized by cytolytic T lymphocytes on a human head and neck carcinoma. J Exp Med 1997;186:785–793.

32   Barratt-Boyes SM: Making the most of mucin: A novel target for tumor immunotherapy. Cancer Immunol Immunother 1996;43:142–151.

33   Gimmi CD, Morrison BW, Mainprice BA, Gribben JG, Boussiotis VA, Freeman GJ, Park SY, Watanabe M, Gong J, Hayes DF, Kufe DW, Nadler LM: Breast cancer-associated antigen, DF 3/MUC 1, induces apoptosis of activated human T cells. Nat Med 1996;2:1367–1370.

34   De Plaen E, Arden K, Traversari C, Gaforio JJ, Szikora JP, De Smet C, Brasseur F, van der Bruggen P, Lethe B, Lurquin C: Structure, chromosomal localization and expression of twelve genes of the MAGE family. Immunogenetics 1994;40:360–369.

35   De Smet C, De Backer O, Faraoni I, Lurquin C, Brasseur F, Boon T: The activation of human gene MAGE-1 in tumor cells is correlated with genome-wide demethylation. Proc Natl Acad Sci USA 1996;93:7149–7153.

36   Kast WM, Offringa R, Peters PJ, Voordouw AC, Meloen RH, van der Eb AJ, Melief CJ: Eradication of adenovirus E1-induced tumors by E1A specific cytotoxic T lymphocytes. Cell 1989;59:603–614.

37   Sogn JA: Tumor immunology: The glass is half full. Immunity 1998;9:757–763.

38   Albelda SM: Role of integrins and other cell adhesion molecules in tumor progression and metastasis. Lab Invest 1993;68:4–17.

39   Pals ST, Horst E, Ossekoppele GJ, Figdor CG, Scheper RJ, Meijer CJ: Expression of lymphocyte homing receptors as a mechanism of dissemination in non-Hodgkin's lymphoma. Blood 1989;73:885–888.

40   Dejana E, Bertocchi F, Bortolami MC, Regonesi A, Tonta A, Breviario F, Giavazzi R: Interleukin-1 promotes tumor cell adhesion to cultured human endothelial cells. J Clin Invest 1988;82:1466–1470.

41   Thomas L: Discussion of paper by P.B. Medawar; in Lawrence HS (ed): Cellular and Humoral Aspects of the Hypersensitivity State. New York, Hoeber-Harper, 1959, pp 1–529.

42   Burnet FM: The concept of immunological surveillance. Prog Exp Tumor Res 1970;13:1–27.

43   Bretscher PA: A two-step, two-signal model for the primary activation of precursor helper T cells. Proc Natl Acad Sci USA 1999;96:185–190.

44   Matzinger P: An innate sense of danger. Semin Immunol 1998;10:399–415.

45   Fuchs EJ, Matzinger P: Is cancer dangerous to the immune system? Semin Immunol 1996;8:271–280.

46   Trauth BC, Klas C, Peters AM, Matzku S, Moller P, Falk W, Debatin KM, Krammer PH: Monoclonal antibody-mediated tumor regression by induction of apoptosis. Science 1989; 245:301–305.

47   Scaffidi C, Fulda S, Srinivasan A, Friesen C, Li F, Tomaselli KJ, Debatin KM, Krammer PH, Peter ME: Two CD95 (APO-1/Fas) signaling pathways. EMBO J 1998;17:1675–1687.

48   Krammer PH: CD95 (APO-1/Fas)-mediated apoptosis: Live and let die. Adv Immunol 1999;71:163–210.

49   Krammer PH: The tumor strikes back: New data on expression of the CD95 (APO-1/Fas) receptor/ligand system may cause paradigm changes in our view on drug treatment and tumor immunology. Cell Death Differ 1997;4:362–364.

50   O'Connell J, Bennett MW, O'Sullivan GC, Collins JK, Shanahan F: The Fas counterattack: A molecular mechanism of tumor immune privilege. Mol Med 1997;3:294–300.

51   Miyashita T, Reed JC: Bcl-2 oncoprotein blocks chemotherapy-induced apoptosis in a human leukemia cell line. Blood 1993;81:151–157.

52   Krajewski S, Blomqvist C, Franssila K, Krajewska M, Wasenius VM, Niskanen E, Nordling S, Reed JC: Reduced expression of proapoptotic gene Bax is associated with poor response rates to combination chemotherapy and shorter survival in women with metastatic breast adenocarcinoma. Cancer Res 1995;55:4471–4478.

53   Owen-Schaub LB, van Golen KL, Hill LL, Price JE: Fas and Fas ligand interactions suppress melanoma lung metastasis. J Exp Med 1998;188:1717–1723.

54   Fulda S, Sieverts H, Friesen C, Herr I, Debatin KM: The CD95 (APO-1/Fas) system mediates drug-induced apoptosis in neuroblastoma cells. Cancer Res 1997;57:3823–3829.

55   Muller M, Wilder S, Bannasch D, Israeli D, Lehlbach K, Li-Weber M, Friedman SL, Galle PR, Stremmel W, Oren M, Krammer PH: Drug induced apoptosis in hepatoma cells is medi-

ated by the CD95 (APO-1/Fas) receptor/ligand system and involves activation of wild-type p53. J Clin Invest 1997;99:403–413.

56 Fulda S, Friesen C, Los M, Scaffidi C, Mier W, Benedict M, Nunez G, Krammer PH, Peter ME, Debatin KM: Betulinic acid triggers CD95 (APO-1/Fas) and p53-independent apoptosis via activation of caspases in neuroectodermal tumors. Cancer Res 1997;57:4956–4964.

57 Walczak H, Miller RE, Ariail K, Gliniak B, Griffith TS, Kubin M, Chin W, Jones J, Woodward A, Le T, Smith C, Smolak P, Goodwin RG, Rauch CT, Schuh JC, Lynch DH: Tumoricidal activity of tumor necrosis factor-related apoptosis-inducing ligand in vivo. Nat Med 1999;5:157–163.

58 Krammer PH, Galle PR, Moller P, Debatin KM: CD95 (APO-1/Fas)-mediated apoptosis in normal and malignant liver, colon and hematopoetic cells; in Vande Wonde GF, Klein G (eds): Advances in Cancer Research. New York, Academic Press, 1998, pp 252–273.

59 Hojo M, Morimoto T, Maluccio M, Asano T, Morimoto K, Lagman M, Shimbo T, Suthanthiran M: Cyclosporin induces cancer progression by a cell autonomous mechanism. Nature 1999;397:530–534.

Dr. Sören T. Eichhorst, Deutsches Krebsforschungszentrum Heidelberg, Abteilung Immungenetik, Im Neuenheimer Feld 280, D–69120 Heidelberg (Germany)
E-mail s.eichhorst@dkfz-heidelberg.de

Rüther U, Nunnensiek C, Schmoll H-J (eds): Secondary Neoplasias following Chemotherapy, Radiotherapy, and Immunosuppression. Contrib Oncol. Basel, Karger, 2000, vol 55, pp 117–138

Malignant Lymphomas and Lympho-proliferative Disorders following Organ Transplantation and Immunomodulatory Therapy

H. K. Müller-Hermelink, T. Rüdiger

Pathologisches Institut der Universität Würzburg, Deutschland

Introduction

In the early days of modern immunology, Sir Macfarlane Burnet published his concept of immunosurveillance. He postulated a major role for the immune system in the rejection and elimination of ubiquitous cancer stem cells such that an even greater occurrence of malignant tumors was prevented. Suggesting this theory were a rough calculation of mutational events in the human body over time; the rise in tumor frequencies as immunocompetence decreases with age, and other conditions of immune malfunction. Researchers soon realized, moreover, that in well-defined states of immunodeficiency, certain types of malignant tumors appeared more frequently than others. There was a preponderance of malignant lymphomas and lymphoproliferative diseases, rather than of the carcinomas dominating in sporadic cancer [43].

To find out why, two clinical settings were studied: congenital immunodeficient disorders and medical immunosuppression after solid-organ transplantation. In both situations, an astonishing frequency of malignant lymphomas was observed [29, 36, 41]. In these two patient collectives, the relative risk of developing malignant lymphoma was far above that of the general population – especially where young age groups were considered. In time, the developing field of viral carcinogenesis revealed that immunosurveillance does not target the tumor cell itself, but rather human tumor viruses (e.g. Epstein-Barr virus, or EBV). In immunodeficiency and under immunosuppression, this leads to uncontrolled proliferation of latently infected cells, which accounts for the increased tumor risk.

Solid-organ transplantation studies then showed that some clinically malignant lymphoproliferations did regress after reduction of immunosuppressive treatment and restoration of immunologic competence. Unfortunately, this beneficial effect was found in only some of the cases. Consequently, a major clinical problem remains unresolved to this day: How should one best treat these patients? Without immunosuppressive therapy, such patients risk acute allograft rejection. On the other hand, by administering immunosuppressive therapy and waiting for a positive response, we risk delaying effective tumor treatment.

Although still rare, these types of malignant lymphomas and lymphoproliferative disorders have become more important as similar tumors increasingly appear in AIDS [45–47]. About 10% of HIV-infected individuals will eventually die of malignant lymphoma – which means hundreds of thousands of lymphoma cases the world over. Recently, Kamel [21] and Natkunam et al. [32] added a new facet to this problem when they reported an increased frequency of malignant lymphomas and of certain types of lymphoproliferative disorders after immunomodulatory treatment for chronic autoimmune diseases.

Malignant lymphomas in the immunosuppressed patient represent a specific spectrum of tumors that differ from sporadic lymphomas. Furthermore, they can be considered, at least in organ transplantation, as a model for lymphoma genesis and progression since grafting and disease origin are so closely linked chronologically. Unfortunately, classification and diagnosis of these tumors are difficult, and treatment options restricted.

In this chapter, we will review the clinical and pathological features and the classification and pathogenic concepts of malignant lymphoma arising after organ transplantation and/or immunomodulatory treatment.

Lymphoproliferative Diseases (LPD) after Allogenic Organ Transplantation

Clinical Correlation

In 1994, Penn [35] estimated the total frequency of cancer in transplantations to be at least 6%, of which posttransplant lymphoproliferative disorders (PTLDs) comprised approximately 23%, resulting in an overall estimate of at least 1.4%. This mean value is modified by many factors, of which allograft type and immunosuppressive regimen are the most important. The incidence of PTLD is approximately 1% for renal and 2% for hepatic transplants, but varies from 2 to 10% for heart, heart-lung and bone marrow transplants.

These differences appear to be related more to the different degrees of immunosuppression than to the organ itself. However, with increasing organ mass and types of tissue involved, entirely different factors move into the foreground, such as the number of allogenic passenger lymphocytes, frequency of allograft rejection, and graft-versus-host reaction. Under conventional immunosuppression (antilymphocyte globulin serum and azathioprine), PTLDs occur in about 1–5% of cardiac transplants. After the introduction of cyclosporine, much higher frequencies of PTLD were initially observed (9–13%). However, by reducing the dose and monitoring serum levels of the drug, frequencies have recently dropped to 1–2%. Other immunosuppressive regimens must also be taken into careful consideration. For example, in one series, cardiac transplant recipients receiving a cumulative dose of at least 75 mg of OKT3 showed a 37.5% incidence of PTLD – compared to 6.2% for those patients who received lesser amounts.

The majority of PTLDs occurs shortly after transplantation, in most instances at a mean time of 6 months after transplantation. However, a small but steady number of PTLDs continues to occur throughout the following years. In one series of pediatric liver transplants, the actual risk was 2.8% per year, resulting in a cumulative frequency of 20% at 7 years [28]. Whereas EBV-positive cases are seen early after transplantation, EBV-negative PTLDs and T-cell lymphomas tend to occur in the later posttransplant period (see below).

Clinical presentations of PTLDs vary considerably. In younger patients in particular, the disease very often commences with mononucleosis-like symptoms (tonsillar enlargement and cervical lymphadenopathy), and rapidly transforms into general lymphadenopathy. In about half of these patients in a survey conducted by the University of Minnesota [19], the disease was rapidly fatal, whereas in the other half, it was self-limited. In another type of presentation, localized tumor masses very often occur at extranodal sites, such as the gastrointestinal tract or the central nervous system, or at unusual sites (liver, lung, oral cavity skin, or uterus). Multiple gastrointestinal tumors are not uncommon. Involvement of the allograft itself is rare (10–15%). Involvement of the allograft and early development after transplantation are, in some cases, related to donor-cell origin of the tumor [44]. Donor-cell origin is especially frequent in bone marrow transplantation. It is more likely if isolated T-cell depletion of the graft has been performed to prevent graft-versus-host disease. Most other PTLDs are of host-cell origin, involving a generalized recurrence or de novo infection by EBV, or localized EBV-associated multiclonal or monoclonal proliferations.

In the early days, PTLDs were considered frankly malignant diseases and were treated (mostly without success) with antitumoral, combined cytostatic regimens. This view was challenged when Starzl et al. [42] demonstrated that many PTLDs regressed spontaneously when immunosuppressive therapy was reduced or discontinued.

Thirty-one percent of PTLDs respond favorably. Early-onset lesions and polymorphic, rather than monomorphic, pathological histologies (see below) are more likely to respond. However, exact predictive diagnosis must take into account morphological, molecular, karyotypic and virological data.

Pathological Classification of PTLDs

The WHO committee on PTLDs and malignant lymphoma in immuno-deficiency syndromes has not yet issued its final recommendations for their classification. However, comparison of the four existing proposals for PTLD classification reveals a high degree of concordance. The term 'posttransplant lymphoproliferative disease' (PTLD) is now used for all malignant lymphomas and lymphoma-like proliferations developing after organ transplantation. Hence, PTLDs include benign self-limiting disease that regresses after reduction of immunotherapy, as well as progressive tumors that are overtly malignant. The first classification of PTLDs was proposed by Frizzera et al. [15]. They distinguished PTLDs from reactive hyperplasia as being histologically invasive, destroying follicular areas, and possessing a very prominent large-cell component closely imitating a malignant lymphoma. Two major categories were recognized: polymorphic diffuse B-cell hyperplasia (PBCH) and polymorphic diffuse B-cell lymphoma (PBCL). In time, Shapiro et al. [40] added the term 'atypical lymphoid hyperplasia' (ALH) to denote a polymorphic paracortical or interstitial proliferation that lacks the invasive, destructive nature of PBCH, and overt lymphoma fulfilling the criteria of B-immunoblastic lymphoma as defined in the Lukes and Collins or KIEL classifications.

Nalesnik et al. [30] described diffuse plasma cell hyperplasia without architectural effacement that was seen in lymph nodes of patients with concurrent or subsequent PTLD. They recognized only one category of polymorphic PTLD, which included both the PBCH and PBCL of the Frizzera classification [15]. In their opinion, the distinguishing criteria as described by Frizzera et al. (amount of necrosis and atypia of immunoblasts) were not of prognostic value, and were difficult to diagnose consistently. Monomorphic PTLD, in turn, exhibits uniform lymphoid cell proliferation at one stage of differentiation and usually evinces proliferations of large or small blastic B immunoblasts and/or plasmoblasts.

Drawing on the categories from Nalesnik et al. [30], Knowles et al. [23] correlated a morphological approach to PTLD. Knowles et al. differentiated between plasmacytic hyperplasia; polymorphic lymphoproliferative disorder comprising the PBCH and PBCL described by Frizzera et al. [15], and the immunoblastic lymphoma and multiple myeloma of the group's monomorphic PTLD.

Summarizing the results of a workshop conducted by the Society of Haematopathology, Harris et al. [20] used the term 'early lesions' for reactive plasmacytic hyperplasia and an infectious mononucleosis-like pattern. Polymorphic PTLDs were divided into rare polyclonal and more frequent monoclonal cases. Monomorphic PTLDs were divided into B-cell non-Hodgkin's lymphoma of immunoblastic, centroblastic, anaplastic and Burkitt's and Burkitt's-like lymphoma types, as well as peripheral T-cell lymphoma and others (table 1).

Table 1. Categories of PTLD recognized at the Workshop of the Society for Haematopathology

---

Early lesions
   Reactive plasmacytic hyperplasia
   Infectious mononucleosis-like lesions

PTLD – Polymorphic
   Polyclonal (rare)
   Monoclonal

PTLD – Monomorphic
B-cell lymphoma
   Diffuse large B-cell lymphoma (immunoblastic, centroblastic, anaplastic)
   Burkitt's lymphoma, Burkitt-like lymphoma
T-cell lymphoma
   Peripheral T-cell lymphoma, unspecified type (usually large-cell)
   Anaplastic large-cell lymphoma (T or null)
   Other types (hepatosplenic γ-δ, T-NK)
Other
   T-cell-rich/Hodgkin's disease-like large B-cell lymphoma
   Plasmacytoma-like
   Plasma cell myeloma

Pathological Features of PTLDs
Early Lesions

This term is used for PTLDs occurring soon after organ transplantation (mean time 3–4 months) and frequently involving adenoids, tonsils and superficial nodes, but also extranodal localizations in children or young adults. The histologic pattern is overlapping, exhibiting plasmocytic hyperplasia without destruction of the underlying architecture of lymphoid tissue or organ tissue (fig. 1); atypical lymphoid hyperplasia involving the interfollicular-type tissue of the lymph nodes and tonsils, and features merging with histologic and clinical signs of infectious mononucleosis-like PTLD (fig. 2). Plasma cells do not show light chain restriction. EBV can be demonstrated in most instances, showing either a polyclonal, oligoclonal or monoclonal type of infection. These lesions tend to regress spontaneously or after reduction of immunosuppressive treatment. In rare cases, they may progress to higher histological grades and be accompanied by more aggressive clinical behavior. They may even be fatal, as can infectious mononucleosis in certain conditions.

Polymorphic PTLDs

Polymorphic PTLDs are invasive, destructive lesions that efface underlying normal architecture of lymphoid tissues or involved organs (fig. 3). In contrast to 'sporadic' B-cell lymphomas, these tumor masses consist of a mixture of cell types. This mixture includes the full range of B-cell maturation – from immunoblasts to plasma cells – and a 'background' inflammatory component of different T-cell subpopulations. There may be areas of necrosis – which can be prominent – and dispersed large blast cells superficially resembling Hodgkin's cells or anaplastic large cells. Proliferation is pronounced. In addition to the polymorphic areas, small monomorphic foci of blast cells are often present. Given the high degree of polymorphism and microheterogeneity, a distinction between polymorphic B-cell hyperplasia and polymorphic B-cell lymphoma as suggested by Frizzera et al. [15] appears neither practical nor necessary [20].

Immunophenotyping on paraffin sections reveals monotypic light chain restriction and immunoglobulin secretion in some cases, but no immunoglobulin production in others. Proliferation markers such as Ki67 reveal active proliferation, which may include some of the reactive T cells. EBV may be detected in most cases by the demonstration of LMP1, and in almost all cases by EBER in situ hybridization, suggesting EBV latency types 2 or 3 (see below).

Polymorphic PTLD may regress partially or completely after discontinuation of immunosuppressive treatment. With surgery, radiation therapy or chemotherapy, it may resolve, although less frequently. Other cases may progress despite therapy.

Monomorphic PTLDs

Most cases of monomorphic PTLDs fulfill all of the criteria for diagnosing aggressive lymphoma on morphological grounds. Most evince a B-cell phenotype (fig. 4). These lymphomas should be designated and classified according to the criteria contained in recent proposals (REAL classification, WHO classification), and should include the term 'PTLD' for clinical and prognostic reasons. Monomorphic PTLDs involve aggressive, invasive tumors that destroy the architecture of the lymphoid or extranodal tissues. These lymphomas are most frequently composed of large transformed immunoblasts, with large round to oval nuclei and prominent nucleoli, as well as basophilic cytoplasm showing only few or no signs of B-cell maturation or differentiation toward plasma cells. The term may also be used in cases exhibiting bizarre or multinucleated nuclear features (as are also seen in usual types of diffuse, large B-cell lymphomas). According to the cytologic criteria of the KIEL classification, most cases may be classified as immunoblastic; some as centroblastic, and certain rare cases as anaplastic or Burkitt-like. Immunophenotyping reveals B-cell antigen in most cases. CD20 may be negative in plasmoplastic lymphomas or anaplastic myelomas, which are rarely seen as PTLDs. If immunoglobulin production is detected, it shows light chain restriction. The proliferation fraction is very high: usually over 90% of tumor cells stain with the Ki67 antigen. Most monomorphic PTLDs representing malignant non-Hodgkin's lymphomas or multiple myelomas after organ transplantation tend to occur in an older age group (> 50 years). Most do not regress after discontinuation of immunosuppressive treatment, or in fact will progress despite cytostatic treatment.

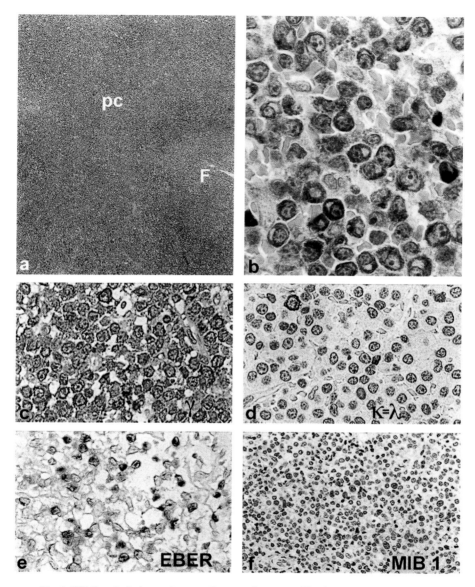

Fig. 1. PTLD early lesion – plasma cell type. **a** Low magnification showing an ill-defined follicle (F) and a diffuse increase of mature plasma cells in the interfollicular area. **b** High magnification of mature plasma cells (Giemsa staining). **c** Immunohistologic detection of γ heavy chain staining all plasma cells. **d** Identical immunohistologic detection of κ (or λ) showing only individual plasma cell staining. **e** EBER in situ hybridization showing a high percentage of plasma cells containing latent EBV. **f** MIB-1 immunohistochemical staining detecting the Ki67 antigen showing a high proliferation of plasma cells.

The Role of EBV in PTLDs

EBV is the most important human γ herpesvirus latently infecting lymphocytes and inducing cellular proliferation [3]. In vitro, EBV is able to infect only human B lymphocytes via the CD21 membrane receptor. Most human adults are infected, and carry latently infected B lymphocytes in the peripheral blood and lymphoid organs. In non-immunosuppressed persons, 1 out of 10 B lymphocytes is infected latently by EBV. In these lymphocytes, EBV expresses at least 11 genes: 2 encode for small non-polyadenylated RNAs (EBER1 and EBER2); 6 code for nuclear proteins (EBNA1, -2, -3A, -3B, -3C and leader protein LP), and 3 for membrane proteins (Latent Membrane Protein LMP-1, LMP-2A and LMP-2B). Based on an observed variable expression of these genes in latently infected tumor cells, Rickinson's group [37b] has defined three different types of latent infections, designated as latency type I, II and III (table 2). Latency type I was originally observed in endemic EBV-associated African Burkitt's lymphoma evincing the expression of EBER1 and EBER2 as well as the transcription of EBNA1. No other EBV-associated nuclear antigen or membrane protein is expressed. Latency type II is observed in the cells of undifferentiated nasopharyngeal carcinoma and Hodgkin's disease showing the expression of EBER1 and EBER2, activation of EBNA1 transcription, and expression of one or more membrane antigens leading to the expression of LMP1 and/or LMP2A or B. Latency type III is seen in vitro in transformed lymphoblastoid cell lines and in many immunodeficiency-associated lymphomas showing the expression of EBER1 and 2, all nuclear antigens, and the main latent membrane proteins of EBV.

Transition to lytic infection is initiated after transcription of the ZEBRA immediate early protein, which can be seen in some latency type-III-infected cells, and very frequently in immunodeficiency-associated malignant lymphomas.

EBV usually presents an episomal extrachromosomal nuclear DNA ring, which is completed by the terminal repeats. The number of these repeats is characteristic of individual virions. Consequently, the clonality of EBV infection can be detected by Southern blot analysis using probes detecting these terminal repeats [9, 33, 34]. Monoclonal EBV integration in tumors (meaning EBV infection of the clonal tumor stem cell) is evidenced by one band in the Southern blot gels. Polyclonal integration (meaning polyclonal infection of tumor cells after tumor formation – which is very rare – or, more frequently, polyclonal lymphoproliferation) is demonstrated by multiple bands or a smear.

EBV infection is detected in 90% of PTLDs by EBER in situ hybridization techniques. Plasmacytic hyperplasia and mononucleosis-like early lesions usually show polyclonal EBV patterns involving elevated numbers of EBV-positive small lymphocytes or activated blast cells. Polymorphic PTLD and monomorphic PTLD show monoclonal EBV integration, and a positive result of EBER in situ hybridization in most, if not all, tumor cells. These cases usually also show LMP1 expression

Table 2. Latency types of EBV

Latency type	Expressed genes	Associated diseases
I	EBNA1	Burkitt's lymphoma
II	EBNA1 LMP1	Hodgkin's lymphoma Nasopharyngeal carcinoma Peripheral T-cell lymphoma
III	EBNA 1–6 LMP1, 2A, 2B	Posttransplant lymphoproliferations Peripheral T-cell lymphoma

in at least some tumor cells, but in far fewer cells than detected by EBER1 hybridization. Half of the cases of polymorphic PTLD also evince expression of EBNA2, suggesting that these cases are of type III latency, while the others are of type II latency. Latency type I, lacking the expression of EBNA2 and LMP1, is seen in some of the malignant lymphomas or monomorphic PTLDs [1].

Two strains of EBV, type A and B, which vary genetically, have been identified. Type A is found in peripheral blood B cells of immunocompetent patients the world over. Type B was initially found in individuals in Central Africa, and frequently appears in immunosuppressed patients, particularly in HIV-infected persons. Every case of PTLD investigated for the presence of type A or type B EBV contained only type A, although an increased incidence of type B EBV was found in peripheral blood B cells in organ transplant recipients [6, 14, 39].

Molecular Studies on PTLDs

Clonality

Southern blot hybridization techniques or PCR-based amplification of the CDR3 region of the immunoglobulin heavy chain in early lesions of PTLDs usually show a polyclonal smear or, in rare cases, a slight clonal predominance. Analysis of the T-cell receptor by PCR-based amplification of the γ-chain gene shows polyclonal results. In polymorphic PTLDs, Southern blot analysis of JH, as well as PCR-based amplification of the CDR3 region of the immunoglobulin heavy chain gene, shows a monoclonal or oligoclonal result. Investigation of multiple tumor nodules within one organ, such as the gastrointestinal tract, may show different clones in each lesion. The T-cell receptor is polyclonal. Using Southern blot analysis or PCR for the immunoglobulin heavy chain gene, malignant lymphoma occurring as PTLD shows monoclonal proliferations.

Molecular Detection of Altered Tumor Suppressor Genes and Oncogenes

Knowles and co-workers [2, 4–8, 22, 23, 39] extensively studied the status of proto-oncogenes and tumor suppressor genes. Early lesions and polymorphic PTLDs characteristically lack evidence of BCL1, BCL2, C-myc, H-K-N-ras and p53 gene alterations [23]. On the other hand, monomorphic lymphomas after organ transplantation consistently contain structural alterations of one or more proto-oncogenes or tumor suppressor genes. Most commonly involved here are the ras, c-myc or p53 genes. More recently, bcl6 gene mutation in these disorders was analyzed [4]. It showed bcl6 gene mutations in 43% of the polymorphic PTLDs and in 90% of the non-Hodgkin's lymphomas diagnosed as PTLDs. bcl6 gene mutations predict shorter survival, as well as refractoriness to reduced immunosuppression and/or surgical excision.

These findings suggest that the mutational status of the bcl6 gene is a reliable indicator for the stratification of polymorphic PTLDs into the biological categories of hyperplastic lesions and malignant lymphoma. This will, of course, also guide therapeutic decisions.

Donor/Recipient Status of PTLD

Early investigation of PTLD occurring after bone marrow transplantation frequently shows involvement of donor lymphocytes and early fatal generalized lymphoproliferative disease [25, 26, 48]. The derivation of malignant lymphomas and PTLDs may be detected by sex chromosome analyses or by polymorphic markers, which are also used in forensic medicine to identify individual probes [44]. PTLDs occurring after solid-organ transplantation are most often of host cell origin.

However, PTLDs occurring soon after transplantation (3–6 months) and involving the allografted organ may be of donor cell origin. A review of publications shows that PTLDs of *donor* origin appear to offer a greater likelihood of freedom from disease after treatment [24, 44].

Karyotypic Alterations in PTLD

Karyotypic studies have been conducted in individual cases of polymorphic and monomorphic PTLDs [11, 12]. In early lesions of PTLD, no clonal chromosomal aberrations have been found. However, polymorphic and monomorphic PTLDs present distinctive abnormalities that can lead to very complex karyotypes. Although more aberrant karyotypes are found in monomorphic PTLDs associated with a rapid and often fatal clinical course, the finding of abnormal karyotypes itself does not automatically predict an unfavorable course. In fact, there are several reports of complete regression in cases with documented clonal cytogenetic aberrations [10, 18].

Rare Types of PTLDs
EBV-Negative B-Cell-Related PTLDs

Although 90% of PTLDs are associated with EBV, about 10% turn out negative even when the most sensitive in situ hybridization techniques for EBER1 and EBER2 are used. EBV-negative PTLDs tend to occur later after transplantation;

---

often only after 5–7 years. While no clear-cut morphologic correlations or conclusions can be drawn, it is known that some of them involve plasma-cell-rich proliferations (PTLD workshop summary); diffuse large B-cell centroblastic lymphomas, or Burkitt's lymphomas [1]. Although the number of reported cases is rather small,

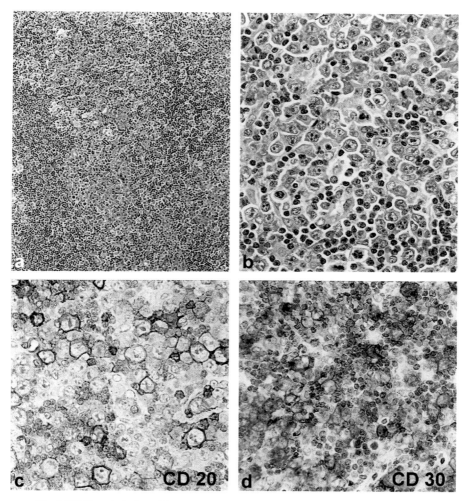

Fig. 2. PTLD early lesion with mononucleosis-like features (polymorphic B-cell hyperplasia). **a** Low magnification showing interfollicular infiltration of the pulp area by activated lymphoid cells. **b** Higher magnification of this area, showing mostly immunoblasts with some small lymphoid sites admixed, as well as some plasmoblasts and plasma cells. **c** Immunohistologic detection of CD20 showing that most activated cells in the interfollicular pulp are staining with different intensities. Also found, however, are negative cells that are detected by CD3 (not shown). **d** Immunohistologic detection of CD30 showing that most of the activated cells express CD30.

similar categories of PTLDs are said to be present in the absence of EBV involving other viruses (such as HHV8) [13] or other mutagenic events related to the drugs used for immunosuppression. The type of PTLDs appearing in the absence of EBV association does not support the view that these cases are coincidental 'sporadic' malignant lymphomas.

Hodgkin's Disease

Classical Hodgkin's disease is not considered to be a typical complication of organ transplantation. Cases have been observed so rarely that some of them may involve coincidental lymphoma rather than PTLDs [16, 31, 38]. However, in the PTLD workshop [20], 1 case showed features of T-cell-rich B-cell lymphoma with Hodgkin's disease-like aspects. This regressed after discontinuation of immunosuppression and, by expression of EBNA2, evinced type III latency rather than the type II latency typical for Hodgkin's disease. All of the cases of Hodgkin's disease in our material, as well as those reported by Anagnostopoulos [1], did exhibit EBV in Hodgkin's cells.

Peripheral T-Cell Lymphoma as a PTLD

Fewer than 20 cases of T-cell lymphoma occurring in solid-organ transplant recipients have been described [17]. They tend to (1) occur much later following transplantation. T-cell proliferations (2) occur at extranodal sites, and (3) only rarely involve the allograft tissue. Only half of the reported cases are associated with EBV infection. According to established diagnostic criteria for peripheral T-cell lymphomas, the cases observed fit into different categories. The few cases of lymphoblastic lymphoma are considered to be coincidental. Other cases are found in the categories of extranodal cytotoxic lymphomas; nasal lymphoproliferations; cytotoxic nodal lymphomas, and hepatosplenic γ-δ lymphoma. A few cases of type T/O anaplastic large-cell lymphoma have been reported. In the series of natural killer-like T-cell lymphomas observed at Vanderbilt University Medical Center [27], 3 of 6 reported cases occurred after organ transplantation. The 1998 EAHP workshop on peripheral T-cell lymphomas, held in Leiden, reported on 7 cases of posttransplant cytotoxic T/NK-cell lymphomas, of which half were associated with EBV. All of these lymphomas occurred in the late posttransplantation period, with a medium latency of 19 months. Clinically, the lymphomas manifested primarily in extranodal localizations involving the intestinal tract (2), the skin (2), the mediastinum (1), two hepatosplenic lymphomas, and one nasal-type peripheral T-cell lymphoma involving the nose and lymph node (1). All of these cases appear to have followed an aggressive course. Immunophenotyping showed positive staining for cytotoxic granula-associated proteins (TIA1 and granzyme B). Four of the 7 cases expressed CD56; 5/7 cases were CD8+; only 1 was CD4+, and all were CDS-cytoplasmic-positive. Five of the 7 cases were of the α/β receptor type; 1 case showed a TCR γ phenotype (table 3).

Table 3. Immunophenotypes and molecular studies in patients with posttransplant lymphoma

No.	CD2	CD3	βF1	CD5	CD4	CD8	CD45R0	TIA1	GrB	CD56	CD30	ALK1	CD20	CD79a	EMA	LMP1	EBER	Molecular studies	Others
9	nd	+	–	(+)	+	–	+	+	+	+	(+)	–	–	–	–	+	+	GL nd	
26	nd	+	+	+	+	+	+	+	+	+	–	–	–	–	–	–	–	nd	
32	–	+	+	–	–	+	+	+	nd	nd	–	nd	–	+	–	–	–		Cytogenetic abberations
33	+	+	+	–	–	+	–	+	+	–	–	–	–	–	–	–	–	CβR	
54	+	+	+	–	–	+	+	+	+	+	+	+	–	–	+	+	nd	CβR TCR G	
62	nd	+	+	nd	–	+	+	+	+	–	–	–	–	–	–	+	+	CβR TCR G	
100	nd	+	–	nd	–	–	+	(+)	–	(+)	–	–	–	–	–	–	+	TCR R	

nd = Not determined.

Most T-cell lymphomas occurring after organ transplantation appear to be of the cytotoxic phenotype of T/NK lineage. This suggests a malignant transformation of effector T cells in transplant rejection and virus infections.

Conclusions

Chronology, clinical pathologic features and molecular data suggest that PTLDs involve a multistep, discontinuous process of transformation. There are different ages at which the various lesions manifest, and a lack of clear-cut transitions from one step to the other. However, when immunosuppression is reduced or discontinued, clinical response suggests that mutagenic events alter the immunologically responsive phase of this EBV-related lymphoproliferative process such that a nonresponsive lymphoma can develop. The pathogenesis of this process is still unclear. EBV-related hyperproliferation may also increase mutability of the bcl6 gene, which is normally found already mutated in germinal-center hyperproliferation. What is more, inhibition of apoptosis by BCL2-like proteins may favor the persistence of mutated clones, while medical treatment may increase hypermutation. Finally, all of these effects and others may coexist.

Post-organ-transplantation immunosuppression in children and young adults most likely favors the development of a prolonged, less regulated phase of primary or reactivated EBV infection correlating to some of the early lesions, including plasma cell hyperplasia and mononucleosis-like features. Polymorphic lesions involve clonal overgrowth and tumor formation, which can sometimes be actively counterregulated by cytotoxic T cells against EBV antigens. This process includes polymorphic PTLDs. If such proliferation is complicated by endogenous alterations of proto-oncogenes and tumor suppressor genes where the bcl6 gene may play a pacemaker role, immunosurveillance of viral antigens may be weakened, so that it can no longer induce complete tumor regression. An overview of these findings is summarized in table 4.

Table 4. Molecular genetic features of PTLD according to Knowles [22]

Category	IgH clonality	EBV clonality	Oncogene/tumor suppressor gene alterations	Clinical course
Plasma cell hyperplasia	Polyclonal	Absent Multiple infectious events Clonal	None	Non-aggressive
Polymorphic PTLD	Monoclonal	Clonal	None	?
Monomorphic PTLD	Monoclonal	Clonal	Yes	Aggressive

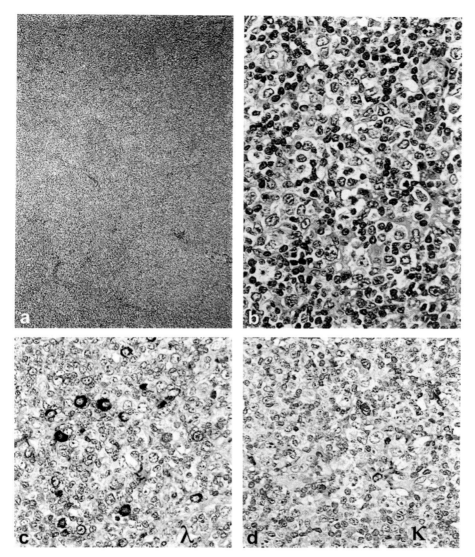

Fig. 3. PTLD (polymorphic B-cell lymphoma). **a, b** Low magnification showing total efface-ment of lymph node architecture with large areas of necrosis. **c** Higher magnification showing atypical polymorphic blast cells expressing the CD20 antigen (not shown) and some plasma cells. **d** Light chain restriction for κ in plasma cells of this case.

Iatrogenic Lymphoproliferative Disorders after Immunomodulatory Treatment

Iatrogenic lymphoproliferative disorders that were not induced by transplantation have been recognized as such only very recently [21]. The most common clinical setting for these disorders is methotrexate treatment for rheumatologic diseases, especially rheumatoid arthritis. This in itself presents a problem: in solid-organ transplant recipients, PTLD is most likely related to the state of medical immunosuppression. However, for patients with rheumatoid arthritis receiving methotrexate therapy, the extent and activity – if any – of immunosuppression is usually unknown. Clearly, not all malignant lymphomas that occur in patients with rheumatologic disease are related to immunomodulatory treatment. Lymphoproliferative disorders related to immunosuppressive or immunomodulatory treatment appear to comprise only a minority of lymphomas in these patients. Most of these lymphomas are probably coincidental with rheumatologic disease, and are not induced by immunosuppression. As for other autoimmune diseases, most lymphomas in patients with rheumatoid arthritis involve malignant lymphomas that are EBV-negative and histologically similar to lymphomas seen in patients without rheumatologic disease. It is crucial that one recognizes iatrogenic lymphoproliferative disease after immunomodulatory treatment for rheumatoid arthritis because such disorders affect therapeutic management and prognosis. Unfortunately, the paucity of specific diagnostic criteria makes its difficult to objectively assess the frequency of iatrogenic lymphoproliferative disorders. What *is* known, though, is that most iatrogenic lymphoproliferative disorders are EBV-positive, which makes inclusion of EBV studies key to such assessments.

There are three main categories of morphological features of the iatrogenic lymphoproliferative disorders reported: (1) atypical polymorphic lymphoproliferative disorder; (2) diffuse aggressive non-Hodgkin's lymphomas (different cell types), and (3) Hodgkin's disease and lymphoproliferations resembling Hodgkin's disease.

Atypical Polymorphic Lymphoproliferative Disorder

These tumor lesions, occurring in lymph nodes or extranodal tissues, efface the organ architecture. They comprise a mixture of lymphoid cells at various stages of activation and maturation, and include small mature lymphocytes, immunoblasts, plasmocytoid lymphocytes, plasma cells, and a varying degree of T-cell infiltration. With Southern blot or PCR analysis, or by immunohistochemical detection of immunoglobulin light chains, these cases reveal clonal immunoglobulin rearrangement or clonal light chain restriction. Nevertheless, many of them regress when immunosuppressive treatment is stopped.

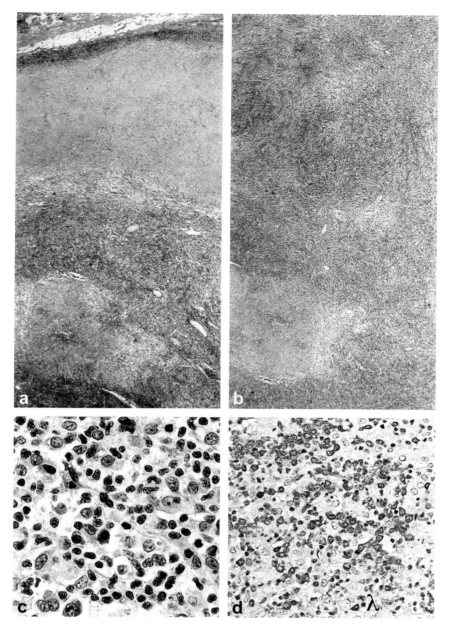

Fig. 4. PTLD – monomorphic type (monomorphic B-cell lymphoma). **a** Low magnification showing complete effacement of the lymph node architecture. **b** Monomorphic infiltration of large blast cells admixed with reactive small lymphocytes. **c, d** Immunological detection of light chain restriction (λ in many of the blast cells and early plasma cell differentiation in tumorous plasmoblasts).

Diffuse Aggressive Non-Hodgkin's Lymphomas

This category of iatrogenic lymphoproliferative disorders evinces cytologically different types of diffuse large B-cell lymphomas of either the large-cell type or the Burkitt-like type. Some of these proliferations have pleomorphic features and focally show Reed-Sternberg-like cells. EBV can usually be detected by EBER in situ hybridization in almost all tumor cells, or – by immunohistochemical detection of LMP1 – in many tumors. Even so, to our knowledge, a detailed analysis of EBV latency types has not been published. Most of these tumors contain EBV strain type A, a situation which resembles that of PTLDs.

Hodgkin's Disease and Lymphoproliferations Resembling Hodgkin's Disease

These cases have the most intriguing morphology in the group of iatrogenic lymphoproliferative disorders. Diagnosis of these tumors is very difficult, since lymphomas may show features of Hodgkin's disease at one site, and diffuse large B-cell lymphoma at others. The phenotype of Hodgkin's cells is very often positive for CD20 and CD30. This makes it difficult to differentiate between classical Hodgkin's disease and lymphoproliferations resembling it. Hodgkin's disease in iatrogenic lymphoproliferative disorders may show diagnostic features of mixed cellularity, or the nodular sclerosing variant of classical Hodgkin's lymphoma, including a typical phenotype of Hodgkin's cells. Exact diagnosis requires morphologic and immunophenotypic examinations, as well as detailed studies on EBV status that include the definition of latency type.

'Sporadic' Atypical Lymphoproliferative Disorders

The pathologic features of lymphoproliferative disorders after organ transplantation and/or immunomodulatory treatment differ from those of sporadic cases of malignant lymphoma. However, their respective morphologies are by no means specific. Clinical experience in treating malignant lymphoma suggests that similar, if not identical, cases are also seen without a clinical report of these conditions.

A further well-researched clinical picture is that of secondary B-cell-derived lymphoproliferations in peripheral T-cell lymphomas after treatment [37a, Zettl, A.: Pers. commun., 1999]. The tumors observed are usually EBV-associated, and exhibit all of the morphologic and immunophenotypic features of PTLDs. EBV is also found in 5–10% of aggressive non-Hodgkin's lymphomas in the general population. Moreover, polymorphic lymphoproliferations associated with EBV – with or without Hodgkin's disease-like features – are definitely found outside of manifest immunosuppression or immunomodulatory treatment.

The question therefore remains whether PTLDs and iatrogenic lymphoproliferations meet the well-defined conditions that enable recognition of a morphology specific to immunodeficiency-related lymphoma and lymphoproliferative disorders – and in contrast to that found in less well-defined states of immunodeficiency or in postchemotherapeutic immunosuppression in elderly patients predisposing to an undefined type of 'sporadic' lymphoproliferative disorder.

References

1 Anagnostopoulos I: Epstein-Barr-Virus in benignen und malignen Lymphknotenproliferationen. Berlin, Institut für Pathologie. Freie Universität, 1999, p 184.
2 Ballerini P, Gaidano G, Gong JZ, Tassi V, Saglio G, Knowles DM, Dall-Favera R: Multiple genetic lesions in acquired immunodeficiency syndrome-related non-Hodgkin's lymphoma Blood 1993;81:166–176.
3 Brooks L, Thomas JA: The significance of Epstein-Barr virus in the pathogenesis of lymphoid and epithelial neoplasia. Curr Diagn Pathol 1995;2:163–174.
4 Cesarman E, Chadburn A, Liu YF, Migliazza A, Dalla-Favera R, Knowles DM: BCL-6 gene mutations in posttransplantation lymphoproliferative disorders predict response to therapy and clinical outcome. Blood 1998;92:2294–2302.
5 Cesarman E, Moore PS, Rao PH, Inghirami G, Knowles DM, Chang Y: In vitro establishment and characterization of two acquired immunodeficiency syndrome-related lymphoma cell lines (BC-1 and BC-2) containing Kaposi's sarcoma-associated herpesvirus-like (KSHV) DNA sequences. Blood 1995;86:2708–2714.
6 Chadburn A, Cesarman E, Knowles DM: Molecular pathology of posttransplantation lymphoproliferative disorders. Semin Diagn Pathol 1997;14:15–26.
7 Chadburn A, Cesarman E, Liu YF, Addonizio L, Hsu D, Michler RE, Knowles DM: Molecular genetic analysis demonstrates that multiple posttransplantation lymphoproliferative disorders occurring in one anatomic site in a single patient represent distinct primary lymphoid neoplasms. Cancer 1995;75:2747–2756.
8 Chadburn A, Chen JM, Hsu DT, Frizzera G, Cesarman E, Garrett TJ, Mears JG, Zangwill SD, Addonizio LJ, Michler RE, Knowles DM: The morphologic and molecular genetic categories of posttransplantation lymphoproliferative disorders are clinically relevant. Cancer 1998;82:1978–1987.
9 Cleary ML, Nalesnik MA, Shearer WT, Sklar J: Clonal analysis of transplant-associated lymphoproliferations based on the structure of the genomic termini of the Epstein-Barr virus. Blood 1988;72:349–352.
10 Cohen JI: Epstein-Barr virus lymphoproliferative disease associated with acquired immunodeficiency. Medicine (Baltimore) 1991;70:137–160.
11 Delecluse HJ, Rouault JP, French M, Dureau G, Magaud JP, Berger F: Post-transplant lymphoproliferative disorders with genetic abnormalities commonly found in malignant tumours. Br J Haematol 1995;89:90–97.
12 Delecluse HJ, Rouault JP, Jeammot B, Kremmer E, Bastard C, Berger F: Bcl6/Laz3 rearrangements in post-transplant lymphoproliferative disorders. Br J Haematol 1995;91:101–103.
13 Dotti G, Fiocchi R, Motta T, et al: Primary effusion lymphoma after heart transplantation: A new entity associated with human herpesvirus-8. Leukemia 1999;13:664–670.
14 Franco A, Munoz C, Aranda I, Cabezas A, Perdiguero M, Prados C: Immunological aspects of a case of posttransplant lymphoproliferative disorder. Am J Nephrol 1995;15:137–141.

15 Frizzera G, Hanto DW, Gajl-Peczalska KJ, et al: Polymorphic diffuse B-cell hyperplasias and lymphomas in renal transplant recipients. Cancer Res 1981;41:4262–4279.

16 Gattuso P, Castelli MJ, Peng Y, Reddy VB: Posttransplant lymphoproliferative disorders: A fine-needle aspiration biopsy study. Diagn Cytopathol 1997;16:392–395.

17 Hanson MN, Morrison VA, Peterson BA, Stieglbauer KT, Kubic VL, McCormick SR, McGlennen RC, Manivel JC, Brunning RD, Litz CE: Posttransplant T-cell lymphoproliferative disorders – an aggressive, late complication of solid-organ transplantation. Blood 1996;88:3626–3633.

18 Hanto DW, Gajl-Peczalska KJ, Frizzera G, Arthur DC, Balfour HH Jr, McClain K, Simmons RL, Najarian JS: Epstein-Barr virus induced polyclonal and monoclonal B-cell lymphoproliferative diseases occurring after renal transplantation. Clinical, pathologic, and virologic findings and implications for therapy. Ann Surg 1983;198:356–369.

19 Hanto DW, Najarlan JS: Advances in the diagnosis and treatment of EBV-associated lymphoproliferative diseases in immunocompromised hosts. J Surg Oncol 1985;30: 215–220.

20 Harris NL, Ferry JA, Swerdlow SH: Posttransplant lymphoproliferative disorders: Summary of Society for Hematopathology Workshop. Semin Diagn Pathol 1997;14:8–14.

21 Kamel OW: Iatrogenic lymphoproliferative disorders in nontransplantation settings. Semin Diagn Pathol 1997;14:27–34.

22 Knowles DM: Immunodeficiency-associated lymphoproliferative disorders. Mod Pathol 1999;12:200–217.

23 Knowles DM, Cesarman E, Chadburn A, Frizzera G, Chen J, Rose EA, Michler RE: Correlative morphologic and molecular genetic analysis demonstrates three distinct categories of posttransplantation lymphoproliferative disorders. Blood 1995;85:552–565.

24 Larson RS, Scott MA, McCurley TL, Vnencak-Jones CL: Microsatellite analysis of post-transplant lymphoproliferative disorders: Determination of donor/recipient origin and identification of putative lymphomagenic mechanism. Cancer Res 1996;56:4378–4381.

25 Lones MA, Lopez-Terrada D, Shintaku IP, Rosenthal J, Said JW: Posttransplant lymphoproliferative disorder in pediatric bone marrow transplant recipients; disseminated disease of donor origin demonstrated by fluorescence in situ hybridization. Arch Pathol Lab Med 1998;122:708–714.

26 Lucas KG, Pollok KE, Emanuel DJ: Post-transplant EBV-induced lymphoproliferative disorders. Leuk Lymphoma 1997;25:1–8.

27 Macon WR, Williams ME, Greer JP, Hammer RD, Glick AD, Collins RD, Cousar JB: Natural killer-like T-cell lymphomas; aggressive lymphomas of T-large granular lymphocytes. Blood 1996;87:1474–1483.

28 Malatack JF, Gartner JC Jr, Urbach AH, Zitelli BJ: Orthotopic liver transplantation, Epstein-Barr virus, cyclosporine, and lymphoproliferative disease: A growing concern. J Pediatr 1991;118:667–675.

29 McKhann C: Primary malignancy in patients undergoing immunosuppression for renal transplantation. Transplantation 1969;8:209–212.

30 Nalesnik MA, Jaffe R, Starzl TE, Demetris AJ, Porter K, Burnham JA, Makowka L, Ho M, Locker J: The pathology of posttransplant lymphoproliferative disorders occurring in the setting of cyclosporine-prednisone immunosuppression. Am J Pathol 1988;133:173–192.

31 Nalesnik MA, Randhawa P, Demetris AJ, Casavilla A, Fung JJ, Locker J: Lymphoma resembling Hodgkin disease after posttransplant lymphoproliferative disorder in a liver transplant recipient. Cancer 1993;72:2568–2573.

32	Natkunam Y, Elenitoba-Johnson KS, Kingma DW, Kamel OW: Epstein-Barr virus strain type and latent membrane protein 1 gene deletions in lymphomas in patients with rheumatic diseases. Arthritis Rheum 1997;40:1152–1156.

33	NerI A, Barriga F, Inghirami G, Knowles DM, Neequaye J, Magrath IT, Dalla-Favera R: Epstein-Barr virus infection precedes clonal expansion in Burkitt's and acquired immunodeficiency syndrome-associated lymphoma. Blood 1991;77:1092–1095.

34	Patton DF, Wilkowski CW, Hanson CA, Shapiro R, Gajl-Peczalska KJ, Filipovich AH, McClain KL: Epstein-Barr virus-determined clonality in posttransplant lymphoproliferative disease. Transplantation 1990;49:1080–1084.

35	Penn I: Occurrence of cancers in immunosuppressed organ transplant recipients. Clin Transplant 1994;99–109.

36	Penn I, Hammond W, Brettschneider L, Starzl TE: Malignant lymphomas in transplantation patients. Transplant Proc 1969;1:106–112.

37a	Quintanilla-Martinez L, Fend F, Moguel LR, et al: Peripheral T-cell lymphoma with Reed-Sternberg-like cells of B-cell phenotype and genotype associated with Epstein-Barr virus infection. Am J Surg Pathol 1999;23:1233–1240.

37b	Rowe M, Lear AL, Croom-Carter D, Davies AH, Rickinson AB: Three pathways of Epstein-Barr virus gene activation from EBNA1-positive latency in B lymphocytes. J Virol 1992;66:122–131.

38	Rowlings PA, Curtis RE, Passweg JR, Deeg HJ, Socie G, Travis LB, Kingma DW, Jaffe ES, Sobocinski KA, Horowitz MM: Increased incidence of Hodgkin's disease after allogeneic bone marrow transplantation. J Clin Oncol 1999;17:3122–3127.

39	Scheinfeld AG, Nador RG, Cesarman E, Chadburn A, Knowles DM: Epstein-Barr virus latent membrane protein-1 oncogene deletion in post-transplantation lymphoproliferative disorders. Am J Pathol 1997;151:805–812.

40	Shapiro RS, McClain K, Frizzera G, Gajl-Peczalska KJ, Kersey JH, Blazar BR, Arthur DC, Patton DF, Greenberg JS, Burke B, et al: Epstein-Barr virus associated B cell lymphoproliferative disorders following bone marrow transplantation. Blood l988;71:1234–1243.

41	Specter BD, Perry GS, Kersey JH: Genetically determined immunodeficiency diseases and malignancy: Report from the immunodeficiency-cancer registry. Clin Immunol Immunopathol 1978;11:12–29.

42	Starzl TE, Nalesnik MA, Porter KA, Ho M, Iwatsuki S, Griffith BP, Rosenthal JT, Hakala TR, Shaw BW Jr, et al: Reversibility of lymphomas and lymphoproliferative lesions developing under cyclosporin-steroid therapy. Lancet 1984;i:583–587.

43	Swerdlow SH: Classification of the posttransplant lymphoproliferatlve disorders: From the past to the present. Semin Diagn Pathol 1997;14:2–7.

44	Weissmann DJ, Ferry JA, Harris NL, Louis DN, Delmonico F, Spiro I: Posttransplantation lymphoproliferative disorders in solid organ recipients are predominantly aggressive tumors of host origin. Am J Clin Pathol 1995;103:748–755.

45	Ziegler JL: Lymphomas and other neoplasms associated with AIDS. Immunol Ser 1989;44:359–370.

46	Ziegler JL, Beckstead JA, Volberding PA, Abrams DI, Levine AM, Lukes RJ, Gill PS, Burkes RL, Meyer PR, Metroka CE, et al: Non-Hodgkin's lymphoma in 90 homosexual men. Relation to generalized lymphadenopathy and the acquired immunodeficiency syndrome. N Engl J Med 1984;311:565–570.

47	Ziegler JL, Bragg K, Abrams D, Beckstead J, Cogan M, Volberding P, Baer D, Wilkinson L, Rosenbaum E, Grant K, et al: High-grade non-Hodgkin's lymphoma in patients with AIDS. Ann NY Acad Sci 1984;437:412–419.

48   Zutter MM, Martin PJ, Sale GE, Shulman HM, Fisher L, Thomas ED, Dumam DM: Epstein-Barr virus lymphoproliferation after bone marrow transplantation. Blood 1988;72:520–529.

Prof. Dr. med. H.K. Müller-Hermelink, Pathologisches Institut der Universität Würzburg, Joseph-Schneider-Straße 2, D–97080 Würzburg (Germany)
Tel. +49 931 2013-776, Fax -440, E-mail path062@mail.uni-wuerzburg.de

Rüther U, Nunnensiek C, Schmoll H-J (eds): Secondary Neoplasias following Chemotherapy, Radiotherapy, and Immunosuppression. Contrib Oncol. Basel, Karger, 2000, vol 55, pp 139–146

....

Chromosomal Aberrations and Molecular Changes in Therapy-Related Leukemias

A. Staratschek-Jox, J. Bullerdiek

Center for Genetics and Genetic Counselling, University of Bremen, Germany

With combined treatment modalities including high-dose chemotherapy followed by autologous stem cell support, many patients suffering from lymphomas, leukemias or solid tumors can achieve long-term remission. However, the risk of developing therapy-related secondary neoplasms markedly increases with the use of certain chemotherapeutic agents. Leukemia secondary to chemotherapy and environmental toxins now accounts for 10–20% of all acute myeloid leukemias (AML) [1]. In fact, leukemia related to alkylating agents was described as far back as 1975 [2]. A second type of leukemia was soon related to therapy regimens including doxorubicin or teniposide, two agents that target DNA topoisomerase II [3]. Two years later, etoposide was identified as the cause of leukemia with monoblastic features [4]. Thus, by the late 1980s, some causative agents of secondary leukemias had been clearly identified, necessitating elucidation of the molecular mechanisms leading to cell transformation.

Technical Advances in Cancer Cytogenetics

Although early attempts to demonstrate the chromosomal complement of cancer cells date back to the 1800s, the first examples of specific chromosomal aberrations in cancer cells were not described until the 1960s [5]. Subsequently, the introduction of chromosome-banding techniques not only facilitated the precise identification of each chromosome based on its unique banding pattern [6], but also enabled the characterization of structural chromosomal alterations [7]. More recently, conventional cytogenetic analyses of cancer cells have been supplemented by the development of molecular cytogenetic techniques, such as fluorescent in situ hybridization (FISH), and FISH-based comparative genomic hybridization (CGH). These can shed additional light on unusual findings, and detect chromosomal imbalances in

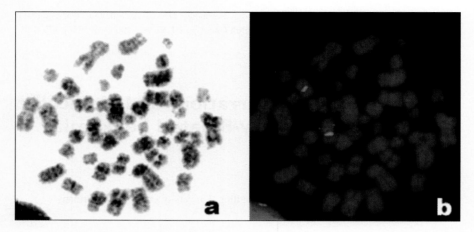

Fig. 1. Detection of a 5q– aberration in a metaphase spread obtained from myelodysplastic bone marrow (MDS). The chromosomes were visualized either by DAPI fluorescent dye *(b)* or by inverted DAPI staining in gray scales *(a)*. To identify both chromosomes 5, a fluorescent probe hybridizing to the telomeric region of the chromosome (D5S23, 5p15.2) was used. A green signal was detected on the short arm of each chromosome 5. The distal fragment of the long arm of chromosome 5 was stained using the probe LSI EGR 1 hybridizing to 5q31 *(b)*. While this probe detected orange signals on one of the chromosomes 5, no staining was obtained on the other chromosome 5, indicating a deletion affecting the long arm.

samples not suited to conventional cytogenetic analyses [for review, see 8]. With FISH, fluorescent-labeled specific DNA probes are used to detect submicroscopic deletions, amplifications or rearrangements of particular chromosomal regions that comprise 3 kb or even less. FISH can also detect certain chromosomal alterations in nondividing cells, although a preliminary diagnosis of the aberration must be made so that the appropriate FISH probe can be selected.

With CGH, tumor cell DNA labeled with a fluorochrome is hybridized on metaphase chromosomes of normal lymphocytes. In addition, DNA obtained from normal autologous lymphocytes is labeled with a different fluorescent dye and is cohybridized on the same metaphase. Thus, in this assay, both DNA probes compete for hybridization on the same metaphase. Imbalances such as DNA amplification or deletion in the tumor cells can be detected by image analysis of the different fluorescent signals resulting from DNA binding. Like FISH, CGH can analyze nondividing cells, thereby eliminating the laborious and often unsuccessful step of preparing tumor-cell metaphases. However, chromosomal aberrations of < 10 megabases may be missed by CGH. Fortunately, these can be detected by cytogenetic analysis. The best cytogenetic technique to use thus depends not only on its inherent strengths and weaknesses, but also on the type of tumor and the specimens available.

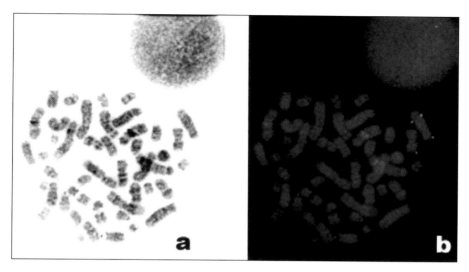

Fig. 2. Presence of a 7q– aberration in a metaphase spread obtained from myelodysplastic bone marrow (MDS). The chromosomes were visualized either by DAPI fluorescent dye *(b)* or by inverted DAPI staining in gray scales *(a)*. Both chromosomes 7 were identified by FISH analysis using a centromeric probe hybridizing to D7Z1 *(b,* green signals). A second probe hybridizing to 7q21 revealed orange staining on one of the chromosomes 7, while the absence of orange staining on the other chromosome 7 indicated a deletion affecting 7q *(b).*

The detection of many typical or even specific chromosomal aberrations has resulted in karyotypic alterations becoming valuable diagnostic and prognostic tools. What is more, these instruments provide new insights into the pathogenesis of the corresponding neoplasms.

Secondary Leukemias Induced by Alkylating Agents

Leukemia caused by alkylating agent therapy was first observed as a recurrent complication of intensive treatment for Hodgkin's disease [9–11]. Patients have a high risk of developing secondary leukemia when they receive a large cumulative dose of the alkylating agent or additional radiation therapy. Splenectomy and older age are also risk factors [for review, see 12]. The mean latency period for developing this leukemia is 5–7 years. Generally, progression from pancytopenia with myelodysplastic changes to myelodysplastic syndrome (MDS) and on to AML is observed [13].

Characteristic of leukemic cells is complete or partial deletion of chromosome 5 (fig. 1) or 7 (fig. 2), respectively [14–16]. Deletion of IRF-1 mapping to chromosome 5q31.1 has been frequently observed in leukemic cells, suggesting that alterations of this gene may contribute to leukemia development [17]. Even in leukemic cells lacking 5q deletions, a truncated IRF-1 protein – resulting from accelerated exon skipping of IRF-1 mRNA – was detected that lost DNA binding capacity [18]. Moreover, granulocyte-macrophage colony-stimulating factor (GM-CSF) as well as interleukins IL-3, IL-4 and IL-5 map to the long arm of chromosome 5 [19–21], and deregulated expression of these genes might lead to enhanced growth of myeloid cells. In addition to chromosomal alteration of chromosomes 5 and/or 7, multiple segmental jumping translocations – characterized by multiple copies of the ABL and/or MLL oncogenes – occur in treatment-related leukemias [22]. This suggests that the altered expression of one or both of these genes contributes to the malignant phenotype of leukemic cells. Furthermore, germline mutations of p53 have been frequently correlated to additional translocations [23], providing evidence of a possible genetic predisposition to genomic instability in therapy-related AML blasts.

Secondary Leukemias Induced by DNA Topoisomerase II-Targeted Drugs

The second form of treatment-related AML is caused by drugs targeting DNA topoisomerase II. Such drugs include etoposide and teniposide, antineoplastics frequently used to inhibit DNA topoisomerase II [24]. Also, anthracyclines, dactinomycin, mitoxantrone and amsacrine intercalate with DNA topoisomerase II, thereby reducing its activity [25–27].

The significant feature of topoisomerase II activity here is that it leads to transient cleavage and religation of double-strand DNA [24, 28], with the aim of promoting relaxation of supercoiled DNA. Antineoplastic agents that interfere with topoisomerase II activity enhance cleavage of double-strand DNA lacking religation [29]. This, in turn, results in chromosomal fragmentation and sister chromatid exchanges [30], DNA deletions and insertions [31], and cell death by apoptosis [32]. The induction of chromosomal translocations appears to be a critical step in leukemogenesis associated with topoisomerase-targeting drugs. These leukemias are often characterized by chromosomal translocations affecting 11q23 (fig. 3) [33] harboring the MLL gene [34]. Within this chromosomal region, topoisomerase II-mediated cleavage is a specific event [35], which strongly supports the view that chromosomal translocation involving 11q23 arises during alteration of topoisomerase II activity. Less frequent chromosomal translocation t(8;21), t(3;21), inv(16), t(15;17) or t(9;22) also occurs, whereby most of the leukemias harboring these translocations present as myelomonoblastic variants [12].

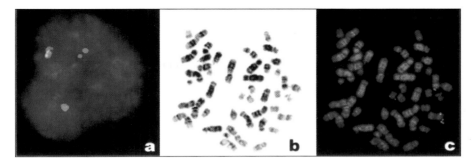

Fig. 3. Presence of t(11;19)(q23;p13) in blast cells of AML. FISH was performed on an interphase nucleus *(a)* and on a metaphase spread *(c)*. Chromosomal DNA was visualized either by DAPI fluorescent dye *(a, c)* or by inverted DAPI staining in gray scales *(b)*. Two probes (PAC 4746, green signals; PAC 4746, orange signals), both hybridizing to 11q23 and in close proximity to each other, were used in FISH analysis *(a, c)*. The location of green and orange signals on one of the chromosomes 11 in the metaphase spread or in close proximity to each other in the interphase nucleus indicated a normal chromosome 11. The detection of green signals on the other chromosome 11, with simultaneous absence of an orange signal in the same region, pointed to a translocation involving this chromosomal band. The detection of orange signals on one of the chromosomes 19 provided further evidence that material of one of the chromosomes 11 was translocated to one of the chromosomes 19. Chromosomes 11 and 19 were identified by inverted DAPI staining *(b)*.

The Role of the MLL Gene in Therapy-Related Leukemias

The breakpoint cluster region of most of the chromosomal translocations affecting the long arm of chromosome 11 maps to a region of the MLL gene located on 11q23 [36]. The MLL gene contains 36 exons, and encodes a 3,969 amino acid protein [37]. Defects in yolk sac hematopoiesis in MLL-null murine embryos [38], as well as in the differentiation block of MLL double knockout hematopoietic stem cells [39], suggest that expression of the MLL gene is critical for hematopoiesis. Reciprocal translocations involving the MLL gene lead to disruption of the gene and to the establishment of novel fusion genes. Today, more than 30 different partner genes have been described. Half of them are cloned, representing transcription factors in a substantial proportion of cases [12]. Altered expression of an MLL fusion protein most probably leads to a lack of differentiation of leukemic cells.

Outlook

Secondary leukemias most often occur in conjunction with the administration of either alkylating or topoisomerase II-targeting drugs. In order to prevent therapy-related leukemias, it is essential to understand the differences between cytotoxic versus leukemogenic effects of these drugs. The risk of developing secondary leukemia increases with dose incrementation and repeated administration [33]. The challenge to cancer treatment now and in the near future will be to develop new regimens that minimize the risk of contracting secondary leukemia – but without decreasing remission rates.

Acknowledgement

We wish to thank Dr. A. Hagemeijer and Dr. S. Franke, Center for Human Genetics, K.U. Leuven, Belgium, for kindly providing us with figures 1–3.

References

1   Smith MA, McCaffrey RP, Karp JE: The secondary leukemias: Challenges and research directions. J Natl Cancer Inst 1996;88:407–418.
2   Kyle RA, Pierre RV, Bayrd ED: Multiple myeloma and acute leukemia associated with alkylating agents. Arch Intern Med 1975;135:185–192.
3   Secker-Walker LM, Stewart EL, Todd A: Acute lymphoblastic leukaemia with t(4;11) follows neuroblastoma: A late effect of treatment? Med Pediatr Oncol 1985;13:48–50.
4   Ratain MJ, Kaminer LS, Bitran JD, Larson RA, Le Beau MM, Skosey C, Purl S, Hoffman PC, Wade J, Vardiman JW: Acute nonlymphocytic leukemia following etoposide and cisplatin combination chemotherapy for advanced non-small-cell carcinoma of the lung. Blood 1987;70:1412–1417.
5   Van Steenis H: Chromosomes and cancer. Nature 1966;209:819–821.
6   Caspersson T, Zech L, Johansson C: Differential binding of alkylating fluorochromosomes in human chrosomes. Exp Cell Res 1970;60:315–319.
7   Yunis JJ: High resolution of human chromosomes. Science 1976;191:1268–1270.
8   Popescu NC, Zimonjic DB: Molecular cytogenetic characterization of cancer cell alterations. Cancer Genet Cytogenet 1997;93:10–21.
9   Coltman CA Jr, Dixon DO: Second malignancies complicating Hodgkin's disease: A Southwest Oncology Group 10-year follow-up. Cancer Treat Rep 1982;66:1023–1033.
10 Tester WJ, Kinsella TJ, Waller B, Makuch RW, Kelley PA, Glatstein E, DeVita VT: Second malignant neoplasms complicating Hodgkin's disease: The National Cancer Institute experience. J Clin Oncol 1984;2:762–769.
11 Kaldor JM, Day NE, Clarke EA, Van Leeuwen FE, Henry-Amar M, Fiorentino MV, Bell J, Pedersen D, Band P, Assouline D: Leukemia following Hodgkin's disease. N Engl J Med 1990;322:7–13.
12 Felix CA: Secondary leukemias induced by topoisomerase-targeted drugs. Biochim Biophys Acta 1998;1400:233–255.
13 Michels SD, McKenna RW, Arthur DC, Brunning RD: Therapy-related acute myeloid leukemia and myelodysplastic syndrome: A clinical and morphologic study of 65 cases. Blood 1985;65:1364–1372.

14   Pedersen-Bjergaard J, Haahr S, Philip P, Thomsen M, Jensen G, Ersboll J, Nissen NI: Abolished production of interferon by leucocytes of patients with the acquired cytogenetic abnormalities 5q– or –5 in secondary and de-novo acute non-lymphocytic leukaemia. Br J Haematol 1980;46:211–223.

15   Van den Berghe H, Vermaelen K, Mecucci C, Barbieri D, Tricot G: The 5q– anomaly. Cancer Genet Cytogenet 1985;17:189–255.

16   Whang-Peng J, Young RC, Lee EC, Longo DL, Schechter GP, DeVita VT Jr: Cytogenetic studies in patients with secondary leukemia/dysmyelopoietic syndrome after different treatment modalities. Blood 1988;71:403–414.

17   Willman CL, Sever CE, Pallavicini MG, Harada H, Tanaka N, Slovak ML, Yamamoto H, Harada K, Meeker TC, List AF: Deletion of IRF-1, mapping to chromosome 5q31.1, in human leukemia and preleukemic myelodysplasia. Science 1993;259:968–971.

18   Harada H, Kondo T, Ogawa S, Tamura T, Kitagawa M, Tanaka N, Lamphier MS, Hirai H, Taniguchi T: Accelerated exon skipping of IRF-1 mRNA in human myelodysplasia/ leukemia; a possible mechanism of tumor suppressor inactivation. Oncogene 1994;9: 3313–3320.

19   Pettenati MJ, Le Beau MM, Lemons RS, Shima EA, Kawasaki ES, Larson RA, Sherr CJ, Diaz MO, Rowley JD: Assignment of CSF-1 to 5q33.1: Evidence for clustering of genes regulating hematopoiesis and for their involvement in the deletion of the long arm of chromosome 5 in myeloid disorders. Proc Natl Acad Sci USA 1987;84: 2970–2974.

20   Le Beau MM, Epstein ND, O'Brien SJ, Nienhuis AW, Yang YC, Clark SC, Rowley J: The interleukin-3 gene is located on human chromosome 5 and is deleted in myeloid leukemias with a deletion of 5q. Proc Natl Acad Sci USA 1987;84:5913–5917.

21   Le Beau MM, Lemons RS, Espinosa R 3rd, Larson RA, Arai N, Rowley JD: Interleukin-4 and interleukin-5 map to human chromosome 5 in a region encoding growth factors and receptors and are deleted in myeloid leukemias with a del(5q). Blood 1989;73:647–650.

22   Tanaka K, Arif M, Eguchi M, Kyo T, Dohy H, Kamada N: Frequent jumping translocations of chromosomal segments involving the ABL oncogene alone or in combination with CD3-MLL genes in secondary leukemias. Blood 1997;89:596–600.

23   Felix CA, Megonigal MD, Chervinsky DS, Leonard DG, Tsuchida N, Kakati S, Block AM, Fisher J, Grossi M, Salhany KI, Jani-Sait SN, Aplan PD: Association of germline p53 mutation with MLL segmental jumping translocation in treatment-related leukemia. Blood 1998;91:4451–4456.

24   Corbett AH, Osheroff N: When good enzymes go bad: Conversion of topoisomerase II to a cellular toxin by antineoplastic drugs. Chem Res Toxicol 1993;6:585–597.

25   Zunino F, Capranico G: DNA topoisomerase II as the primary target of anti-tumor anthracyclines. Anticancer Drug Des 1990;5:307–317.

26   Wassermann K, Markovits J, Jaxel C, Capranico G, Kohn KW, Pommier Y: Effects of morpholinyl doxorubicins, doxorubicin, and actinomycin D on mammalian DNA topoisomerases I and II. Mol Pharmacol 1990;38:38–45.

27   Malonne H, Atassi G: DNA topoisomerase targeting drugs: Mechanisms of action and perspectives. Anticancer Drugs 1997;8:811–822.

28   Wang JC: DNA topoisomerases. Annu Rev Biochem 1996;65:635–662.

29   Osheroff N: Effect of antineoplastic agents on the DNA cleavage/religation reaction of eukaryotic topoisomerase II: Inhibition of DNA religation by etoposide. Biochemistry 1989;28:6157–6160.

30 Gupta RS, Bromke A, Bryant DW, Gupta R, Singh B, McCalla DR: Etoposide (VP16) and teniposide (VM26): Novel anticancer drugs, strongly mutagenic in mammalian but not prokaryotic test systems. Mutagenesis 1987;2:179–186.

31 Han YH, Austin MJ, Pommier Y, Povirk LF: Small deletion and insertion mutations induced by the topoisomerase II inhibitor teniposide in CHO cells and comparison with sites of drug-stimulated DNA cleavage in vitro. J Mol Biol 1993;229:52–66.

32 Bertrand R, Kerrigan D, Sarang M, Pommier Y: Cell death induced by topoisomerase inhibitors. Role of calcium in mammalian cells. Biochem Pharmacol 1991;42:77–85.

33 Pui CH, Behm FG, Raimondi SC, Dodge RK, George SL, Rivera GK, Mirro J Jr, Kalwinsky DK, Dahl GV, Murphy SB: Secondary acute myeloid leukemia in children treated for acute lymphoid leukemia. N Engl J Med 1989;321:136–142.

34 McCabe NR, Burnett RC, Gill HJ, Thirman MJ, Mbangkollo D, Kipiniak M, van Melle E, Ziemin-van der Poel S, Rowley JD, Diaz MO: Cloning of cDNAs of the MLL gene that detect DNA rearrangements and altered RNA transcripts in human leukemic cells with 11q23 translocations. Proc Natl Acad Sci USA 1992;89:11794–11798.

35 Stanulla M, Wang J, Chervinsky DS, Thandla S, Aplan PD: DNA cleavage within the MLL breakpoint cluster region is a specific event which occurs as part of higher-order chromatin fragmentation during the initial stages of apoptosis. Mol Cell Biol 1997;17:4070–4079.

36 Thirman MJ, Gill HJ, Burnett RC, Mbangkollo D, McCabe NR, Kobayashi H, Ziemin-van der Poel S, Kaneko Y, Morgan R, Sandberg AA: Rearrangement of the MLL gene in acute lymphoblastic and acute myeloid leukemias with 11q23 chromosomal translocations. N Engl J Med 1993;329:909–914.

37 Rasio D, Schichman SA, Negrini M, Canaani E, Croce CM: Complete exon structure of the ALL1 gene. Cancer Res 1996;56:1766–1769.

38 Hess JL, Yu BD, Li B, Hanson R, Korsmeyer SJ: Defects in yolk sac hematopoiesis in Mll-null embryos. Blood 1997;90:1799–1806.

39 Fidanza V, Melotti P, Yano T, Nakamura T, Bradley A, Canaani E, Calabretta B, Croce CM: Double knockout of the ALL-1 gene blocks hematopoietic differentiation in vitro. Cancer Res 1996;56:1179–1183.

Jörn Bullerdiek, Zentrum für Humangenetik und Genetische Beratung, Universität Bremen, Leobener Straße, ZHG, D–28359 Bremen (Germany)
Tel./Fax +49 421 2184239

Rüther U, Nunnensiek C, Schmoll H-J (eds): Secondary Neoplasias following Chemotherapy, Radiotherapy, and Immunosuppression. Contrib Oncol. Basel, Karger, 2000, vol 55, pp 147–164

Secondary Tumorigenesis after Radiotherapy

Jürgen Ammon

Aachen, Deutschland

Introduction

Today's curative radiotherapy enables many patients to achieve a normal life span, especially when the newest methods of adjuvant chemotherapy are also part of the therapeutic regimen. Unfortunately, these longer survival times are also bringing to light late sequelae of radiotherapy; in particular, radiotherapy-induced secondary malignancy. This phenomenon is, luckily, very rare, and not surprisingly also difficult to trace, as Jablon's [1984] calculation illustrates: out of 1,000,000 persons, 160,000 will evince a malignancy in the course of their lives, meaning an incidence of 16%. An increased incidence of malignancy due to exposure to radiation would be, for example, a frequency of 0.5%. 0.5% of the 160,000 persons equals 800. Accordingly, the 'normal' incidence of malignancies occurring during the course of the collective's lives would be raised to 160,800. This reveals how difficult it is to separate those very rare tumors that may have been caused by irradiation, from tumors of other etiologies.

Despite the minimal frequency of radiation-induced secondary malignancies, many individual reports of tumors arising in previous radiation fields began to appear right after the discovery of x-rays [Upton, 1986]. But it was not until survivors of the atomic bomb in Hiroshima and Nagasaki were examined on a large scale that enough reliable data became available on the frequency and type of secondary tumors occurring after ionizing radiation [Preston et al., 1987]. These studies also spurred research on patients who, for example, had received radiotherapy for tumors in their childhood, or for Hodgkin's disease or breast cancer. As a result, we can now make concrete statements on the role of dosage, the interval between irradiation and secondary tumorigenesis, and on possible additional effects of cytostatic agents.

It is difficult to analyze secondary tumors developing after ionizing radiation since patients may have been exposed to very different sources of radiation. These include radiation from their surroundings, from outer space, and from incorporated natural radionuclides. Taking the entire population into consideration, the use of ionizing radiation in medicine – especially in diagnostics – accounts for half of the natural exposure to radiation. It is assumed that 3% of all cases of cancer-induced mortality can be traced to natural radiation exposure. One-half of these, or 1.5%, are assumed to stem from the use of ionizing radiation in medicine [Jablon, 1984]. Neoplasms can also develop after the therapeutic use of ionizing radiation. They are found either in the previous radiation field or in its immediate vicinity. Secondary carcinomas can also develop outside of the previous radiation field when particularly susceptible tissue is subjected to scatter radiation.

Incidence and Histology

Certain criteria must be fulfilled to diagnose a postirradiation secondary tumor as such. Fajardo [1986] established correlating guidelines, which are still valid today: (1) the tumor must have arisen within a previous radiation field (fig. 1); (2) the secondary malignancy should differ histologically from the primary, irradiated tumor; (3) if the secondary tumor is leukemic, the latency period should be more than 2 years, and if it is a solid tumor, more than 6 years, and (4) the amounts of statistical data should be large enough so that a possible association can be reasonably assumed.

Generally speaking, persons exposed to ionizing radiation should be expected to develop radiation-induced tumors significantly more often than the nonirradiated population. On the basis of several studies, Levitt [1995] found that the following types of tumors can be induced by radiation: osteo- and soft-tissue sarcomas; mesotheliomas; paranasal tumors; basal cell and squamous epithelial carcinomas of the skin; bronchial and esophageal carcinomas; gastric carcinomas; colon carcinomas; thyroid cancer; leukemias; malignant lymphomas; multiple myelomas; breast cancer, and hepatocellular cancers. These types of tumors have been found not only in survivors of the atomic bomb. Boice [1988] also discovered that these tumors can develop in patients irradiated for benign (table 1) or malignant (table 2) disease. Many studies of patients irradiated for benign skeletal diseases or for mammary gland, gynecological or dermal disease, found that such patients evinced a higher incidence of the above-mentioned secondary tumors.

The clinical picture is similar for patients who had, many years before, been irradiated for a malignancy with a favorable prognosis. Such malignancies included gynecological tumors of the cervix, ovary or breast; Hodgkin's and non-Hodgkin's lymphomas, and childhood tumors.

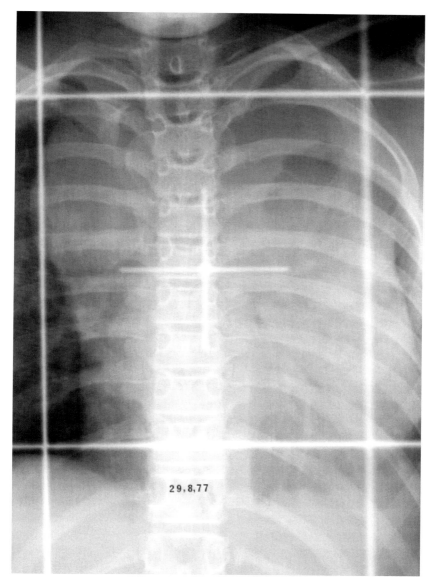

29,8,77

Fig. 1. Example of a secondary tumor. The female patient, born in 1964, received emergency radiotherapy for acute dyspnea (6×100 cGy) in 1977. This resulted in complete remission of the mediastinal tumor. Histologic biopsy of a supraclavicular lymph node confirmed a lymphoblastic lymphoma in a supraclavicular lymph node. The patient was referred at the end of 1998 for a lobular mammary carcinoma on the right side. This tumor may be radiation-induced, since all criteria are met: the tumor developed in a previous field of irradiation; it differs histologically from the primary tumor, and the latency period is 21 years.

Table 1. Histologic types of secondary tumors after radiotherapy for benign diseases; from Boice [1988]

Population	Excess cancers
Spondylitis	Leukemia, lymphomas, lung, esophagus, stomach, central nervous system
Tinea capitis	Thyroid, brain, skin
Thymus enlargement	Thyroid, breast, skin
Benign head and neck disease	Thyroid, salivary gland, neural tumors
Benign breast conditions	Breast
Benign gynecological disease	Leukemia, intestine, rectum, uterus, urinary organs

Table 2. Histologic types of secondary tumors after radiotherapy for malignant diseases; from Boice [1988]

Population	Excess cancers
Cervical cancer	Leukemia, bladder, rectum, uterus, ovary, stomach, breast, connective tissue, thyroid, kidney
Childhood cancer	Bone, thyroid, connective tissue, breast, possibly brain, no leukemia
Hodgkin's disease	Possibly breast, stomach, thyroid, oral cavity, lung, no leukemia
Non-Hodgkin's lymphoma	Leukemia
Uterine corpus cancer	Rectum, leukemia
Ovarian cancer	Colon, rectum, bladder
Breast cancer	Uterus; possibly leukemia, lung, second breast

Periods of Latency

The interval between irradiation and detection of a secondary tumor varies. Levitt [1995] found that differentiation must be made between leukemias and solid tumors. Leukemias may develop as early as 2 years postradiation, with incidence peaking 5–10 years after radiotherapy. Thereafter, risk decreases with time [Coleman and Tucker, 1989]. For solid tumors, intervals of at least 6 years are usual. Recent studies (fig. 2) support these findings, and include observation periods of up to 25 years. In particular, follow-up of patients with Hodgkin's disease shows that leukemia is a risk as early as 2 years after radiotherapy [Tucker et al., 1988].

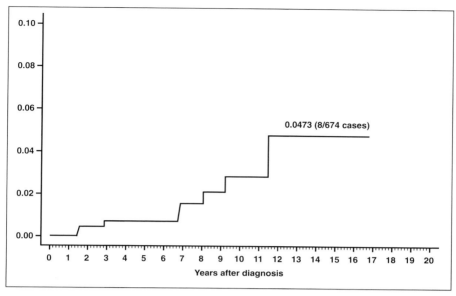

Fig. 2. Development of secondary tumors in children after treatment for Ewing's sarcoma. From Dunst et al. [1998].

It is interesting to note that in these studies on chronological associations, tumors outside of the radiation fields were also detected – albeit with lower frequency. Accordingly, Nyandoto et al. [1998] were able to demonstrate that most tumors found within the radiation fields had developed after radiotherapy for Hodgkin's disease. About one-fourth of the tumors developed in the immediate vicinity of the field boundaries. The distribution of types of tumors and their correlating time intervals were the same, however (fig. 3), so that latency period does not appear to depend on dosage.

Problems Arising after Irradiation of Specific Tumor Types

Total-Body Irradiation and Bone Marrow Transplantation
Total-body irradiation is conducted in conjunction with bone marrow transplantation. Initially, patients thus treated were primarily those with systemic malignant disease. In the meantime, however, there are also several solid tumors for which bone marrow transplantation can be considered after total-body irradiation and chemotherapy. Although little is known about possible late sequelae, especially the induction of secondary tumors, there is a new and very comprehensive analysis based on data of the International Bone Marrow Transplant Registry from 1964 to 1992 [Curtis et al.,

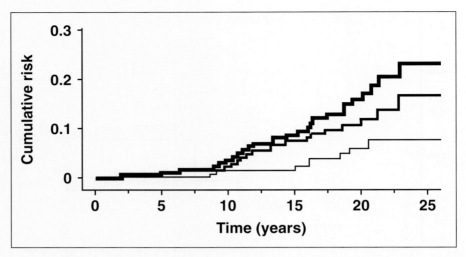

Fig. 3. Development of secondary tumors after treatment for Hodgkin's disease. The top curve depicts the risk of developing any secondary tumor; the middle curve shows the risk of developing a secondary tumor within the previous field of irradiation, and the bottom curve shows the risk of developing a secondary tumor outside of the field of irradiation. From Nyandoto et al. [1998].

1997]. In this study, the data on 19,229 cases from 235 treatment centers were evaluated. The majority of these patients had been treated for leukemia (75%); 11.2% for severe aplastic leukemia, and the rest for other diseases, such as Hodgkin's and non-Hodgkin's lymphomas, myelodysplastic syndromes, or solid carcinomas.

For the 9,501 patients surviving at least 1 year after bone marrow transplantation, the median follow-up period was 3.5 years. 104 patients were followed up for more than 15 years. For conditioning treatment, 73% were administered total-body irradiation, primarily in combination with cyclophosphamide and other cytostatic agents, and 3.4% received limited-field radiation, also in combination with cytostatic agents. The remaining patients were given only cytostatic agents. About one-fourth of the patients received radiation in a single dose; the rest were given fractionated radiation. Radiation doses were 10 Gy in single-dose application, and up to 14 Gy in fractionated administration. The findings of this study permit more precise forecasts of the risk of secondary malignancy.

Of the 19,229 transplantees, 80 developed a solid secondary carcinoma. Compared to 30 – the number of cases to be expected among the normal population – the statistically significant ratio (p < 0.001) of observed vs. expected cases is 2.7. Of these 80 patients, 36 died, and 26 of these 36 deaths were due to the secondary tumor. Findings for the individual tumors were quite varied. For example, the risk of developing typical adult malignomas was only slightly increased. This applied to tumors of the gastrointestinal system, the breast, the respiratory system and the urogenital tract.

On the other hand, the risk of contracting certain rare tumors was significantly higher, especially for carcinomas of the oral cavity, the liver and the thyroid gland, and for melanomas, tumors of the central nervous system, the skeleton and the connective tissue. In addition, the risk of contracting secondary malignancy increased over time during follow-up.

Also of interest is dose dependency. A multivariant analysis showed that increasing the radiation dose increased the risk of developing a solid tumor. Fractionation did not play a significant role here. The risk for doses of 10 Gy was 2.7, and for doses of 14 Gy, 4.1. Age dependency was very pronounced: compared to adults, the risk for children was higher by a factor of 10. With increasing age, risk decreased progressively to only 1.4 for patients over 30 years of age. Limited-field radiation was found to entail a very high risk, averaging 16.1 instead of 2.7.

It must be noted, however, that despite the very large collectives, statistical analysis is very difficult since only a few patients develop a solid secondary tumor. Other study groups [Bathia et al., 1996; Witherspoon et al., 1989] report similar findings, so that the risk after total-body irradiation can be assumed to have the factor 3 (ratio of cases observed vs. cases expected). Also making evaluation difficult is the influence of cytostatic substances in chemotherapy, with their high mutagenic potential. An analysis of the impact of such preparatory treatments on induction of secondary malignomas would be very useful. Be that as it may, all of the authors warn of overrating the risk of secondary tumors after total-body radiation. And since most of these therapeutic regimens aim to cure the patient, the benefits clearly outweigh the possible risks. This is of key importance to follow-up care: in no case should follow-up be stopped – not even after 10 years of tumor-free observation. This especially applies to patients treated with limited-field irradiation.

Irradiation of Hodgkin's Disease

A growing number of publications have reported an increased risk of solid secondary tumors in patients who had been therapied successfully for Hodgkin's disease. Today, this increased incidence of secondary solid malignancies is considered to be the primary long-term complication after successful treatment of Hodgkin's disease, especially now that other therapies – such as newer chemotherapeutic regimens – have reduced the risk of leukemia from about 10% after MOPP (often including maintenance therapy) to less than 1% with ABVD. In addition, improved techniques have nearly eliminated cardiac risk from mediastinal radiation [Glanzmann, 1998]. In 1997, Swerdlow et al. published a study on 1,039 patients treated for Hodgkin's disease at Royal Marsden Hospital. Here, the relative risk of developing a secondary solid tumor after radiation therapy alone was 2.6 (ratio of cases observed to cases expected); after chemotherapy only, 2.1, and after combined radiotherapy and chemotherapy, 3.1. The long-term risk is thus comparable to that of total-body irradiation. Also to be taken into account is the risk of contracting leukemia: leukemia is present in about one-third of all of the cases of secondary tumors developing after therapy for Hodgkin's disease [Tucker et al., 1988].

The same group studied 1,507 patients at Stanford for over 15 years. The patients were divided into four categories for evaluation: those receiving only radiation therapy; those administered only adjuvant chemotherapy; those given only chemotherapy, and those who had received radiation therapy plus radioactive gold in the context of lymphography. Table 3 lists the findings, including the ratio of tumor cases observed vs. tumor cases expected. Analysis revealed statistically significant increases in the incidence of all tumor types. These include the leukemias; carcinomas of the bronchial system and the gastrointestinal tract; non-Hodgkin's lymphomas; melanomas, and tumors of the skeleton and connective tissue. Starting 5 years after therapy, the risk of secondary tumorigenesis remained quite constant over time. The risk of secondary solid tumors peaked at 10 years. By contrast, the risk of leukemia had almost completely disappeared after 10 years.

As expected, most of the tumors observed were found within the previous irradiation fields. Only for melanomas were three found within, and three outside of, the irradiation fields; while two could not be classified precisely. These findings have been confirmed by a more recent study by Nyandoto et al. [1998], where 76% of all secondary tumors were found within the previous irradiation fields or on their peripheries. Accordingly, those authors established a certain dose dependency. For example, patients who had received >40 Gy had roughly twice the risk of developing a secondary tumor as did patients who had received a cumulative dose of about 30 Gy.

However, based on the analysis conducted by Tucker et al. [1988], the overall risk of a secondary tumor is calculated to be 17.6%. Given a follow-up period of 15 years, tumor risk in the normal population would be 2.6%, making it roughly 7 times higher for the patient collective. Figure 4 shows that risk is greatest for solid tumors. By contrast, the risk of contracting leukemia is 3.6%, or relatively slight, and after 9 years of follow-up, no new cases of leukemia developed. Compared to the group that received radiotherapy alone, leukemia risk was significantly higher for those groups that had received radiotherapy plus chemotherapy or only chemotherapy. It should also be noted that leukemias were found only in those patients who had received MOPP.

Blayney et al. reported on the chronology of leukemia risk in 1987. Their study group examined 192 patients who had been therapied for Hodgkin's disease and who had been followed up for more than 15 years. The bone marrow examination conducted on 63 of these patients showed that 11 years after primary treatment, no cases of leukemia could be detected. In addition, the incidence of solid tumors and malignant lymphomas followed roughly the same chronology, whether patients had received radiotherapy only or had had combination treatment.

Table 3. Development of secondary tumors depending on the type of treatment administered for Hodgkin's disease; from Tucker et al. [1988]

Type of second cancer and treatment	Observed cases	Observed/ expected (95% CI)*	% Actuarial risk (± SE at 15 years)
Leukemia			
Radiotherapy	2	11 (1.2–38.4)	0.6 (0.5)
Adjuvant chemotherapy	18	117 (69–185)	4.9 (1.2)
Salvage chemotherapy			
After radiotherapy	2	58 (6.5–210)	1.8 (1.3)
After radiotherapy and gold	3	253 (28–915)	12.3 (6.8)
Chemotherapy only	3	150 (26–380)	11.5 (6.6)
Lymphoma			
Radiotherapy	5	21 (6.7–48.6)	3.5 (1.8)
Adjuvant chemotherapy	4	22 (5.9–56.3)	0.9 (0.5)
Solid tumors			
Radiotherapy	16	2.8 (1.4–4.3)	7.0 (1.9)
Adjuvant chemotherapy	16	4.4 (2.8–6.7)	11.7 (3.8)
Salvage chemotherapy			
After radiotherapy	4	3.7 (1.0–9.7)	16.5 (10.4)
After radiotherapy and gold	5	22 (7.0–50.7)	35.7 (16.3)
Radiotherapy and gold	4	7.0 (1.9–18.3)	21.9 (10.5)
Chemotherapy only	1	1.1 (0.01–6.3)	5.5 (4.2)

* CI = Confidence interval.

Several study groups also consider breast carcinoma as a secondary tumor when it develops after irradiation to treat Hodgkin's malignoma in female patients. Tinger et al. [1997] recently analyzed 152 female patients who had been given upper-body irradiation at any time between 1966 and 1985. Ten of these patients developed breast cancer. However, the risk of breast carcinoma decreased with increasing age. It peaked when patients under 20 years of age were treated for Hodgkin's disease, and was nearly nonexistent when the patient was over 30 when treated [Hancock et al., 1993]. The average relative risk factor was 5.1 (ratio of cases observed vs. cases expected), given a median age of 25 years at the time of first treatment. Median age at detection of the secondary tumor was 40 years. A correlation was seen between tumor incidence and dose: in the Hancock analysis, risk was doubled with doses of > 40 Gy. Tinger et al. [1997] were not able to confirm these findings, although they did observe an increased incidence when the anterior and axillary doses were higher as part of upper-body irradiation. The analyses by Tinger et al. [1997] discovered a further sign of dose dependency, namely that 80% of the carcinomas detected were found in the up-

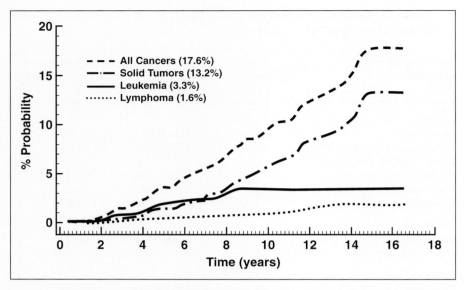

Fig. 4. Risk of developing a secondary tumor charted for 1,507 patients after therapy for Hodgkin's disease. From Tucker et al. [1988].

per outer quadrant, meaning at least on the perimeter, if not within, the area of upper-body irradiation.

To reduce tumor risk, the study groups cited above recommend protecting the gland body wherever possible with appropriate lead shields and other measures. During follow-up, mammography should be conducted every year for at least 10 years after radiotherapy for Hodgkin's disease, in order to detect and treat early any secondary tumor.

An additional late risk is the gastrointestinal tumor. Birdwell et al. [1997] monitored 2,441 patients who had received radiotherapy between 1961 and 1994 for Hodgkin's disease. Given a median follow-up period of 10.9 years, 25 cases of gastrointestinal tumors were detected. At the greatest risk were patients who had received combination therapy, meaning radiation and chemotherapy. Those patients who had had only radiotherapy or only chemotherapy had a slight risk, but not significantly increased. In all, the relative risk (ratio of cases observed vs. cases expected) was 2.5. As was the case for other types of tumors, the risk was higher for younger patients. Risk did not appear to lessen as follow-up time increased. Even after 20 years of follow-up, incidence was still raised. Two-thirds of the tumors detected were found within the previous irradiation fields. Most of these tumors were in the gastric, pancreatic or colorectal regions. There were also 2 cases of small-intestine tumor, which is otherwise extremely rare. In all, however, in terms of incidence, latency, dose and age dependency, the risk of developing gastrointestinal tumors after therapy for

Hodgkin's disease did not differ from that of other solid tumors. Here, too, lifelong follow-up is recommended in order to detect and treat any secondary tumors early on.

It can be concluded that the risk of secondary tumors recognized today primarily applies to patients who were treated in the 1970s, and often with very intensive regimens [Glanzmann, 1998]. But even for those groups, the survival advantages associated with the new therapy outweighed the original risk of contracting a secondary tumor. In the early 1980s, therapy regimens, particularly for early and middle stages, became less intensive, but without sacrificing tumor control. We may therefore expect to see fewer therapy-induced secondary tumors. Accordingly, the Stanford teams [Hancock and Hoppe, 1996] have already reported a tendency towards lower secondary tumor risk in the patients they treated in the 1980s.

Problems after Tumor Irradiation in Children

Hawkins [1990] published a large-scale analysis of the anamneses of 9,279 children who had been therapied for malignancy. The relative risk factor of developing a secondary tumor (ratio of cases observed vs. cases expected) was 4 for children who had received only surgical treatment. After irradiation, the factor rose to 6, and after combination therapy (radiotherapy and chemotherapy), it rose to 9. Thus, on the basis of this and earlier investigations, an increased risk for secondary malignancy after irradiation of pediatric tumors could not be excluded. This finding is also supported by earlier investigations of children with Ewing's sarcoma. Although these children survived after irradiation of their malignancy, it was reported that up to 35% of them developed secondary tumors 10 years later [Strong et al., 1979]. Risk thus appeared greater than for other tumors appearing in childhood and youth. It is therefore understandable that radiotherapy is no longer indicated as often for Ewing's sarcoma, and that more and more patients elect local surgery instead.

On the other hand, the most recent studies appear to indicate that the risk of secondary tumor is much lower than originally thought. The reason for this discrepancy is that most reports on secondary neoplasia have been based on analyses of children who were irradiated 20 or more years ago. Such studies show that after radiotherapy, children have a greater risk of developing secondary tumors, primarily leukemias, lymphomas and solid tumors. Children who were treated for Ewing's sarcoma, however, have an even greater secondary neoplasia risk. In the meantime, the new findings of a CESS study have been published [Dunst et al., 1998], and relativize the risk of secondary carcinoma. This study is based on the evaluation of 674 patients who were treated primarily for Ewing's sarcoma between 1981 and 1991. 162 of the children received only surgical therapy; 212 received precisely targeted radiotherapy, and 274 children were given radiotherapy and chemotherapy. For 26 children, advanced disease made it impossible to conduct therapy precisely as planned. During a mean follow-up of 5.1 years, only 8 secondary malignancies were detected. Five of these were acute myeloid leukemias which had developed after a latency period of 17–78 months. The remaining 3 were solid tumors: an osteosarcoma, a malignant fibrous histiocytoma, and a fibrosarcoma. These 3 tumors were detected after a latency period of 82–136 months. These sarcomas developed within, or in the immediate vicinity of, the previous radiation fields. Comparison with other types of tumors showed that here, too, the leukemias appeared earlier than the solid tumors. Compared with other childhood malignancies, however, children with Ewing's sarcoma must be assumed to have a greater risk of developing a sarcoma as the secondary tumor. The same holds true for children with retinoblastoma.

Thus, it can no longer be assumed that the risk of developing a secondary tumor is extreme. This is also confirmed by a recent American study [Kuttesch et al., 1996] evaluating 266 children with long survival times after therapy for Ewing's sarcoma. The study found 16 secondary tumors, of which 10 were sarcomas that were all found in children who had been irradiated. The correlating risk of radiation-induced sarcoma was stated as 3% after 10 years, and 6.5% after 20 years. Of special note in this study is dose dependency: 20 years after primary therapy, the nonirradiated children did not evince any sarcomas as secondary tumors, nor did the children who had received < 48 Gy. Sarcomas were most common in children who had received doses of > 60 Gy. In summary, even children with Ewing's sarcoma are considered to be at such low risk of developing a sarcoma as a secondary tumor that it has little effect on charting therapeutic strategy.

In conclusion, one must ask whether there really is a definite postradiotherapy tumor. Tucker et al. [1987] tackled this question by examining 9,170 patients who had been treated for a tumor in childhood. They found 64 bone sarcomas, of which 48 were classified as osteosarcomas. In a normal population, 0.4 bone sarcomas would have been expected. Thus, the relative risk of this group (ratio of cases observed vs. cases expected) is 133. The primary tumor also evinced peculiarities. For example, the relative risk for children with retinoblastomas was 999; for children with Ewing's sarcoma, 649; with rhabdomyosarcoma, 297; with Wilm's tumor, 127, and with Hodgkin's disease, 106. The *kind* of primary tumor involved therefore plays a key role in the incidence of bone sarcoma as a secondary tumor. Three percent of the sarcomas were within the previous irradiation fields, and the rest were in the immediate vicinity. This leads one to assume dosage dependency, and further analyses have shown that the incidence of bone tumors increases significantly with progressive doses > 10 Gy.

These facts apply only to pediatric tumors; adults have only a minimal risk of contracting a bone sarcoma as a secondary tumor. Thus, in 68,000 patients irradiated for cervical carcinoma, only 11 bone sarcomas were observed, so that the relative risk for this group was 1.9 [Boice et al., 1985].

According to today's statistics, therefore, radiotherapy can have a carcinogenic effect on children. This risk, however, is so slight that dispensing with radiotherapy cannot be justified if such irradiation can be curative. This also applies to patients who must be administered radiotherapy plus chemotherapy, even though combination therapy is known to increase the risk of a secondary tumor. Here, too, regular follow-up may enable detection and therapy of a secondary tumor at an early stage. Nevertheless, the risk of developing a secondary tumor is not expected to decrease markedly anytime soon. On the other hand, smaller and better-adapted planning volumes, better dosage distribution, and moderate cumulative doses, such as 45 Gy for children, may soon prove beneficial.

Problems after Breast Cancer Irradiation

In the past few years, radiotherapy has assumed an important role in the curative therapy of breast cancer. This applies primarily to radiotherapy after conservative breast surgery. Today's modern radiation techniques and the exclusive use of linear accelerators enable treatment without recognizable late sequelae. This raises the question, therefore, as to what extent a secondary carcinoma is of significance as a late development. Complicating the situation is that x-ray imaging diagnostic procedures are thought to be carcinogenic. It is estimated that in the United States, 788 mammary carcinomas are caused by diagnostic measures each year – albeit out of a total of 119,900 new cases registered annually [Evans et al., 1986]. Female patients who have been x-rayed more frequently for diagnosing tuberculosis also evince an increased breast cancer risk. The same holds true for female patients who were irradiated for mastitis, and for long-term survivors of the atomic bomb [Boice et al., 1992]. This would mean that nearly 1% of all mammary carcinomas may be the result of x-ray diagnostic measures. In light of these findings, the possible risk for the contralateral gland body and for leukemia are under consideration.

Complicating such analyses is that long-term female survivors of breast cancer have a significantly increased risk of developing contralateral breast cancer. Boice et al. [1992] therefore studied 41,109 cases of breast cancer from between 1935 and 1982. 1,927 of these female patients evinced tumors in the contralateral breast. All patients who had developed a secondary tumor within 5 years (995 patients) were excluded from the study. In the final analysis, only 449 cases that involved radiotherapy could be evaluated. Using thermoluminescence dosimeters, the average dose in the region of the contralateral gland body was determined to have averaged 2.5 Gy. In all, this evaluation showed a relative risk of 1.19 compared to the nonirradiated control group. However, the difference for patients who had been observed for more than 10 years was significant, at 1.33. These irradiated patients evinced a 22.7% frequency of contralateral carcinomas, compared to 18.2% for the nonirradiated female patients. Age also appeared to play a role. Patients < 45 years had a relative risk of 1.59. Overall, however, the risk of developing radiation-induced malignancy in the contralateral gland body is low, and should not be seen as a reason to exclude radiotherapy.

Findings were similar for female patients who evinced leukemia as a secondary malignancy. To see whether there was an association, Curtis et al. [1992] studied

82,700 female patients who had undergone treatment between 1973 and 1985 for breast cancer. A total of 80 patients with leukemia were found. These patients were divided into four groups. One group received neither radio- nor chemotherapy, and had a relative risk factor of 1.0. The group that had received irradiation only had a relative risk factor of 2.4. Those patients who had had chemotherapy with alkylating agents had a relative risk factor of 10, and the group with combined therapy had the highest risk factor, 17.4. This study also looked into dose dependency, and was able to calculate the mean exposure to radiation for the red bone marrow. Patients with a mean dose of 7 Gy had a relative risk factor of 2.4; those with doses > 9 Gy evinced a significantly higher relative risk factor of 11. Altogether, however, the risk of leukemia is so slight – even after combined therapy with cyclosphosphamide – that it need not affect the choice of therapy. As noted above, the patients involved had been treated between 1973 and 1985. Since then, techniques have been improved such that the tissues adjacent to the planning volume are exposed to less radiation. As a result, mean doses to the red bone marrow are lower. In addition, cyclophosphamide-free chemotherapeutic regimens are on the rise, so that future analyses will certainly show a lower risk of contracting leukemia.

In concluding, we want to discuss the very rare problem of ataxia telangiectasia. Carriers of the ataxia telangiectasia gene evince a significantly higher tendency towards malignant tumors. Here, the relative risk factor, compared to that of the normal population, is between 61 and 184 [Swift et al., 1991]. In heterozygous carriers, the relative risk factor is lower, being estimated at 2–6. It is assumed that in the United States about 1% of the white population are heterozygous gene carriers. It is therefore postulated that this group accounts for 9–18% of all mammary carcinomas in the United States. It is important for radiotherapists to know that carriers of the ataxia telangiectasia gene are extremely sensitive to radiation. They have a 4-fold higher risk of acute irradiation reactions, particularly of the skin and the mucosa of the small intestine. Just using ionizing rays for diagnostic measures makes their relative risk of developing breast cancer higher than that of the normal population. Ataxia telangiectasia syndrome should be suspected if a moist epitheliolytic skin reaction develops after just 1–2 weeks of radiotherapy. In this case, radiotherapy must be stopped immediately.

Problems after Pelvic-Tumor Irradiation

Twenty years ago, it was standard therapy to administer precisely targeted radiotherapy to patients with cervical carcinoma. As a result, there is no lack of statistical information today on the incidence of secondary tumors. Boice et al. [1988] evaluated data on what is probably the largest such collective – 150,000 – of female patients. They detected various secondary tumors that may have been associated with the original radiotherapy. However, it was unusual that despite the high doses of radiation administered, certain tumors did not appear with greater frequency, such as colon carcinomas, tumors of the small intestine, of the vulva, Hodgkin's disease, multiple myeloma and chronic lymphocytic leukemia. Most likely, the high doses administered rendered the cells unable to transform. Of special note were the breast carcinomas observed. The irradiated patients were found to have a dose of scatter radiation averaging 0.31 Gy, which ought to have led to an increased incidence of tumors. But since no increased risk was detected, we assume that pelvic irradiation rendered the ovaries nonfunctional and thus reduced the risk of carcinoma.

There was increased incidence, however, of bladder and kidney carcinomas. Also, the risk of developing gastric carcinoma was twice as high due to the dose of scatter radiation, which averaged 2 Gy. Chronologically, the risk of a secondary tumor peaked 20 years after radiotherapy. The risk of developing leukemia peaked 1–4 years after radiotherapy, as is usual. In all, however, only a few radiation-induced tumors could be found. Of all the secondary tumors that were seen in this study, only 5% fulfilled all of the criteria of a radiation-induced secondary tumor.

Now that prostate carcinoma can be treated better with radiotherapy, more attention is being paid to the possibility of secondary tumors developing in male patients. Accordingly, Movsas et al. [1998] conducted a large-scale analysis of 18,135 patients with prostate cancer. In all, 1,053 secondary carcinomas were detected. In the entire collective were 543 patients who had received radiotherapy only. In this group, 31 secondary carcinomas were observed. Closer analysis showed, however, that not all of the criteria for a radiation-induced secondary tumor had been met. For example, 30 carcinomas were found within 3 years after radiotherapy, and 26 outside of the previous irradiation fields. For these reasons, one cannot speak of an increased risk for developing a secondary tumor after radiotherapy for a prostate carcinoma.

Among younger patients, a common indication is irradiation of the lumbar lymph node groups after surgery for testicular tumor. Unfortunately, there are not enough statistics to unambiguously answer the question of radiation-induced secondary tumors. Complicating this situation is that about 5% of all patients who had testicular cancer risk developed a tumor in the contralateral testicle. Leeuwen et al. [1993] examined 1,909 patients, and found a 2.6-fold higher incidence of gastrointestinal tumors. Median latency till appearance of the secondary tumor was 12.5 years. Leukemia incidence was not found to be increased. The above-described risks of developing secondary malignancy are, however, much lower than the relapse rates after primary therapy, even if the relapse rate – over a 10-year period – is merely about 1%. This is why discussions about posttherapy secondary neoplasia should not lead the physician to dispense with a highly effective form of therapy – such as radiotherapy – in favor of a wait-and-see approach with its risk of later relapse, or in favor of an uncertain chemotherapy using carboplatin.

Summary

Secondary tumors can result as sequelae to radiotherapy. As a rule, they are found within the previous irradiation field or in its immediate vicinity. It is also possible, however, that scatter radiation causes tumors to develop outside of the previous irradiation field. By definition, a postradiotherapy secondary tumor is present only if it differs histologically from the primary tumor. Otherwise, it is a relapse. There are two basic kinds of secondary tumors: the leukemias and the solid tumors. They differ not only in their appearance, but also in their latency period. Leukemias usually appear 1–3 years after radiotherapy, with incidence decreasing thereafter. After 10 years, there is no longer a risk of developing leukemia. Solid tumors have a longer latency period, of at least 5 years, and this risk increases over time. Compared to that of the normal population, the relative risk for secondary tumors (ratio of tumors observed vs. tumors expected) is 3. Higher risks are found in some special types of pediatric tumors. In the future, the incidence of postradiotherapy secondary malignancies should lessen. This is because correlations between secondary malignancy and the size of the planning volumes, the dose administered and the extent of scatter radiation have now been ascertained. Modern irradiation techniques enable better delineation and limitation of the planning volumes and a reduction in scatter radiation. In any case, the therapeutic benefit of radiotherapy outweighs the possible later risk of developing secondary malignancy, so that an indication for radiotherapy should not be made to depend on such considerations. In conclusion, the following criteria ascertain the diagnosis of secondary malignancy: (1) the histology of the secondary tumor must differ from that of the primary tumor; (2) the secondary tumor is usually within the previous field of radiation, or in its immediate vicinity; (3) the latency period for the secondary tumor should be 1–3 years for leukemia, and for a solid tumor at least 5 years, and finally (4) there should be sufficiently large amounts of statistical data to support a possible association.

References

Bathia S, Ramsay NKC, Steinbuch M: Malignant neoplasms following bone marrow transplantation. Blood 1996;87:3633–3639.

Birdwell SH, Hancock SL, Varghese A, Cox RS, Hoppe RT: Gastrointestinal cancer after treatment of Hodgkin's disease. Int J Radiat Oncol Biol Phys 1997;37:67–73.

Blayney DW, Longo DL, Young RC, Greene MH, Hubbard SM, Postal MG, Duffey PL, De Vita VT Jr: Decreasing risk of leukaemia with prolonged follow-up after chemotherapy and radiotherapy for Hodgkin's disease. N Engl J Med 1987;316:710–714.

Boice JD Jr: Carcinogenesis: A synopsis of human experience with external exposure in medicine. Health Phys 1988;55:621–630.

Boice JD Jr, Day NE, Andersen A: Second cancers following radiation treatment for cervical cancer: An international collaboration among cancer registries. J Natl Cancer Inst 1985;74:955–975.

Boice JD Jr, Engholm G, Kleinerman RA: Radiation dose and second cancer risk in patients treated for cancer of the cervix. Radiat Res 1988;116:3–55.

Boice JD Jr, Harvey EB, Blettner M, Stovali M, Flannery J: Cancer in the contralateral breast after radiotherapy for breast cancer. N Engl J Med 1992;326:781–785.

Coleman C, Tucker MA: Secondary cancers; in De Vita VT Jr, Hellmann S, Rosenberg SH (eds): Cancer, Principles and Practice of Oncology, ed 3. Philadelphia, Lippincott, 1989.

Curtis RE, Boice JD, Stovali M, Bernstein L, Greenberg RS, Flannery JT, Schwartz AG, Weyer P, Moloney WC, Hoover RN: Risk of leukemia after chemotherapy and radiation treatment for breast cancer. N Engl J Med 1992;326:1745–1751.

Curtis RE, Rowlings PA, Deeg HJ, Shriner DA, Socie G, Travis LB, Horowitz MM, Witherspoon RP, Hoover RN, Sobocinski KA, Fraumeni JF Jr, Boice JD Jr: Solid cancers after bone marrow transplantation. N Engl J Med 1997;336:897–904.

Dunst J, Ahrens S, Paulussen M, Rübe C, Winkelmann W, Zoubeck A, Harms D, Jürgens H: Second malignancies after treatment for Ewing's sarcoma: A report from the CESS studies. Int J Radiat Oncol Biol Phys 1998;42:379–384.

Evans JS, Wennberg JE, McNeil BJ: The influence of diagnostic radiography on the incidence of breast cancer and leukaemia. N Engl J Med 1986;315:810–815.

Fajardo LF: Ionizing radiation and neoplasia; in Fenoglio-Preiser M, Weinstein A, Kaufmann B (eds): New Concepts in Neoplasia as Applied to Diagnostic Pathology. Baltimore, Williams & Wilkins, 1986.

Glanzmann C: Maligne Zweittumoren bei Patientinnen nach Therapie eines Morbus Hodgkin am Royal Marsden Hospital. Strahlenther Onkol 1998;174:224–225.

Hancock SL, Tucker MA, Hoppe RT: Breast cancer after treatment of Hodgkin's disease. J Natl Cancer Inst 1993;85:25–31.

Hancock SL, Hoppe RT: Long-term complications of treatment and causes of mortality after Hodgkin's disease. Semin Radiat Oncol 1996;6:225–242.

Hawkins MM: Second primary tumors following radiotherapy for childhood cancer. Int J Radiat Oncol Biol Phys 1990;19:1297–1301.

Jablon S: Epidemiologic perspectives in radiation carcinogenesis; in Boice JD Jr, Fraumeni JF Jr (eds): Radiation Carcinogenesis: Epidemiology and Biologic Significance. New York, Raven Press, 1984, vol. 26.

Kuttesch JF, Wexler LH, Marcus RB: Second malignancies after Ewing's sarcoma: Radiation dose-dependency of secondary sarcomas. J Clin Oncol 1996;14:2818–2825.

Leeuwen FE, Stiggelbout AM, van den Belt-Dusebout AW: Second cancer risk following testicular cancer: A follow-up study of 1,909 patients. J Clin Oncol 1993;11:415–424.

Levitt SH: Secondary malignancies after radiotherapy; in Dunst J, Sauer R (eds): Late Sequelae in Oncology. Springer, Berlin, 1995.

Movsas B, Hanlon AL, Pinover W, Hanks GE: Is there an increased risk of second primaries following prostate irradiation? Int J Radiat Oncol Biol Phys 1998;41:251–255.

Nyandoto P, Muhonen T, Joensuu H: Second cancer among long-term survivors from Hodgkin's disease. Int J Radiat Oncol Biol Phys 1998;42:373–378.

Preston DL, Kato H, Kopecky KJ: Studies of the mortality of A-bomb survivors. Radiat Res 1987;111:151–178.

Strong LC, Herson J, Osborne BM: Risk of radiation-related subsequent malignant tumors in survivors of Ewing's sarcoma. J Natl Cancer Inst 1979;62:1401–1406.

Swerdlow AJ, Barber JA, Horwich A: Second malignancy in patients with Hodgkin's disease treated at the Royal Marsden Hospital. Br J Cancer 1997;75:116–123.

Swift M, Morrell D, Massey RB, Chase CL: Incidence of cancer in 161 families affected by ataxia-telangiectasia. N Engl J Med 1991;325:1831–1836.

Tinger A, Wasserman TH, Klein EE, Miller EA, Roberts T, Piephoff JV, Kucik NA: The incidence of breast cancer following mantle field radiation therapy as a function of dose and technique. Int J Radiat Oncol Biol Phys 1997;37:865–870.

Tucker MA, Coleman CN, Cox RS,Varghese A, Rosenberg SA: Risk of second cancers after treatment for Hodgkin's disease. N Engl J Med 1988;318:76–81.

Tucker MA, D'Angio GJ, Boice JD Jr, Strong LC, Li FP, Stovali M, Stone BJ, Green DM, Lombardi F, Newton W, Hoover RN, Fraumeni JF: Bone sarcomas linked to radiotherapy and chemotherapy in children. N Engl J Med 1987;317:588–593.

Upton AC: Historical perspectives on radiation carcinogenesis; in Upton AC, Albert RE, Burns FJ, Shore RE (eds): Radiation Carcinogenesis. New York, Elsevier, 1986.

Witherspoon RP, Fisher LD, Schoch G: Secondary cancers after bone marrow transplantation for leukaemia or aplastic anemia. N Engl J Med 1989;321:784–789.

Prof. J. Ammon, Muffeter Weg 11, D–52072 Aachen (Germany)
Tel. +49 241 879 9406-0, Fax -2

Rüther U, Nunnensiek C, Schmoll H-J (eds): Secondary Neoplasias following Chemotherapy, Radiotherapy, and Immunosuppression. Contrib Oncol. Basel, Karger, 2000, vol 55, pp 165–202

Secondary Primary Cancers after Cancer and Immunosuppressive Chemotherapy and Radiotherapy

John Roelianto Soedirman

Afdeling Humane Toxicologie, Faculteit Farmacie, Universiteit Utrecht, Utrecht en Afdeling Urologie, Academisch Ziekenhuis Vrije Universiteit, Amsterdam, Nederland

Over the past several decades, advances in cancer treatment have substantially increased the survival of certain patients, especially those with testicular cancer, Hodgkin's disease, and some childhood cancers. At the same time, radiotherapy and chemotherapy are carcinogens and exposure to these therapies results in an increased risk of secondary primary malignancy. Well-known examples of such secondary primary malignancies are leukemias after the use of alkylating agents or podophyllotoxins, urinary bladder cancer after cyclophosphamide, and solid tumors including breast and thyroid cancer arising in radiation fields. Patients with immunodeficiency diseases and those receiving immunosuppressive therapies for organ transplants are prone to develop cancer.

Estimates are that secondary malignancies make up about 5–10% of all new cases of cancers. Two primary malignancies in the same individual may not only be due to therapies, but may – and far more frequently so – also be due to chance, to genetic susceptibility, to a clustering of different risk factors within the same individual, to lifestyle and/or environmental factors, or to some combination of these.

With the remarkable technical advancements in molecular biology, analytical chemistry and computer sciences, many of the interactions between genes, other intrinsic factors, and the environment can now be elucidated, so that future research promise lies in understanding the actual molecular and genetic bases of environmentally caused disorders. This is crucial, because secondary primary cancers are notoriously difficult to treat.

Risk Assessment

The definition of secondary cancers is two or more independent cancers in the same patient, which excludes a local recurrence of the original cancer or cancers that are metastases from the first. But certain metastases may be incorrectly classified as new primary tumors, and lung metastases may be especially difficult to classify as primary or metastatic.

Estimates are that secondary malignancies make up about 5–10% of all new cases of cancers. Cancer patients have a 31% excess risk of developing a second cancer compared to the average risk of a person developing a first cancer. The risk of secondary cancers increases over time. For the first 20 years, women have about twice the risk as men (41 vs. 18%). Thereafter, the rates increase for both, but the differences even out (51 vs. 45%). In children under 15 years, relative risks are 8.02, compared with 3.5 for ages 15–29; and 1.08 for above 30 [157].

Current Methods of Risk Assessment

Initial publications described the carcinogenic effects of radiation and chemotherapeutic agents by reporting on studies of laboratory animals and on single cases or small patient series. Today, larger population bases are the subject of studies, employing proper epidemiological and statistical techniques.

Determining the relative contribution of different causes of cancer in a population is difficult. Secondary malignancies may be due to factors other than the therapies used for cancer patients who, like the general population, are exposed to environmental and occupational carcinogens that can affect multiple sites. In addition, some single-gene disorders, chiefly autosomal dominant diseases, predispose to more than one form of cancer.

The combination of these factors varies so much worldwide that cancer risks derived from a single population may be of limited value when applied to an individual from a different setting. With the great variation in cancer incidence among various human populations, using animal data to calculate carcinogenic risk in humans leads to very uncertain results. According to Ames [8], carcinogens differ in their potency in rodents by a factor of more than a million-fold, and the levels of particular carcinogens to which humans are exposed can vary in carcinogenicity by more than a billion-fold.

The immune system is unquestionably important for one's susceptibility to cancer. This is relevant to the study of therapy-related malignancies, since the primary disease and its treatment can lead to permanent defects in the immune system. Genetically determined immunodeficiency states have been associated with secondary neoplasms [46]. More importantly, organ transplantation with iatrogenic immunodeficiency [4, 24, 46, 53, 176] and acquired immunodeficiency syndrome [69] is associated with increased risk of developing specific cancers. A common malignancy observed in these settings is intermediate or high-grade non-Hodgkin's lymphoma, almost universally of the B-cell type. These lymphomas are similar to those seen after treatment for Hodgkin's disease [46].

Traditional epidemiologic studies, designed to assess suspected carcinogens' impact on health, are often handicapped by our inability to determine individual exposure levels or to account for individual differences in uptake and distribution of toxicants, and by our inability to identify hazardous exposures before adverse health effects are evident clinically. In short, current risk assessment schemes relate risk to the general population, not to individuals or subpopulations.

Future Methods of Risk Assessment

Future research aims to determine the extent to which individuals vary in their intrinsic sensitivity to mutagenic carcinogens. It consequently also seeks to develop sensitive and practical diagnostic methods for identifying high-risk individuals or high-risk subpopulations [164]. With the new tools of molecular biology, efforts are under way to develop highly sensitive and specific techniques for detecting early damage associated with carcinogenesis. The identification of host intrinsic factors that modify individual susceptibility to genotoxic carcinogens, through the use of biomarkers, is one approach to improve cancer risk assessment. As information emerges on the specific features that lead to increased susceptibility, risk assessment can be calculated to protect the most vulnerable members of the population rather than the average individual.

Methods in Clinical Epidemiology

Formal epidemiology studies compare two or more groups of people. With a case-control design, the comparison is between people who have a disorder and those who do not. In such a study, cancer incidence or cancer deaths are retrospectively reviewed and compared with age- and sex-matched controls. Determining a risk factor by the case-control method is more difficult. Participants are selected based upon having a disease, and thus it is not possible to calculate the likelihood of development of that disease based upon the presence or absence of exposure. In general, what is obtained is an odds ratio (OR), which gives the odds of having an effect based on exposure, relative risk (RR), or excess relative risk (ERR). In some instances, the OR can be used as an approximation of RR.

A number of factors should be analyzed when RR estimates for cancer are considered. Firstly, an increased RR does not necessarily mean that a given exposure has had an effect. If the control group has a lower disease or mortality rate than is normally expected, the RR will be > 1.0, even though there is not an excess of disease or mortality in the exposed population [142].

Age at exposure is to be considered in general evaluation of epidemiologic studies. If one ignores the effect of age at exposure, the ERR of leukemia in atomic bomb survivors increases by 3.5% per year, but when correction is made for age at exposure, the excess RR actually decreases by 0.9% per year [142].

Another point to be considered in the assessment of RRs is that if the incidence of cancer in the reference population changes, as has occurred in the United Kingdom, where the incidence of basal cell carcinoma has risen by 240% in 14 years [119], then comparison should be made with calendar-specific incidence rates.

Cohort or follow-up designs compare people who were exposed to radio- and chemotherapy and those who were not exposed, and followed for the type of malignancy of interest. As with all designs, the fundamental principle is that the comparison groups are at equal risk of developing the outcome disorder irrespective of drug or radiation treatment exposure.

Because human exposure does not take place on a prospective experimental basis, each epidemiologic study will have its strengths and weaknesses. Even when these items are examined and a 'statistically significant' result is obtained, there should be a search for consistency with similar studies, dose-response relationships, and plausible underlying biologic mechanisms. Another problem that generally goes unrecognized is that of reporting bias. Often, an investigator will not report a study in which no link with drug or radiation treatment was found. This probably occurs even more often with editors of journals who wish to reserve their space for positive findings. Whether this is appropriate is not at issue, but the public is often left with a distorted view of scientific reality caused by selective reporting of statistical chance associations [142].

Chemotherapy Studies

Before the mid-1980s, most drug epidemiology studies used the case-control design because of its ease and low cost [105]. Cases were defined, identified, and validated by reviewing the original clinical record. Relevant information about the individuals and their exposure to drugs was generally obtained from interviews. People who did not have the disease in question were the controls, and the same information was obtained by the same procedures as for the cases.

Today, information about drug exposure and identification of cases and noncases is obtained in a different manner. Long-term follow-up studies are used as the source from which drug epidemiological research is initiated. Most of these studies have limited information about drug exposure – sometimes only that at the beginning of follow-up – since drug effects are not their primary objective. Such limited information about exposure may compromise the interpretation of the results since accurate and complete information on drug exposure is essential to drug epidemiological studies.

Another relatively new source of data for drug epidemiological studies is computer-based medical information. When these sources are used, it is essential that the information about drug exposure and illness be shown to be reasonably accurate and complete. Furthermore, case definition and clinical-record validation of potential cases is also essential. Information about potential confounders that are not recorded on the computer can often be obtained by questionnaires to patients' physicians or telephone interviews with patients.

Radiotherapy Studies

Most of the epidemiologic data on human radiation carcinogenesis concern doses in excess of 0.1 Gy (10 rad) and usually in excess of 1 Gy (100 rad). Although exposure levels > 1 Gy (100 rad) are relatively rare, there have been sufficient studies to indicate the general magnitude of radiation carcinogenesis associated with such exposures [142]. For radiation levels < 0.1 Gy (10 rad), there is no proven body of data that establishes an increase in human cancer [238]. With the limited amount of human epidemiologic data on low doses, various statistical procedures are employed to extract as much information from the data as possible. The statistical precision of a risk estimate depends upon the expected number of cases, the true number of excess cases, and the standard deviation. The application of valid statistical methods has been outlined and discussed by Land [124]. The sample size needed to find or project an increased health risk in a population depends on the size of the risk already present in the population. Thus, to find an excess of an effect that occurs rarely in a population, only a small number of cases may be needed. However, to find a small increased incidence of cancer (which occurs spontaneously in 30% of people), a large exposed population group is needed. The following example is from Land: Let us examine the risk of breast cancer from 10 mGy (1 rad) and assume the number of excess cases annually to be approximately 6 cases/1 million women exposed, after a latent period of 10 years. Then, if a study of the effect of performing a single high-dose mammographic examination (delivering 1 rad to both breasts) were undertaken, 50 million women would be required in the exposed group and 50 million in a control group. If, on the other hand, we wish to examine the radiation risk with respect to leukemia, a smaller sample is required because of the relative rarity of leukemia in the general population. In this case, if 0.01 Gy (1 rad) bone marrow dose were applied, with a follow-up of 15 years, the number of cases required would be 1/15 of that of the breast cancer example.

Strengths and Weaknesses of Clinical Epidemiology

Studies of radiotherapy of malignant diseases have the advantages of well-defined dose, known type of radiation, and a localized field. The disadvantages are the possibility of concurrent or other therapies that may confound analysis, selection bias due to the disease, the possibility of cell killing rather than cancer induction, and a shortened lifespan for follow-up due to the malignant disease [142].

Many groups have attempted to derive tables assigning the probability of carcinogenesis following a given radiation exposure [154]. Unfortunately, such tables cannot be individualized and may lead to serious errors in individual cases, particularly if individual age and smoking habits are not considered. Predicting the number of cases of cancer that may be produced in a given population by radiation exposure is entirely different from assuming that radiation caused a specific adverse effect such as cancer in a specific individual [104].

Many of the current controversies about epidemiological studies are based on information from long-term follow-up studies or on computer-based medical data.

There are complex analytical difficulties if a cohort analysis on long-term observational follow-up studies is attempted. This is because the drug exposure of interest is often highly variable over time due to changes to drug regimens – either in dose, duration or interval – and concomitant drug use. One example is a study where the contribution of cisplatin to the development of secondary cancers could not be determined although the cohort of 29,000 survivors of testicular cancer was large and the initial treatment modality was known (radiotherapy vs. chemotherapy or both), but not the subsequent treatment courses, the specific drugs or dose schedules [219].

In some cases, a particular drug is no longer en vogue, or the patient population substantially differs from that treated in earlier studies. Beginning in 1971, the National Surgical Adjuvant Breast and Bowel Project (NSABP) initiated a series of randomized, controlled adjuvant trials of melphalan (L-PAM) for 2 years in over 8,000 node-positive breast cancer patients. In 1985, a 10-year analysis of treatment-related leukemias was presented [73]. Despite the importance of this study, it is of little relevance to current treatment practices. Nowadays, adjuvant chemotherapy regimens no longer contain L-PAM, the typical duration is substantially shorter than 2 years, and node-negative patients are the group for whom treatment-related events are of most concern [199].

Reports from population-based registries have limitations that may incorrectly represent the risk of subsequent cancers. For example, the regular follow-up of patients with testicular cancer and an increased awareness of cancer in these patients may produce lead-time bias or the early diagnosis of potentially insignificant cancers (as may be produced by screening for prostate cancers using tests for prostate-specific antigen). It is more likely, however, that these registry studies underestimate the risk of secondary cancers. The incidence of secondary cancers may be falsely low because of miscoding of patients who experience a recurrence of their primary cancer. In addition, estimates may not be accurate in a young, mobile population that may move from the area encompassed by the registry. It is equally problematic to attempt to assign causality in patients who are not specifically followed as part of a clinical trial. Such patients have inadequate data regarding specific details of treatment (i.e., types of treatment, doses and duration of radiation therapy or chemotherapy). The study by Travis et al. [219] mentioned earlier exemplifies this difficulty by including patients from two registries without any information regarding treatment.

Also, none of the patients in the study had specific information concerning the type or duration of primary or secondary therapy [162].

Identical study results may be interpreted differently by different observers. The main issues which lead to disagreement often relate to the validity of the study design, and sometimes to the weight applied to the degree of unmeasured residual confounding – a factor that is present in all observational studies. Principles that apply to interpretation relate to the definition and measurement of drug exposure, the validity and relevance of the case definition, the strength of the association found, the confidence limits around the point estimate of the RR, and the presence or absence of dose and duration effects. In general, the stronger the association – i.e., the higher the RR estimate and the shorter the confidence intervals – the less probable that a finding can be completely annulled because of lack of adjustment for a confounding variable. The presence of dose, duration effects, or both, adds credibility to a causal hypothesis. Finally, several independent, properly designed studies with similar results are needed to confirm that a putative association is valid.

Methods in Molecular Epidemiology

One initial step in identifying a susceptible population is to identify whether there is heterogeneity within the population in the mutagenic burden incurred following cancer treatments. Two tests that have been applied to measuring somatic cell genetic damage following cancer therapy are the HPRT (hypoxanthine phosphoribosyl transferase) mutant frequency assay and the glycophorin A somatic mutation assay [2, 3, 22, 23, 79]. For both tests, increases in mutant frequency are observed in cancer patients following treatment with cytotoxic agents [9, 23, 80, 116, 150, 177, 212].

The HPRT mutation assay and molecular genetic analysis of mutant clones have demonstrated that spontaneously occurring mutations are most often point mutations [3], that ionizing radiation tends to cause large deletions [2, 148], and that mutations occurring in infants typically involve translocations at VDJ recombinase recognition sites [75].

Accepting that variations in mutagenic burden following treatment with cytotoxic agents are likely, it becomes important to identify pathogenetic mechanisms for the variation in mutagenic burden. One hypothesis is that higher levels of carcinogen activation (or lower levels of carcinogen detoxification) lead to higher levels of DNA adduct formation, higher levels of persistent mutations, and increased risk of cancer development following exposure to environmental carcinogens (or to increased risk of leukemia following exposure to cancer therapies). Increased frequencies of mutated lymphocytes have been observed up to 490 days after cessation of therapy in patients treated with various combinations of cytostatic agents [212]. Also, in testicular cancer patients who had been successfully treated with cisplatin-containing regimens, significantly increased levels of chromosomal damage could be demonstrated up to 9 years after cessation of chemotherapy [166].

Another method that may be useful in identifying cancer patients at risk for subsequently developing secondary acute myeloid leukemia (AML) – the most frequent malignant complication of cancer treatment – is identification and quantitation of known leukemogenic translocations in hematopoietic cells following chemotherapy. Here, polymerase chain reaction assays can detect translocations involving the MLL gene in peripheral blood or bone marrow cells (detection limit of approximately 1 abnormal cell among 100,000 normal cells). Evaluations of large numbers of patients treated with topo-II-active agents are still necessary to define a relationship between the level of MLL translocation events during and after chemotherapy and the subsequent risk of developing AML. If a relationship can be demonstrated, then detection of these molecular lesions could identify individuals at particular risk for leukemogenesis from topo-II-active agents, and alternative chemotherapy agents could be considered for these patients.

The use of mutagen hypersensitivity as a biomarker of genetic predisposition to carcinogenesis is yet another indication that environmental health science has advanced to the stage where knowledge of mechanisms can now be applied to predict or document injury. Clinical and epidemiologic studies can be designed to measure human impacts directly, circumventing the difficulties and uncertainties in risk assessment associated with interspecies extrapolation.

Strengths and Weaknesses of Molecular Epidemiology

Cytogenetic monitoring is a relatively inexpensive, sensitive, and rapid approach to evaluating individual carcinogen susceptibility. Lymphocytes with chromosome aberrations are relatively easy to observe and quantify. Tests have repeatedly shown that the assay results of bleomycin-induced chromosome breakage are highly reproducible, and methodologic confounders have been shown not to present a problem. Also, chromosome breakage at fragile or DNA replication sites is an early event in tumor progression and genomic instability associated with exposure to carcinogens. Thus, mutagen hypersensitivity should become a highly useful biomarker of risk to genotoxic carcinogens, as some individuals are more likely to be hypersensitive to chemical induction of chromosome aberrations. Small but important differences in sensitivity are likely to account for increased cancer risk in environmental and occupational exposures.

While useful, the mutagenicity assay monitors only one aspect of the carcinogenic event that occurs in vivo. Cancer is known to be a complex multimechanistic, multistage disease involving mutations, gene rearrangements, gene amplifications, and hypomethylation of DNA. These successive steps of tumor promotion and progression may be caused by agents other than those responsible for the initial genetic damage [164].

Secondary Primary Cancers after Cancer and Immunosuppressive Treatment

Secondary cancers occur more frequently after treatment of primary cancer with either radiotherapy, chemotherapy, or a combination than they would in a control group [58, 97]. In general, chemotherapy appears to be far more potent than radiotherapy in inducing some cancers, particularly leukemia [32, 196]. But while radiation tends to pose a smaller risk, it causes a wider range of neoplasms. Acute nonlymphocytic leukemia (ANLL) is the most common malignancy associated with chemotherapy. Bone marrow (leukemia other than chronic lymphocytic leukemia, CLL), breast (female), salivary glands, and thyroid (more common in females) have a high comparative susceptibility to radiation-induced cancer. Leukemia often appears to be disproportionately increased, because it is otherwise a relatively rare cause of death.

On the basis of epidemiologic literature and secondary tumor induction, the interaction between chemotherapeutic agents and radiation is difficult to determine because of the differences in time of administration with regard to radiation and because of uncertainty about the actual dose delivered to the cells or organ of interest [142]. In a large series of 82,700 patients treated for breast cancer, 90 secondary leukemia cases were reported. The risk was higher when patients were treated with radiotherapy and alkylating agents (RR 17.4) than with radiotherapy alone (RR 2.4) or with chemotherapy alone (RR 10.0) [51]. In some studies of Hodgkin's disease, there is no increase of chemotherapeutic leukemia risk due to subsequent radiation [111, 225], but at least one other study finds opposite results [233]. Breast cancer risk following radiotherapy for Hodgkin's disease may be increased by chemotherapy with alkylating agents. Studies of patients treated for ovarian cancer and Hodgkin's disease have reported that combined treatment with radiotherapy and chemotherapy is not associated with a greater risk of leukemia than is chemotherapy alone [81, 111, 112, 130, 179, 225].

Secondary Primary Cancers after Radiotherapy

After initial reports of excess leukemia in radiologists early in the last century [137, 198], epidemiologic studies of atomic bomb survivors and other groups have clearly shown a relationship between high-dose radiation exposure and the subsequent risk of many tumors, particularly leukemia, lung, breast, stomach, and thyroid.

The effects observed stem from doses > 0.1 Gy (10 rad). The exact form of the dose-response curve below this level remains uncertain, but a linear-quadratic dose-effect relationship appears reasonable [142]. This means that risk estimation at low doses based on a linear extrapolation is likely to be an overestimation. Epidemiologic studies performed to evaluate the possibility of radiation carcinogenesis at doses of < 0.1 Gy (10 rad) require a sample size of at least 100,000 persons exposed to 0.1 Gy (10 rad) and a similar group of sex-matched controls to detect radiogenic cancers at these dose levels [125]. At doses > 4 Gy (400 rad), an analysis of radiation-induced leukemia in patients with cervical cancer showed decreasing risk [28]. Land [124] indicates that depending on the mathematical model used to extrapolate lower doses, the risk estimates for leukemia may vary substantially.

The mean latent period for induction of leukemia by radiation is shorter than for solid tumors, with mean latency to diagnosis generally averaging about 10 years, although the minimal latent period may be as short as 2–3 years.

Secondary Primary Cancers after Chemotherapy

The most important secondary cancer after chemotherapy is ANLL. Epidemiologic studies demonstrated excess leukemia risks after treatment with busulfan, chlorambucil, methyl-CCNU, cyclophosphamide, melphalan, epipodophyllotoxins (etoposide and teniposide), and the combination of mechlorethamine, vincristine, procarbazine, and prednisone (MOPP) [32, 101, 111, 171, 174, 181, 192, 209]. Secondary AML accounts for 10–20% of all cases of AML [78, 145]. A close association between previous treatment with alkylating agents and/or radiotherapy and the development of AML with loss of chromosomes 5 or 7 was first demonstrated by Rowley et al. [192]. This was subsequently confirmed in many studies which also showed that (a) the disease often presented in a stage of myelodysplasia before development of overt AML, (b) deletions of various parts of the long arms of chromosomes 5 or 7 were frequent abnormalities [106, 133], and (c) these patients responded poorly to intensive antileukemic chemotherapy.

Secondary AML is of growing concern because of (a) the increasing arsenal of genotoxic drugs that damage DNA in a variety of ways, (b) the use of these genotoxic agents in combination and at higher dose intensities, and (c) because many patients are surviving longer [203].

Concerns about secondary AML were heightened in 1995 with the detection of 6 cases of AML arising in the NSABP B-25 trial among approximately 2,550 women treated for stage II breast cancer with one of three dose schedules of adjuvant therapy combining cyclophosphamide, doxorubicin, granulocyte colony-stimulating factor, and tamoxifen (for postmenopausal women) [55]. The leukemias occurred in women aged 50–69 years at 10–18 months after they began adjuvant therapy. All of the case subjects with AML had either FAB M4 or FAB M5 morphology, and 2 of the case subjects on whom cytogenetic analysis was performed had 11q23 abnormalities. It is unusual for secondary AML to occur so quickly after the initiation of adjuvant therapy using doxorubicin and cyclophosphamide at standard doses. Thus, concerns were raised that the dose-intensive use of cyclophosphamide in combination with doxorubicin may increase the risk of secondary AML.

In addition to leukemia, chemotherapy may be responsible for a broad spectrum of secondary solid tumors. Except for urinary bladder cancer after cyclophosphamide, the exact extent of its involvement is not clear; partly because chemotherapy is often combined with radiotherapy.

Alkylating Agent-Associated Leukemias

Secondary AML that follows treatment with alkylating agents has a characteristic morphologic and clinical phenotype [133, 174]. Typically, these cases present with a myelodysplastic syndrome that culminates in acute leukemia with a less common phenotype (M6 or M7 with concomitant myelofibrosis). Their peak incidence is 4–6 years following the initiation of cytotoxic therapy for the first malignancy, although they can occur as soon as 12 months or as long as 15–20 years later. Chromosomes 5 and/or 7 are preferentially involved in cases with secondary AML following therapy with alkylating agents.

Topoisomerase-Associated Leukemias

Epipodophyllotoxins and anthracyclines (in addition to their other biochemical activities) cause DNA damage via intranuclear enzyme topoisomerase II and stabilize DNA topoisomerase II covalent linkage. In the late 1980s, a new form of therapy-related AML (t-AML) associated with prior epipodophyllotoxin therapy was recognized [59, 169, 180, 185] and subsequently for anthracyclines [175, 228] as well.

In contrast to alkylating agent-associated secondary AML, epipodophyllotoxin-associated secondary AML exhibits a shorter latent period (median of 2–2.5 years), monocytic phenotypes (FAB M4 or M5 classification), and an acute presentation with substantial blast counts (rather than gradual pancytopenia and fibrosis).

Initially, various abnormalities of the long arm of chromosome 11 – rather than abnormalities of chromosomes 5 or 7 – were reported as characteristic of epipodophyllotoxin-related leukemias [175, 180, 185, 240]. However, there were also instances of abnormality of the long arm of chromosome 21 [169, 180]. Subsequently, it was demonstrated in two larger series of patients with t-AML that there was a highly significant relationship between various balanced translocations to chromosome bands 11q23 and 21q22 and previous therapy with a number of drugs all targeting DNA topoisomerase II, whereas unbalanced aberrations to the same two chromosome bands did not show this association [128, 173].

Based on a 1991 review of the literature [172], it was suggested by Pedersen-Bjergaard and Philip [173] that not only the development of t-AML with balanced translocations to chromosome bands 11q23 and 21q22, but also t-AML with other balanced aberrations such as t(15;17) characteristic of acute promyelocytic leukemia and inv(16) characteristic of AML FAB-subtype M4 with eosinophilia, could be related to a poisoning of DNA topoisomerase II by cytostatic agents. Later reviews and reports [43, 57, 60, 77, 96, 101, 122, 153, 182, 214, 245] support this hypothesis. Cases of t(8;16) [182] and t(6;9) [246] related to therapy with anthracyclines or epipodophyllotoxins have also been observed.

Chemotherapy-Associated Bladder Cancer

Although the first case report linking cyclophosphamide with the development of bladder cancer appeared more than 25 years ago [244], the precise level of risk from this exposure is not known. There are many observations on the occurrence of bladder cancer in patients who received treatment with cyclophosphamide [26, 40, 68, 168, 195, 201, 202], but there are only a few cohort and case-control studies that have investigated this relationship [113, 118, 170, 184]. In a case-control study of 63 cases of bladder tumors and 188 controls among women who received cyclophosphamide therapy for ovarian cancer, there was an approximately fourfold increase in risk for bladder cancer [113]. When 119 patients (76 women and 43 men) with refractory rheumatoid arthritis who were treated with oral cyclophosphamide were compared in a longitudinal cohort study with 119 control patients with rheumatoid arthritis, investigators found 9 bladder tumors in the cyclophosphamide group, compared with no bladder cancers in the control group [184].

The largest cohort study to evaluate the dose-response relationship between cyclophosphamide and bladder cancer included a cohort of over 6,000 2-year survivors of non-Hodgkin's lymphoma. Travis et al. [217] identified 48 patients with secondary cancer of the urinary tract (31 with bladder cancer and 17 with renal cell carcinoma – no transitional cell carcinomas of the renal pelvis or ureter were identified) and 136 matched control subjects. This relatively small number of cancers restricts the inferences that can be drawn from subgroup analyses. Nevertheless, the study clearly indicates that the risk of bladder cancer is closely related to cumulative amount of cyclophosphamide and is likely heightened by radiotherapy that involves a significant dose to the bladder. Based on data from the underlying population with non-Hodgkin's lymphoma, together with the results of this study, an excess of 3 bladder cancers might be expected among 100 patients with non-Hodgkin's lymphoma treated with cumulative doses of cyclophosphamide of between 20 and 50 g and followed for 15 years. At total amounts of 50 g or more, an excess of 7 bladder cancers per 100 patients might result.

Some concerns have been expressed about a possible increase in the risk of new primary malignancy in patients treated with intravesical therapy for superficial bladder cancer. Allen et al. [5] reported a 24% incidence of new malignancies in their series of mitomycin C-treated patients. No further related evidence is reported in literature about intravesical chemotherapy, though similar concerns about BCG-treated patients were reported by Khanna et al. [117]. However, Guinan et al. [84] proved that the incidence of new malignancies in BCG-treated patient sis similar to that observed in the general population.

Secondary Primary Cancers after Treatment for Hodgkin's Disease

Today, at the time of diagnosis approximately 75% of Hodgkin's disease patients have a chance for long-term disease-free survival [12]. This is partly because there is much information on the subject; secondary cancers after Hodgkin's disease have been intensively studied for more than 20 years [13, 27, 31, 92–94, 109, 138, 230].

Boivin et al. [33] studied chemotherapy, radiotherapy and splenectomy in 10,472 patients with Hodgkin's disease, among whom 122 leukemias and 438 solid tumors were observed. Patients treated with chemotherapy, compared with those who did not receive chemotherapy, had statistically significant RRs of 14 for leukemia and 1.4 for solid tumors. Statistically significant increased risk of leukemia was associated with treatment with agents such as chlorambucil, procarbazine and vinblastine, and with the MOPP combination (mechlorethamine, vincristine, procarbazine and prednisone). These findings are remarkable, since vinblastine has not previously been shown to cause cancer, and mechlorethamine and cyclophosphamide, known leukemia-inducing agents, showed no elevated risks in the current study [31]. Neither radiotherapy nor splenectomy was associated with a statistically significant increase in leukemia or solid tumors overall.

According to Mauch et al. [139], leukemia risk is especially increased within the first 10 years after treatment. In their opinion, this is related to the use of chlormethine, vincristine, procarbazine and prednisone (MOPP). Their study involved 794 patients with Hodgkin's disease, stage IA–IIIB. All had undergone staging laparotomy and had been treated with radiotherapy, and with chemotherapy if indicated. Seventy-two patients out of 794 developed a secondary malignancy. RRs were high for leukemia (66.2), non-Hodgkin's lymphoma (18.4) and sarcoma (44.5). Absolute risks (= number of malignancies observed minus number of expected malignancies, divided by person-years' exposition, multiplied by 10,000) were 9.3, 11.1 and 6.9, respectively. RR for leukemia after combined radiotherapy and chemotherapy was 178.5, but after radiotherapy only 25.5. RR for solid tumors was also increased, but to a lesser degree (7.8 and 3.5, respectively). Younger age was also a risk factor. Risk for breast cancer was highly increased in women under 24 years with Hodgkin's disease. RR for solid tumors did not decrease after 15 years of follow-up. However, treatments were so different and numbers so small, that caution is warranted. For more definitive risk estimates, longer follow-up is necessary.

Patients with Hodgkin's disease develop lung cancer at a rate 2–8 times that of the general population [1, 109, 132, 210, 225]. A portion of this increase might be related to thoracic radiotherapy [110, 132] and, possibly, to chemotherapy [110]. Additional quantitative data were provided by Travis et al. [215], who evaluated 13,886 patients with Hodgkin's disease, including more than 3,000 10-year survivors. Secondary lung malignancies developed in 121 patients (119 histologically confirmed), representing a significant excess (observed-to-expected ratio 2.69; 95% CI 2.23–3.21). Risk was elevated at the intervals of 1–4, 5–9 years and ≥ 10 years after Hodgkin's disease (p for trend = 0.014). Significant excesses of lung cancer were evident among patients whose primary therapy included radiation only, chemotherapy only, or both. Long-term survivors treated initially with radiotherapy alone had a fivefold risk of secondary lung cancer (p for trend = 0.0004).

Large significant risks of small-cell lung carcinoma (observed-to-expected ratio 7.12; 95% CI 4.29–11.12) occurred after radiotherapy alone, but not after other types of treatment. In contrast, notable excesses of squamous cell carcinoma and adenocarcinoma occurred within most therapy groups. List et al. [134] previously observed that more than 50% of lung cancers after Hodgkin's disease may be of the small-cell type, although risk could not be quantified. Small-cell lung cancer accounted for approximately 20% of the cases in the series of Travis et al. [215], similar to its representation (16.8%) among primary lung cancers within the SEER database. SEER is a set of geographically defined, population-based central tumor registries in the United States, operated by local nonprofit organizations under contract to the National Cancer Institute (NCI). Each registry annually submits its cases to the NCI on a computer tape. These computer tapes are then edited by the NCI and made available for analysis [221].

Patients who develop lung cancer after Hodgkin's disease typically smoke [1, 132, 134, 225]. Although this lymphoma is generally not considered tobacco-related [17, 61, 103], a later analysis [141] of mortality data among cigarette smokers suggested an excess risk of Hodgkin's disease. Tobacco and radiation may interact in the development of secondary pulmonary neoplasia [102, 132, 158], but the pathogenic mechanisms are not clear. In one small investigation [54], the spectrum of p53 mutations in lung cancers after radiotherapy for Hodgkin's disease did not resemble smoking-related patterns, although all patients had a history of heavy tobacco use.

Because of the lack of detailed information on initial and subsequent therapy, and the absence of data on lung radiation doses and on tobacco use, a causal link between treatment for Hodgkin's disease and lung cancer cannot be conclusively made on the basis of the results of Travis et al. [215]. Furthermore, the significant excesses observed within 5 years after therapy are not consistent with current understanding of latency periods for radiation-induced lung cancer, and instead suggest the action of etiologic co-factors that remain to be identified. Significantly increased risks of lung cancer also appear within 5 years after treatment for non-Hodgkin's lymphoma [216], but not for breast cancer [218]. On the basis of these data, approximately 138 excess lung cancers may be expected to occur among 10,000 Hodgkin's disease patients followed for 15 years after therapy. Their results underscore the need for additional epidemiologic and molecular studies to clarify the relationship between smoking, radiation, chemotherapy, immunologic factors, and other influences in the occurrence of lung cancer among these patients.

Johnson [107] points out that the association between Hodgkin's disease and lung cancer may result from both conditions being caused by the same etiologic agent, citing studies of meat workers in whom excess mortality from both malignancies may have occurred [45, 83, 108]. When shared etiologic factors contribute to the development of multiple primary tumors [30], increased cancer risks are typically reciprocal, i.e., they occur in both directions. Thus, Travis et al. [218] examined the risk of secondary primary Hodgkin's disease among 175,867 2-month survivors of lung cancer reported to the NCI's SEER Program (1973–1992). More than 15,000 patients survived 5 or more years after diagnosis of lung cancer. During 275,253 person-years of follow-up, 6 cases of Hodgkin's disease occurred, compared with 10.80 expected (observed-to-expected ratio 0.56; 95% CI 0.20–1.21). The lack of an elevated risk means that shared etiologic factors probably do not play a major role in the development of lung cancer after Hodgkin's disease in the general population. Moreover, having an uncommon occupation probably does not account for many of the lung cancers observed among men and women with this lymphoma.

Patients undergoing high-dose therapy and autotransplantation have the long-term risks associated with their initial therapy for Hodgkin's disease in addition to the high-dose therapy that preceded the transplant. In one large series, the actuarial risk of developing leukemia was approximately 10% of patients with Hodgkin's disease undergoing autotransplantation [236]. It is difficult to ascertain the contribution of the high-dose regimen to leukemia risk, since these patients had been exposed to MOPP-like regimens before coming to transplant.

Secondary Primary Cancers after Treatment for Hodgkin's Disease in Children

Bhatia et al. [19], representing the Late Effects Study Group, report that secondary cancers developed 18 times more often in patients who received treatment for Hodgkin's disease before the age of 16 than would be expected in the general population (as measured by the standardized incidence ratio or RR). Secondary cancers caused 37 of the 276 deaths in the cohort of 1,380 persons they analyzed. As has been observed in other studies of secondary cancer after Hodgkin's disease [16, 33, 93, 131, 211, 225], leukemia caused the most deaths, had a standardized incidence ratio of 78.8, and, along with secondary non-Hodgkin's lymphoma, was most strongly correlated with the extent of exposure to alkylating agents. Non-Hodgkin's lymphoma had a standardized incidence ratio of 20.9.

Radiation was implicated as the primary factor in the induction of solid tumors. As has been observed in many studies of radiation-induced tumors, the risk increased with prolonged follow-up, and breast and thyroid carcinomas or bone and soft-tissue sarcomas were common tumor types [16, 28, 33, 86, 131, 211, 225, 227, 237]. Although the periods during which patients were at risk were not specified by Bhatia et al. [19] and probably varied according to treatment group, the risks at 15 years were similar after radiation therapy alone (standardized incidence ratio 11, actuarial risk 3.3%) or combined chemotherapy and radiation (standardized incidence ratio 13, actuarial risk 4.6%) and were not increased significantly after chemotherapy alone (standardized incidence ratio 5, actuarial risk 2.9%). The authors report a significantly increased risk of solid tumors within 5 years of therapy, which is not typical of radiation-associated tumors identified in other settings [86, 225, 227]. Whether these early events in children derive from higher radiation doses, concomitant chemotherapy, young age, genetic factors, or the impairment of immune functions by Hodgkin's disease and its therapy, needs clarification [62].

Of special concern is the high risk of secondary breast cancer that Bhatia et al. [19] report among the 483 women treated for Hodgkin's disease during childhood, with a standardized incidence ratio of 75.3 (17 observed cases vs. 0.2 expected) and an actuarial risk projected to reach 55% by the age of 45. High risks of secondary breast cancer were previously reported among 885 women treated for Hodgkin's disease at Stanford University, who had an RR of 4.1 [86]. In that population, the RR was 136 for those treated before the age of 15, decreased with increasing age at treatment, and was not elevated for those treated after the age of 30. However, the absolute risk or annual excess risk of breast cancer after exposure was relatively constant for all women irradiated before the age of 30 years: 30–40 excess cases per 10,000 person-years of observation. The cohort of the Late Effect Study Group appears to have an absolute risk of breast cancer of 10.7 excess cases per 10,000 person-years of observation, assuming a calculation of the standardized incidence ratio based on patients of both sexes [62]. In the Stanford study [86], the breast cancers that arose within 15 years of treatment were associated with the addition of chemotherapy to irradiation, and the absolute risk was markedly higher more than 15 years after therapy, exceeding 160 cases per 10,000 person-years of observation.

Secondary Primary Cancers after Treatment for Non-Hodgkin's Lymphoma

Significant excess of secondary ANLL was linked with prednimustine (RR 13.4; 95% CI 1.1–156) and regimens containing mechlorethamine and procarbazine (RR 12.6; 95% CI 2.0–79) among 11,386 2-year survivors of non-Hodgkin's lymphoma [220]. Cyclophosphamide regimens administered to patients with non-Hodgkin's lymphoma within the cohort were associated with a small, nonsignificant increased risk of secondary ANLL (RR 1.8; 95% CI 0.7–4.9), with most patients receiving relatively low cumulative doses (< 20,000 mg). Elevated risks of leukemia following chlorambucil appeared restricted to patients given cumulative doses of ≥ 1,300 mg (RR 6.5; 95% CI 1.6–26).

Despite the excesses of secondary ANLL associated with specific therapies, secondary leukemia remained a relatively rare event in this multicenter study of non-Hodgkin's lymphoma. Travis et al. [220] estimate that of 10,000 patients with non-Hodgkin's lymphoma treated for 6 months with selected regimens including low cumulative doses of cyclophosphamide and followed for 10 years, an excess of 4 leukemias might be expected.

Secondary Primary Cancers after Treatment for Testicular Cancer

Testicular cancer is now largely curable since the introduction of cisplatin in the early 1970s. The 5-year survival rate is more than 90%. But with life extension, an increased risk of several secondary cancers is being observed, and this elevated risk is maintained for more than two decades following the initial diagnosis [219]. Increases are seen for leukemias and lymphomas, for cancers of the pancreas, urinary bladder, thyroid and connective tissue. Particularly, the observed RRs of leukemia (5.2 for acute lymphoblastic leukemia, 3.07 for ANLL) and connective tissue tumors (3.16) were high. It is unfortunate that Travis et al. [219] provide an incomplete picture of the risk of secondary cancers in patients with testicular cancer. By confining the database to those who received radiation therapy or chemotherapy, the baseline incidence of nontesticular cancers in patients treated with surgery alone is unknown [162]. There are probably common etiologic factors, genetic risks, or prenatal exposures that may be causing a generally higher incidence of cancer in these patients. The recognition of an association between germ cell cancer and disease caused by HIV-1 (human immunodeficiency virus type 1) opens up the possibility of associations with non-Hodgkin's lymphoma, sarcoma, anal cancer and others [187]. An increased risk of melanoma has been reported in patients with testicular cancer [109]. Others have reported an association between acute megakaryocytic leukemia and primary mediastinal germ cell tumors, including the presence of isochromosome 12p in the leukemic cells of patients.

Earlier, Boshoff et al. [36] reported on the incidence of secondary cancer in 679 patients with advanced germ cell cancer treated with etoposide-containing protocols. This is the first report of secondary cancers associated with the POMB/ACE regimen, where a higher incidence might be expected due to the inclusion of an alkylating agent (cyclophosphamide) and another intercalating agent (actinomycin D). They found an RR of 150 of developing t-AML (CI 55–326): 6 of 679 patients developed AML. None of these patients had a primary mediastinal germ cell tumor and only 1 patient had received radiotherapy. The median interval between the onset of cytotoxic treatment and the development of leukemia was 27 months. The FAB M4 morphology was seen in 4 of 6 cases.

Of the 212 patients reported by Pedersen-Bjergaard et al. [169], 84 received > 2,000 mg/m^2 etoposide, and all five secondary hematologic malignancies occurred in this group. The Memorial Sloan-Kettering Cancer Center [14] and Indiana University [160] published the incidence of secondary leukemia in their patients treated with BEP. The incidence was lower here than had been reported by Pedersen-Bjergaard et al. [169]. However, Indiana University only included patients treated with a cumulative dose of < 2,000 mg/m^2 etoposide, while the Memorial Sloan-Kettering

Cancer Center only included patients who had achieved a durable complete remission. Hannover University [34] reported 1 case of acute lymphoblastic leukemia in 221 patients treated with $\leq 2,000$ mg/m^2 etoposide.

In their series of 679 patients with germ cell tumors, Boshoff et al. [36] confirmed the risk associated with etoposide-containing regimens. Although this risk in patients with germ cell cancer is dose-related, t-AML does occur at low cumulative doses of treatment (0.6% of patients treated with $< 2,000$ mg/m^2). Patients with germ cell cancer who receive $> 2,000$ mg/m^2 etoposide are at particular risk of developing t-AML.

Although there have been anecdotal case reports of t-AML following PVB, in large groups of patients treated with PVB no increase in risk was observed [34, 161]. Whether cisplatin, bleomycin or other drugs contribute to the increased incidence of t-AML in etoposide-containing regimens cannot be determined from the current data. However, it seems unlikely, given the incidence of t-AML with similar characteristics in children treated with etoposide regimens for acute lymphocytic leukemia and not exposed to cisplatin and bleomycin [241].

The specific use of radiotherapy and chemotherapy to treat germ cell tumors has evolved during the past few decades. In the 1960s, 1970s and 1980s, classic alkylators used in the treatment of these cancers, such as cyclophosphamide, were also commonly employed in germ cell tumor regimens. These alkylating agents are no longer common in the treatment of advanced germ cell tumors [37]. Furthermore, chemotherapy often ran up to 2 years (even in the adjuvant setting) in the early trials of therapy for testicular cancer, as compared with the 9–12 weeks of treatment now used [66, 67].

Radiation is a well-established and effective therapy for the treatment of early-stage seminoma. Indeed, before cisplatin-based combination chemotherapy, radiation therapy was the only treatment. As was the case for Hodgkin's disease, extended ports (using prophylactic mediastinal radiotherapy) became the standard of care for patients with stage IIB disease.

The issues of secondary leukemia are more complex and more worrisome. Unlike the case for secondary solid tumors, there is little chance for awareness, early diagnosis, or, for the most part, treatment. The contribution of etoposide to the safe and effective management of disseminated germ cell tumors is indisputable. Unfortunately, it is also indisputable that etoposide, in the combination of chemotherapy given for germ cell tumors, is solely responsible for the development of certain subsets of secondary leukemia [172, 185, 186]. Even so, etoposide will, rightfully, remain an essential component of germ cell tumor chemotherapy and will be associated with a very small incidence of secondary leukemias [160].

The realization that any treatment, even two cycles of chemotherapy or low-dose radiation therapy, is likely to be associated with a definable risk of secondary cancers, should cause careful consideration of the relative benefits of such therapy.

This consideration should call into question such practices as primary chemotherapy for stage I disease (50–70% of patients receive unnecessary chemotherapy), automatic administration of chemotherapy for pathologic stage II nonseminoma (50–70% of patients receive unnecessary chemotherapy), and adding radiation therapy to treat persistent masses in seminoma (0–5% benefit). Approaches that reduce the need for chemotherapy or radiation therapy should be considered, such as retroperitoneal lymphadenectomy in early-stage nonseminoma and surveillance in early-stage seminoma [162].

Secondary Primary Cancers after Treatment for Breast Cancer

Of interest are three follow-up studies of women treated for breast cancer that sought to determine the risk of leukemia [29, 50, 206]. Here, as elsewhere, the leukemogenic effects must be interpreted with respect to the volume of bone marrow irradiated and the total dose [49–51, 199], for these effects depend on the treatment techniques and the field arrangements, both of which have markedly changed during the past 40 years. Virtually all studies of ANLL after radiotherapy for breast cancer are of the postmastectomy chest wall and nodal irradiation. In most of these studies, no increase, or perhaps a slight increase in the RR of ANLL, is observed. The risk of ANLL may be overestimated in registry studies due to the unreported use of radiotherapy in the controls and the unreported use of chemotherapy in the patient cases [50]. Higher doses of radiation – in excess of 9 Gy – to the total active bone marrow were associated with statistically significant higher RRs of ANLL, independent of the effect of alkylating agents [51]. However, radiation doses of < 9 Gy to the total active bone marrow were not associated with statistically significant increases in the risk of ANLL.

Seemingly in contrast to these studies, two NSABP trials showed a tenfold increase in ANLL in 1,116 patients treated with radiation alone after surgery [73]. However, this higher RR was based on only 4 cases of ANLL compared with the expected incidence of 0.39 in an age-matched population. Given so few cases, the lower limit of the 95% CI pertaining to the tenfold increased RR reported in the NSABP trials overlaps with the two- to fourfold increase in the RRs of ANLL observed in other studies [50].

The NSABP trials give us the opportunity to contrast the effects of postmastectomy chest wall and nodal irradiation with breast radiotherapy after lumpectomy. All 4 cases of ANLL occurred in 646 patients treated with postmastectomy irradiation (trial B-04), whereas none was observed in the 470 patients treated with breast radiotherapy (trial B-06). This observation is consistent with a lower dose of radiation to a smaller volume of bone marrow after breast radiotherapy, as compared with postmastectomy chest wall and nodal irradiation [199].

The risk of ANLL after breast radiotherapy is likely to be nil or perhaps too small to detect, judging from the low risks of ANLL after postmastectomy irradiation. A more important question is whether the risk of ANLL is higher after combination therapy for adjuvant chemotherapy and radiotherapy. This question has not been covered in most breast cancer studies [199]. The risk of ANLL does not appear to be increased in ovarian cancer and Hodgkin's disease after both treatments, compared with that of chemotherapy alone [81, 130, 179, 225]. In contrast, the RR of ANLL was higher in breast cancer patients who received alkylating agents and postmastectomy irradiation (RR 17.4; 95% CI 6.4–47) than in patients who received alkylating agents alone (RR 10; 95% CI 3.9–25.2) or radiation alone (RR 2.4; 95% CI 1.0–5.8) [51]. However, the differential impact of L-PAM and cyclophosphamide on the risks of ANLL was not considered in this analysis [199].

Adjuvant regimens no longer contain L-PAM, the alkylating agent responsible for the vast majority of treatment-related ANLL in breast cancer patients. Moreover, L-PAM and cyclophosphamide differ in their leukemogenic potential [48, 51, 81, 85]. The RR of ANLL after L-PAM is between 24 and 44, but the risk after cyclophosphamide is only between 1.3 and 3. The latter thus corresponds to between 1 and 10 excess cases of ANLL per 10,000 women treated with cyclophosphamide. Higher cumulative drug doses, which until recently reflected longer treatment durations, also increase the RR of ANLL. In early adjuvant trials, treatment was often for 1 or 2 years. Shorter durations of adjuvant chemotherapy, on the order of 6 months, have been shown to be as therapeutically effective as longer durations [65]. At 10 years, the absolute risk of ANLL associated with a typical 6-month course of standard-dose adjuvant cyclophosphamide, methotrexate and fluorouracil (CMF) is about 5 excess cases per 10,000 treated women [51].

In the cohort of patients with breast cancer reported by Valagussa et al. [232], the 5-year risk of secondary malignancies following CMF ± doxorubicin adjuvant systemic therapy was only 1.7%, and increased to 4.2% only after the 10th year, reaching 6.5% at 15 years. The data reported by Rubagotti et al. [193] show a somewhat higher (4.2%) 5-year cumulative risk of secondary cancers documented after treatment with CMF-based adjuvant systemic therapy.

The risk of ANLL after standard-dose adjuvant cyclophosphamide or postmastectomy chest wall irradiation is exceedingly small and of little clinical relevance. Whether these modalities interact to increase the risk of ANLL is less certain but of potential importance, now that standard treatment practices include breast radiotherapy and adjuvant chemotherapy. It is likely, however, that the risks of ANLL after combined modality treatment will be very small. Concerns about secondary AML were heightened in 1995 when the NSABP B-25 trial detected 6 cases of AML among approximately 2,550 women treated for stage II breast cancer with one of three dose schedules of adjuvant therapy combining cyclophosphamide, doxorubicin, granulocyte colony-stimulating factor and tamoxifen (for postmenopausal women) [55]. The leukemias occurred in women aged 50–69 years at 10–18 months after they began adjuvant therapy. All of the case subjects with AML had either FAB

M4 or FAB M5 morphology, and 2 of the case subjects on whom cytogenetic analysis was performed had 11q23 abnormalities. It is unusual for secondary AML to occur so quickly after the initiation of adjuvant therapy using doxorubicin and cyclophosphamide at standard doses. Thus, concerns were raised that the dose-intensive use of cyclophosphamide in combination with doxorubicin may increase the risk of secondary AML.

Contralateral breast cancer is the most frequent secondary cancer in breast cancer patients. The annual risk of contralateral breast cancer is 0.3–1.0% per year and is constant for at least 15–20 years [95, 140].

Several observations support the biologic plausibility that radiation for breast cancer increases the risk of contralateral breast cancer [199]. Radiation exposes the contralateral breast to low-dose ionizing radiation, which is a breast cancer carcinogen. Postmastectomy irradiation and breast radiotherapy expose the contralateral breast to an average total dose of between 2 and 7 Gy [51, 74, 213]. Women exposed to low-dose radiation under such diverse circumstances as the Nagasaki and Hiroshima bombings, multiple fluoroscopic examinations, irradiation for postpartum mastitis, and mantle irradiation for Hodgkin's disease have elevated risks of subsequent breast cancer [86, 100, 125, 143]. The minimum latency period between radiation exposure and detectable increases in breast cancer risk is about 10 years. Radiation exposure in younger women, particularly those exposed in their teens and 20s, results in the highest risks of subsequent breast cancer. The risks then decrease with advancing age of exposure and are not detectable in women after age 40.

Treatment factors other than radiation may affect the rate of contralateral breast cancers. Adjuvant tamoxifen, and possibly chemotherapy, decrease the risk of contralateral breast cancer [71, 98, 155]. In subsequent studies, the impact of these treatments will need to be considered.

Secondary Primary Cancers after Treatment for Childhood Cancer

A number of studies have examined the risk of secondary tumors after treatment for childhood cancers [226, 228]. In these studies, there was a close correlation between leukemia risk and the dose of alkylating agents. The RR of leukemia reached 23 in the highest dose group. A lower risk was seen for doxorubicin, and radiation dose had no influence on leukemia risk. Another study by Rosenberg and Kaplan [191] examining leukemia risk after MOPP chemotherapy showed an enhanced leukemia risk, but this was largely independent of radiation dose. A report by Hawkins et al. [90], in which over 16,000 survivors of childhood cancer were studied, indicated that radiation, as well as specific chemotherapies involving alkylating agents or epipodophyllotoxins, can induce secondary leukemias.

Radiation doses of < 10 Gy appear to carry, at worst, only a slightly increased risk of subsequent bone cancer, according to a cohort study of 13,175 3-year survivors of childhood cancer diagnosed in Britain between 1940 and 1983 [91]. In contrast to radiotherapy given at doses of ≥ 10 Gy, regimens of chemotherapy to which the present cohort was exposed do not appear to be as important in the development of subsequent bone cancer. However, the numbers of patients exposed to anthracyclines, epipodophyllotoxins, and some other types of drugs were insufficient to satisfactorily assess any relations between cumulative exposure and the risk of subsequent bone cancer.

Secondary Primary Cancers after Transplantation and Immunosuppression

There is growing concern about new cancers as possible late sequelae of compromised immune function and of treatment, particularly total-body irradiation and high-dose chemotherapy used as conditioning regimens for transplantation. A few studies have reported an increased incidence of new cancers after bone marrow transplantation – mainly lymphomas and hematopoietic disorders – which occurred early in the follow-up period [18, 56, 121, 136, 204, 236, 242, 243]. Lymphoproliferative disorders are the most common cancer in the first year after allogeneic bone marrow transplantation; most are related to compromised immune function and Epstein-Barr virus infection [18, 242, 243]. Using a multi-institution database that includes almost 20,000 recipients of allogeneic transplants, including 3,200 who survived for 5 or more years, Curtis et al. [52] determined the risk of new solid cancers after bone marrow transplantation. The transplant recipients were at significantly higher risk of developing new solid cancers than was the general population (observed cases: 80; ratio of observed-to-expected cases 2.7; $p < 0.001$). The risk was 8.3 times higher than expected among those who survived 10 or more years after transplantation. The elevated risks for several solid cancers are consistent with a radiogenic effect, especially for cancers of the thyroid, salivary gland, bone, connective tissue and brain.

In univariate and multivariate analyses, the immunosuppressive drugs used to prevent or treat acute graft-versus-host disease had no apparent effect on the risk of a new solid cancer. The drugs used for pretransplantation conditioning, evaluated singly and in combination, were not significantly related to the risk of solid cancer.

Long-term administration of immunosuppressants is associated with an increased rate of malignant disorders; for example, the link between cancers and cyclosporine is thought to be dose-related. Dantal et al. [53] report the development of cancer in two groups of patients who had been randomly allocated, at 1 year after transplantation, to either a low- or a high-target therapeutic range for cyclosporine. The random allocation of patients to the different immunosuppressive regimens distinguishes this paper from large registry reports of cancers after renal transplantation. Dantal et al. [53] showed that the low-target-range group had fewer cancers, but more episodes of late acute rejection, after an average follow-up of 5.5 years. Two thirds of the cancers were skin cancers.

The pattern of tumors found in renal transplant populations varies geographically. In Japan, renal, thyroid, uterine cancers and lymphomas are the most common [99], whereas in Saudi Arabia, Kaposi's sarcoma predominates [7]. These variations are not explained by differences in immunosuppressive regimens, so they must reflect environmental triggers and genetic susceptibility.

Non-Hodgkin's lymphoma is most common in the first year after transplantation. Incidence then falls and remains reasonably constant thereafter at 0.06–0.08% per year [165]. This pattern suggests that the development of lymphoma after transplantation depends on factors present at the time of exposure to immunosuppressants. In the case of posttransplantation lymphoproliferative disorder, the factor is almost always Epstein-Barr virus infection. For other posttransplant cancers, there is increasing incidence with duration of follow-up. Queensland, Australia, shows a prevalence of skin cancer of 20% at 5 years after transplantation, of 45% at 10 years, and of 75% at 20 years [38]. In the Netherlands, the prevalence of skin cancer after renal transplantation is 10% at 10 years, increasing to 40% at 20 years [88], which is similar to that reported from the north of England [135]. The geographical difference in incidence is probably due to the influence of solar ultraviolet radiation on the pathogenesis of the disease. The increasing incidence with time emphasizes the importance of long follow-up before attribution of a difference in frequency to any particular therapeutic maneuver.

In the examination of the RRs of complications after renal transplantation, the reference population should be patients on dialysis. There is evidence from northern Italy that among patients maintained on dialysis, the incidence of cancer overall is not increased, and that squamous cell carcinoma is less common than among healthy controls [147].

Another point to be considered in the assessment of RRs is that if the incidence of cancer in the reference population changes, as occurred in the UK, where the incidence of basal cell carcinoma had risen by 240% in 14 years [119], then comparison should be made with calendar-specific incidence rates. Even with this kind of analysis, the RR of some cancers in a renal transplant population in Scandinavia was much higher than that of the general population [24]. It was 10–30 times above that expected for cancers of the lip, skin (nonmelanotic), kidney, endocrine glands, cervix and vulvovagina, and for non-Hodgkin's lymphoma. An incredibly high relative risk of 1,000 is seen for a few tumors, such as primary cerebral lymphoma and Kaposi's sarcoma, whereas the incidence of breast carcinoma in women is not increased [4]. Presumably, these variations occur because the immune response plays an important part in the pathogenesis of some tumors but not of others.

In the renal transplant population in Leeds, UK, half of the kidney recipients who received their grafts more than 20 years ago, and half of those now aged over 65 who underwent transplantation more than 10 years ago, have had at least one squamous cell carcinoma. As this population ages and remains on immunosuppressive therapy, the number of nonmelanotic skin cancers seen will inevitably rise. A major clinical problem is how to reduce the morbidity from this type of cancer. There is strong evidence that synthetic retinoids can prevent skin cancer in kidney recipients, albeit with side effects such as dry mouth and hair loss [39].

The preferential localization of skin cancer (and cutaneous warts) on sun-exposed skin strongly suggests that sunlight impacts the pathogenesis of both disorders. High-risk patients need to seek sun protection. Despite verbal advice and written information upon hospital discharge for all newly transplanted patients at St James's Hospital, Leeds, only half of them recall receiving advice, and compliance with sun protection measures is poor [159].

In Summary: Secondary cancers are an ironic and tragic consequence of progress in the treatment of malignancies, and are likely to increase as success with radiation and cytotoxic therapies for solid tumors and hematologic cancers grows. Serial monitoring of the earliest genetic changes of individuals at risk could lead to intervention before cumulative genetic damage and irreversible transformation ensue. Several studies have demonstrated the protective properties of various antioxidants against the mutagenic action of cytostatic drugs such as doxorubicin, cisplatin, mitomycin C, bleomycin and melphalan in vitro or in animals [6, 10, 11, 20, 41, 44, 47, 114, 115, 127, 129, 151,163, 178, 188, 194, 197, 222–224, 239]. But clinical data are lacking on the influence of antioxidants on the incidence of secondary cancer in patients who were treated with cytostatic drugs.

References

1   Abrahamsen JF, Andersen A, Hannisdal E, Nome O, Abrahamsen AF, Kvaloy S, Host H: Second malignancies after treatment of Hodgkin's disease: The influence of treatment, follow-up time, and age. J Clin Oncol 1993;11:255–261.

2   Albertini RJ, Nicklas JA, Fuscoe JC, Skopek TR, Branda RF, O'Neill JP: In vivo mutations in human blood cells: Biomarkers for molecular epidemiology. Environ Health Perspect 1993;99:135–141.

3   Albertini RJ, Nicklas JA, O'Neill JP, Robinson SH: In vivo somatic mutations in humans: Measurement and analysis. Annu Rev Genet 1990;24:305–326.

4   Allen RDM, Chapman JR: Long-term complications: Neoplasia; in Allen RDM, Chapman JR (eds): A Manual of Renal Transplantation. London, Arnold, 1994, pp 241–245.

5   Allen RJ, Johnson DE, Swanson DA: Mitomycin C for superficial bladder cancer: Fate of patients 10 years later. J Urol 1990;143:342A.

6   Al-Shabanah OA: Inhibition of Adriamycin-induced micronuclei by desferrioxamine in Swiss albino mice. Mutat Res 1993;301:107–111.

7   Al-Sulaiman MH, Al-Khader AA: Kaposi's sarcoma in renal transplant recipients. Transplant Sci 1994;4:46–60.

8   Ames BN: Dietary carcinogens and anticarcinogens. Science 1983;221:1256–1264.

9   Ammenheuser MM, Au WW, Whorton EB Jr, Belli JA, Ward JB Jr: Comparison of hprt vari-ant frequencies and chromosome aberration frequencies in lymphocytes from radiotherapy and chemotherapy patients: A prospective study. Environ Mol Mutagen 1991;18:126–135.

10 Anderson D, Basaran N, Blowers SD, Edwards AJ: The effect of antioxidants on bleomycin treatment in in vitro and in vivo genotoxicity assays. Mutat Res 1995;329:37–47.

11 Anderson D, Yu TW, Phillips BJ, Schmezer P: The effects of various antioxidants and other modifying agents on oxygen-radical-generated DNA damage in human lymphocytes in the COMET assay. Mutat Res 1994;307:261–271.

12 Armitage JO: Long-term toxicity of the treatment of Hodgkin's disease. Ann Oncol 1998;9 (suppl 5):133–136.

13 Arseneau JC, Sponzo RW, Levin DL, Schnipper LE, Bonner H, Young RC, Canellos GP, Johnson RE, DeVita VT: Nonlymphomatous malignant tumors complicating Hodgkin's di-sease. Possible association with intensive therapy. N Engl J Med 1972;287:1119–1122.

14 Bajorin DF, Motzer RJ, Rodriguez E, Murphy B, Bosl GJ: Acute nonlymphocytic leukaemia in germ cell tumour patients treated with etoposide containing chemotherapy. J Natl Cancer Inst 1993;85:60–62.

15 Basco VE, Coldman AJ, Elwood JM, Young ME: Radiation dose and second breast cancer. Br J Cancer 1985;52:319–325.

16 Beaty O III, Hudson MM, Greenwald C, Luo X, Fang L, Wilimas JA, Thompson EI, Kun LE, Pratt CB: Subsequent malignancies in children and adolescents after treatment for Hodgkin's disease. J Clin Oncol 1995;13:603–609.

17 Bernard SM, Cartwright RA, Darwin CM, Richards ID, Roberts B, O'Brien C, Bird CC: Hodg-kin's disease: Case control epidemiological study in Yorkshire. Br J Cancer 1987;55:85–90.

18 Bhatia S, Ramsay NKC, Steinbuch M, Dusenbery KE, Shapiro RS, Weisdorf DJ, Robison LL, Miller JS, Neglia JP: Malignant neoplasms following bone marrow transplantation. Blood 1996;87:3633–3639.

19 Bhatia S, Robison LL, Oberlin O, Greenberg M, Bunin G, Fossati-Bellani F, Meadows AT: Breast cancer and other second neoplasms after childhood Hodgkin's disease. N Engl J Med 1996;334:745–751.

20 Bianchi L, Tateo F, Pizzala R, Stivala RA, Grazia Verri M, Melli R, Santamaria L: Carote-noids reduce the chromosomal damage induced by bleomycin in human cultured lym-phocytes. Anticancer Res 1993;13:1007–1010.

21 Bierman PJ, Vose JM, Langnas AN, Rifkin RM, Hauke RJ, Smir BN, Greiner TC: Hodgkin's disease following solid organ transplantation. Ann Oncol 1996;7:265–270.

22 Bigbee WL, Langlois RG, Stanker LH, Vanderlaan M, Jensen RH: Flow cytometric analysis of erythrocyte populations in Tn syndrome blood using monoclonal antibodies to glycophorin A and the Tn antigen. Cytometry 1990;11:261–271.

23 Bigbee WL, Wyrobek AJ, Langlois RG, Jensen RH, Everson RB: The effect of chemotherapy on the in vivo frequency of glycophorin A 'null' variant erythrocytes. Mutat Res 1990;240: 165–170.

24 Birkeland SA, Storm HH, Lamm LU, Barlow L, Blohme I, Forsberg B, Eklund B, Fjeldborg O, Friedberg M, Frodin L, Glattre E, Halvorsen S, Holm NV, Jakobsen A, Jorgensen HE, La-defoged J, Lindholm T, Lundgren G, Pukkala E: Cancer risk after renal transplantation in the nordic countries, 1964-1986. Int J Cancer 1995;60:183–189.

25 Blichert-Toft N, Rose C, Andersen JA, Overgaard M, Axelsson CK, Andersen KW, Mourid-sen HT: Danish randomized trial comparing breast conservation therapy with mastectomy: 6 years of life-table analysis. Natl Cancer Inst Monogr 1992;11:19–25.

26   Boffetta P, Kaldor JM: Secondary malignancies following cancer chemotherapy. Acta Oncol 1994;33:591–598.

27   Boice JD Jr: Second cancer after Hodgkin's disease – The price of success? J Natl Cancer Inst 1993;85:4–5.

28   Boice JD Jr: Carcinogenesis – A synopsis of human experience with external exposure in medicine. Health Phys 1988;55:621–630.

29   Boice JD Jr, Harvey EB, Blettner M, Stovall M, Flannery JT: Cancer in the contralateral breast after radiotherapy for breast cancer. N Engl J Med 1992;326:781–785.

30   Boice JD Jr, Storm HH, Curtis RE, Jensen OM, Kleinerman RA, Jensen HS, Flannery JT, Fraumeni JF Jr: Introduction to the study of multiple primary cancers. Natl Cancer Inst Monogr 1985;68:3–9.

31   Boice JD Jr, Travis LB: Body wars: Effect of friendly fire (cancer therapy). J Natl Cancer Inst 1995;87:705–706.

32   Boivin JF: Second cancers and other late effects of cancer treatment: A review. Cancer 1990;65(suppl 3):770–775.

33   Boivin JF, Hutchison GB, Zauber AG, Bernstein L, Davis FG, Michel RP, Zanke B, Tan CT, Fuller LM, Mauch P: Incidence of second cancers in patients treated for Hodgkin's disease. J Natl Cancer Inst 1995;87:732–741.

34   Bokemeyer C, Schmoll HJ: Secondary neoplasms following treatment of malignant germ cell tumors. J Clin Oncol 1993;11:1703–1709.

35   Bokemeyer C, Schmoll HJ: Treatment of testicular cancer and the development of secondary malignancies. J Clin Oncol 1995;13:283–292.

36   Boshoff C, Begent RH, Oliver RT, Rustin GJ, Newlands ES, Andrews R, Skelton M, Holden L, Ong J: Secondary tumours following etoposide containing therapy for germ cell cancer. Ann Oncol 1995;6:35–40.

37   Bosl GJ, Geller NL, Bajorin D, Leitner SP, Yagoda A, Golbey RB, Scher H, Vogelzang NJ, Auman J, Carey R: A randomized trial of etoposide + cisplatin versus vinblastine + bleomycin + cisplatin + cyclophosphamide + dactinomycin in patients with poor prognosis germ cell tumors. J Clin Oncol 1988;8:1231–1238.

38   Bouwes Bavinck JN, Hardie DR, Green A, Cutmore S, MacNaught A, O'Sullivan B, Siskind V, Van der Woude FJ, Hardie IR: The risk of skin cancer in renal transplant recipients in Queensland, Australia. Transplantation 1996;61:715–721.

39   Bouwes Bavinck JN, Tieben LM, van der Woude FJ, Tegzess AM, Hermans J, ter Schegget J, Vermeer BJ: Prevention of skin cancer and reduction of keratotic skin lesions during acitretin therapy in renal transplant recipients: A double-blind, placebo-controlled study. J Clin Oncol 1995;13:1933–1938.

40   Cannon J, Linke CA, Cos LR: Cyclophosphamide-associated carcinoma of urothelium: Modalities for prevention. Urology 1991;38:413–416.

41   Cederberg H, Ramel C: Modifications of the effect of bleomycin in the somatic mutation and recombination test in *Drosophila melanogaster*. Mutat Res 1989;214:69–80.

42   Chao NJ, Nademanee AP, Long GD, Schmidt GM, Donlon TA, Parker P, Slovak ML, Nagasawa LS, Blume KG, Forman SJ: Importance of bone marrow cytogenetic evaluation before autologous bone marrow transplantation for Hodgkin's disease. J Clin Oncol 1991;9:1575–1579.

43   Cimino G, Moir DT, Canaani O, Williams K, Crist WM, Katzav S, Cannizzaro L, Lange B, Nowell PC, Croce CM: Cloning of ALL-1, the locus involved in leukemias with the t(4;11)(q21;q23), t(9;11)(p22;q23), and t(11;19)(q23;p13) chromosome translocations. Cancer Res 1991;51:6712–6714.

44   Cloos J, Gille JJ, Steen I, Lafleur MV, Retel J, Snow GB, Braakhuis BJ: Influence of the anti-oxidant N-acetyl-cysteine and its metabolites on damage induced by bleomycin in PM2 bacteriophage DNA. Carcinogenesis 1996;17:327–331.

45   Coggon D, Pannett B, Pippard EC, Winter PD: Lung cancer in the meat industry. Br J Ind Med 1989;46:188–191.

46   Coleman CN: Secondary malignancy after treatment of Hodgkin's disease: An evolving picture. J Clin Oncol 1986;6:821–824.

47   Cunningham ML, Ringrose PS, Lokesh BR: Inhibition of the genotoxicity of bleomycin by superoxide dismutase. Mutat Res 1984;135:199–202.

48   Curtis RE, Boice JD Jr, Moloney WC, Ries LG, Flannery JT: Leukemia following chemotherapy for breast cancer. Cancer Res 1990;50:2741–2746.

49   Curtis RE, Boice JD Jr, Shriner DA, Hankey BF, Fraumeni JF Jr: Second cancers after adjuvant tamoxifen therapy for breast cancer. J Natl Cancer Inst 1996;88:832–834.

50   Curtis RE, Boice JD Jr, Stovall M, Flannery JT, Moloney WC: Leukemia risk following radiotherapy for breast cancer. J Clin Oncol 1989;7:21–29.

51   Curtis RE, Boice JD Jr, Stovall M, Bernstein L, Greenberg RS, Flannery JT, Schwartz AG, Weyer P, Moloney WC, Hoover RN: Risk of leukemia after chemotherapy and radiation treatment for breast cancer. N Engl J Med 1992;326:1745–1751.

52   Curtis RE, Rowlings PA, Deeg HJ, Shriner DA, Socie G, Travis LB, Horowitz MM, Witherspoon RP, Hoover RN, Sobocinski KA, Fraumeni JF Jr, Boice JD Jr: Solid cancers after bone marrow transplantation. N Engl J Med 1997;336:897–904.

53   Dantal J, Hourmant M, Cantarovich D, Giral M, Blancho G, Dreno B, Soulillo JP: Effect of long-term immunosuppression in kidney-graft recipients on cancer incidence: Randomised comparison of two cyclosporin regimens. Lancet 1998;351:623–628.

54   De Benedetti VM, Travis LB, Welsh JA, van Leeuwen FE, Stovall M, Clarke EA, Boice JD Jr, Bennett WP: p53 mutations in lung cancers following radiation therapy for Hodgkin's disease. Cancer Epidemiol Biomarkers Prev 1996;2:93–98.

55   DeCillis A, Anderson S, Wickerham D, Brown A, Fisher B: Acute myeloid leukemia in NSABP B-25 (abstract). Proc Annu Meet Am Soc Clin Oncol 1995;14:92.

56   Deeg HJ, Socié G, Schoch G, Henry-Amar M, Witherspoon RP, Devergie A, Sullivan KM, Gluckman E, Storb R: Malignancies after marrow transplantation for aplastic anemia and Fanconi anemia: A joint Seattle and Paris analysis of results in 700 patients. Blood 1996;87: 386–392.

57   Detourmignies L, Castaigne S, Stoppa AM, Harrousseau JL, Sadoun A, Janvier M, Demory JL, Sanz M, Berger R, Bauters F: Therapy-related acute promyelocytic leukemia: A report on 16 cases. J Clin Oncol 1992;10:1430–1435.

58   de Vathaire F, Francois P, Hill C, Schweisguth O, Rodary C, Sarrazin D, Oberlin O, Beurtheret C, Dutreix A, Flamant R: Role of radiotherapy and chemotherapy in the risk of second malignant neoplasms after cancer in childhood. Br J Cancer 1989;59:792–796.

59   DeVore R, Whitlock J, Hainsworth JD, Johnson DH: Therapy-related acute nonlymphocytic leukemia with monocytic features and rearrangement of chromosome 11q. Ann Intern Med 1989;110:740–742.

60   Djabali M, Selleri L, Parry P, Bower M, Young B, Evans GA: A trithorax-like gene is interrupted by chromosome 11q23 translocations in acute leukaemias [published erratum appears in Nat Genet 1993;4:431]. Nat Genet 1992;2:113–118.

61   Doll R, Peto R, Wheatley K, Gray R, Sutherland I: Mortality in relation to smoking: 40 years' observations on male British doctors. Br Med J 1994;309:901–911.

62 Donaldson SS, Hancock SL: Second cancers after Hodgkin's disease in childhood (editorial). N Engl J Med 1996;334:792–794.

63 Donegan WL: Evaluation of a palpable breast mass. N Engl J Med 1992;327:937–942.

64 Doyle T, Venkatachalam K, Maeda K, Saeed SM, Tilchen EJ: Hodgkin's disease in renal transplant recipients. Cancer 1983;51:245–247.

65 Early Breast Cancer Trialists' Collaborative Group: Systemic treatment of early breast cancer by hormonal, cytotoxic, or immune therapy: 133 randomized trials involving 31,000 recurrences and 24,000 deaths among 75,000 women. Lancet 1992;339:1–15, 71–85.

66 Einhorn LH, Williams SD, Loehrer PJ, Birch R, Drasga R, Omura G, Greco FA: Evaluation of optimal duration of chemotherapy in favorable-prognosis disseminated germ cell tumors: A Southeastern Cancer Study Group protocol. J Clin Oncol 1989;7:387–391.

67 Einhorn LH, Williams SD, Troner M, Birch R, Greco FA: The role of maintenance therapy in disseminated testicular cancer. N Engl J Med 1981;305:727–731.

68 Ellis M, Lishner M: Second malignancies following treatment in non-Hodgkin's lymphoma. Leuk Lymphoma 1993;9:337–342.

69 Fauci AS, Macher AM, Longo DL, Lane HC, Rook AH, Masur H, Gelmann EP: Acquired immunodeficiency syndrome: Epidemiologic, clinical, immunologic, and therapeutic considerations. Ann Intern Med 1984;100:92–106.

70 Fisher B, Costantino J, Redmond C, Fisher E, Margolese R, Dimitrov N, Wolmark N, Wickerham DL, Deutsch M, Ore L: Lumpectomy compared with lumpectomy and radiation therapy for the treatment of intraductal breast cancer. N Engl J Med 1993;328:1581–1586.

71 Fisher B, Costantino JP, Wickerham DL, Redmond CK, Kavanah M, Cronin WM, Vogel V, Robidoux A, Dimitrov N, Atkins J, Daly M, Wieand S, Tan-Chiu E, Ford L, Wolmark N: Tamoxifen for prevention of breast cancer: Report of the National Surgical Adjuvant Breast and Bowel Project P-1 Study. J Natl Cancer Inst 1998;90:1371–1388.

72 Fisher B, Redmond C: Lumpectomy for breast cancer: An update of the NSABP experience. Monogr Natl Cancer Inst 1992;11:7–13.

73 Fisher B, Rockette H, Fisher ER, Wickerham DL, Redmond C, Brown A: Leukemia in breast cancer patients following adjuvant chemotherapy or postoperative radiation: The NSABP experience. J Clin Oncol 1985;3:1640–1658.

74 Fraass BA, Roberson PL, Lichter AS: Dose to the contralateral breast due to primary breast irradiation. Int J Radiat Oncol Biol Phys 1985;11:485–497.

75 Fuscoe JC, Zimmermann LJ, Lippert MJ, Nicklas JA, O'Neill JP, Albertini RJ: V(D)J recombinase-like activity mediates HPRT gene deletion in human fetal T-lymphocytes. Cancer Res 1991;51:6001–6005.

76 Garnier JL, Lebranchu Y, Lefrancois N, Martin X, Dubernard JM, Berger F, Touraine JL: Hodgkin's disease after renal transplantation. Transplant Proc 1995;7:1785.

77 Gillis S, Sofer O, Zelig O, Dann EJ, Lotan H, Ben Yehuda D, Isacson R, Rachmilewitz EA, Ben-Bassat I, Polliack A: Acute promyelocytic leukemia with t(15;17) following treatment of Hodgkin's disease – A report of 4 cases. Ann Oncol 1995;6:777–779.

78 Golomb HM, Alimena G, Rowley JD, Vardiman JW, Testa JR, Sovik C: Correlation of occupation and karyotype in adults with acute nonlymphocytic leukemia. Blood 1982;60:404–411.

79 Grant SG, Bigbee WL: In vivo somatic mutation and segregation at the human glycophorin A (GPA) locus: Phenotypic variation encompassing both gene-specific and chromosomal mechanisms. Mutat Res 1993;288:163–172.

80   Grant SG, Bigbee WL: Bone marrow somatic mutation after genotoxic cancer therapy (letter; comment) [published erratum appears in Lancet 1994;344:415]. Lancet 1994;343: 1507–1508.

81   Greene M, Harris E, Gershenson D, Malkasian GD Jr, Melton LJ 3rd, Dembo AJ, Bennett JM, Moloney WC, Boice JD Jr: Melphalan may be a more potent leukemogen than cyclophosphamide. Ann Intern Med 1986;105:360–367.

82   Greene MH, Young TI, Clark WH Jr: Malignant melanoma in renal transplant recipients. Lancet 1981;i:1196–1199.

83   Guberan E, Usel M, Raymond L, Fioretta G: Mortality and incidence of cancer among a cohort of self-employed butchers from Geneva and their wives. Br J Ind Med 1993;50: 1008–1016.

84   Guinan P, Brosman S, deKernion J, Lamm D, Williams R, Richardson C, Reitsma D, Hanna M: Intravesical bacillus Calmette-Guérin and second primary malignancies. Urology 1989; 33:380–381.

85   Haas JF, Kittelmann B, Mahnert WH: Risk of leukaemia in ovarian tumour and breast cancer patients following treatment by cyclophosphamide. Br J Cancer 1987;55:213–218.

86   Hancock SL, Tucker MA, Hoppe RT: Breast cancer after treatment of Hodgkin's disease. J Natl Cancer Inst 1993;85:25–31.

87   Hankey BF, Curtis RE, Naughton MD, Boice JD Jr, Flannery JT: A retrospective cohort analysis of second breast cancer risk for primary breast cancer patients with an assessment of the effect of radiation therapy. J Natl Cancer Inst 1983;70:797–804.

88   Hartevelt MM, Bouwes Bavinck JN, Kootte AM, Vermeer BJ, Vandenbroucke JP: Incidence of skin cancer after renal transplantation in the Netherlands. Transplantation 1990;49: 506–509.

89   Hawkins MM, Draper GJ, Kingston JE: Incidence of second primary tumours among childhood cancer survivors. Br J Cancer 1987;56:339–347.

90   Hawkins M, Wilson L, Stovall M, Marsden HB, Potok MH, Kingston JE, Chessells JM: Epipodophyllotoxins, alkylating agents and radiation and the risk of secondary leukaemia after childhood cancer. Br Med J 1992;304:951–958.

91   Hawkins MM, Wilson LM, Burton HS, Potok MH, Winter DL, Marsden HB, Stovall MA: Radiotherapy, alkylating agents, and risk of bone cancer after childhood cancer. J Natl Cancer Inst 1996;88:270–278.

92   Henry-Amar M: Second cancer after the treatment for Hodgkin's disease: A report from the International Database on Hodgkin's Disease. Ann Oncol 1992;3(suppl 4):117–128.

93   Henry-Amar M, Dietrich PY: Acute leukemia after the treatment of Hodgkin's disease. Hematol Oncol Clin North Am 1993;7:369–387.

94   Henry-Amar M, Hayat M, Meerwaldt JH, Burgers M, Carde P, Somers R, Noordijk EM, Monconduit M, Thomas J, Cosset JM: Causes of death after therapy for early stage Hodgkin's disease entered on EORTC protocols. Int J Radiat Oncol Biol Phys 1990;19:1155–1157.

95   Hislop TG, Elwood JM, Coldman AJ, Spinelli JJ, Worth AJ, Ellison LG: Second primary cancers of the breast: Incidence and risk factors. Br J Cancer 1984;49:79–85.

96   Hoffmann L, Möller P, Pedersen-Bjergaard J, Waage A, Pedersen M, Hirsch FR: Therapy-related acute promyelocytic leukemia with t(15;17)(q22;q12) following chemotherapy with drugs targeting DNA topoisomerase II. A report of two cases and a review of the literature. Ann Oncol 1995;6:781–788.

97   Holm LE: Cancer occurring after radiotherapy and chemotherapy. Int J Radiat Oncol Biol Phys 1990;19:1303–1308.

98 Horn PL, Thompson WD: Risk of contralateral breast cancer: Association with histologic, clinical, and therapeutic factors. Cancer 1988;62:412–424.

99 Hoshida Y, Tsukuma H, Yasunaga Y, Xu N, Fujita MQ, Satoh T, Ichikawa Y, Kurihara K, Imanishi M, Matsuno T, Aozasa K: Cancer risk after renal transplantation in Japan. Int J Cancer 1997;71:517–520.

100 Hrubec Z, Boice JD Jr, Monson RR, Rosenstein M: Breast cancer after multiple chest fluoroscopies: Second follow-up of Massachusetts women with tuberculosis. Cancer Res 1989;49:229–234.

101 Hunger SP, Tkachuk DC, Amylon MD, Link MP, Carroll AJ, Welborn JL, Willman CL, Cleary ML: HRX involvement in de novo and secondary leukemias with diverse chromosome 11q23 abnormalities. Blood 1993;81:3197–3202.

102 Inskip PD, Boice JD Jr: Radiotherapy-induced lung cancer among women who smoke (editorial) [published erratum appears in Cancer 1994;73:2456]. Cancer 1994;73:1541–1543.

103 International Agency for Research on Cancer (IARC): IARC Monographs on the Evaluation of the Carcinogenic Risk of Chemicals to Humans: Tobacco Smoking. Lyon, IARC, 1986, vol 38.

104 Jacobson H: Radioepidemiological table. Report of Council on Scientific Affairs, American Medical Association. JAMA 1987;257:806–809.

105 Jick H, García Rodríguez LA, Pérez-Gutthann S: Principles of epidemiological research on adverse and beneficial drug effects. Lancet 1998;352:1767–1770.

106 Johansson B, Mertens F, Heim S, Kristoffersson U, Mitelman F: Cytogenetics of secondary myelodysplasia (sMDS) and acute nonlymphocytic leukemia (sANLL). Eur J Haematol 1991;47:17–27.

107 Johnson ES: Re: Lung cancer after Hodgkin's disease (letter). J Natl Cancer Inst 1996;88:51–52.

108 Johnson ES, Dalmas D, Noss J, Matanoski GM: Cancer mortality among workers in abattoirs and meat-packing plants: An update. Am J Ind Med 1995;27:389–403.

109 Kaldor JM, Day NE, Band P, Choi NW, Clarke EA, Coleman MP, Hakama M, Koch M, Langmark F, Neal FE: Second malignancies following testicular cancer, ovarian cancer and Hodgkin's disease: An international collaborative study among cancer registries. Int J Cancer 1987;15:571–585.

110 Kaldor JM, Day NE, Bell J, Clarke EA, Langmark F, Karjalainen S, Band P, Pedersen D, Choi W, Blair V: Lung cancer following Hodgkin's disease: A case-control study. Int J Cancer 1992;52:677–681.

111 Kaldor JM, Day NE, Clarke EA, van Leeuwen FE, Henry-Amar M, Fiorentino MV, Bell J, Pedersen D, Band P, Assouline D: Leukemia following Hodgkin's disease. N Engl J Med 1990;322:7–13.

112 Kaldor JM, Day NE, Petterson F, Clarke EA, Pedersen D, Mehnert W, Bell J, Host H, Prior P, Karjalainen S: Leukemia following chemotherapy for ovarian cancer. N Engl J Med 1990;322:1–6.

113 Kaldor JM, Day NE, Kittelman B, Pettersson F, Langmark F, Pedersen D, Prior P, Neal F, Karjalainen S, Bell J: Bladder tumours following chemotherapy and radiotherapy for ovarian cancer: A case-control study. Int J Cancer 1995;63:1–6.

114 Kataoka Y, Perrin J, Hunter N, Milas L, Grdina DJ: Antimutagenic effects of amifostine: Clinical implications. Semin Oncol 1996;23:53–57.

115 Katz AJ: Sodium thiosulfate inhibits cisplatin-induced mutagenesis in somatic tissue of drosophila. Environ Mol Mutagen 1989;13:97–99.

116 Kelsey KT, Caggana M, Mauch PM, Coleman CN, Clark JR, Liber HL: Mutagenesis after cancer therapy. Environ Health Perspect 1993;101(suppl 3):177–184.

117 Khanna OP, Chou RH, Son DL, Mazer H, Read J, Nugent DM, Cottone R, Heeg M, Rezvan M, Viek N: Does bacillus Calmette-Guérin immunotherapy accelerate growth and cause metastatic spread of secondary primary malignancy? Urology 1988;31:459–468.

118 Kinlen LJ: Incidence of cancer in rheumatoid arthritis and other disorders after immunosuppressive treatment. Am J Med 1985;78:44–49.

119 Ko CB, Walton S, Keczkes K, Bury HP, Nicholson C: The emerging epidemic of skin cancer. Br J Dermatol 1994;130:269–272.

120 Kolb HJ, Bender-Götze C: Late complications after allogenic bone marrow transplantation for leukaemia. Bone Marrow Transplant 1990;6:61–72.

121 Kolb HJ, Guenther W, Duell T, Socie G, Schaeffer E, Holler E, Schumm M, Horowitz MM, Gale RP, Fliedner TM: Cancer after bone marrow transplantation. Bone Marrow Transplant 1992;10(suppl 1):135–138.

122 Kudo K, Yoshida H, Kiyoi H, Numata S, Horibe K, Naoe T: Etoposide-related acute promyelocytic leukemia. Leukemia 1998;12:1171–1175.

123 Kurtz JM, Miralbell R: Radiation therapy and breast conservation: Cosmetic results and complications. Semin Radiat Oncol 1992;2:125–131.

124 Land CE: Estimating cancer risks from low doses of ionizing radiation. Science 1980;209:1197–1203.

125 Land CE, Boice JD Jr, Shore RE, Norman JE, Tokunaga M: Breast cancer risk from low-dose exposures to ionizing radiation: Results of parallel analysis of three exposed populations of women. J Natl Cancer Inst 1980;65:353–376.

126 Land CE, Saku T, Hayashi Y, Takahara O, Matsuura H, Tokuoka S, Tokunaga M, Mabuchi K: Incidence of salivary gland tumors among atomic bomb survivors, 1950-1987: Evaluation of radiation-related risk. Radiat Res 1996;146:28–36.

127 Larramendy ML, Bianchi MS, Padron J: Correlation between the anti-oxidant enzyme activities of blood fractions and the yield of bleomycin-induced chromosome damage. Mutat Res 1989;214:129–136.

128 Larson RA, Le Beau MM, Ratain MJ, Rowley JD: Balanced translocations involving chromosome bands 11q23 and 21q22 in therapy-related leukemia. Blood 1992;79:1892–1893.

129 Laughton MJ, Halliwell B, Evans PJ, Hoult JR: Anti-oxidant and pro-oxidant actions of the plant phenolics quercetin, gossypol and myrecetin. Effects on lipid peroxidation, hydroxyl radical generation and bleomycin-dependent damage to DNA. Biochem Pharmacol 1989;38:2859–2865.

130 Lavey RS, Eby NL, Prosnitz LR: Impact on second malignancy risk of the combined use of radiation and chemotherapy for lymphomas. Cancer 1990;66:80–88.

131 van Leeuwen FE, Klokman WJ, Hagenbeek A, Noyon R, van den Belt-Dusebout AW, van Kerkhoff EH, van Heerde P, Somers R: Second cancer risk following Hodgkin's disease: A 20-year follow-up study. J Clin Oncol 1994;12:312–325.

132 van Leeuwen FE, Klokman WJ, Stovall M, Hagenbeek A, van den Belt-Dusebout AW, Noyon R, Boice JD Jr, Burgers JM, Somers R: Roles of radiotherapy and smoking in lung cancer following Hodgkin's disease. J Natl Cancer Inst 1995;87:1530–1537.

133 Levine E, Bloomfield C: Leukemias and myelodysplastic syndromes secondary to drug, radiation, and environmental exposure. Semin Oncol 1992;19:47–84.

134 List AF, Doll DC, Greco FA: Lung cancer in Hodgkin's disease: Association with previous radiotherapy. J Clin Oncol 1985;3:215–221.

135 London NJ, Farmery SM, Will EJ, Davison AM, Lodge JP: Risk of neoplasia in transplant patients. Lancet 1995;346:403–406.

136 Lowsky R, Lipton J, Fyles G, Minden M, Meharchand J, Tejpar I, Atkins H, Sutcliffe S, Messner H: Secondary malignancies after bone marrow transplantation in adults. J Clin Oncol 1994;12:2187–2192.

137 Matanoski GM, Seltser R, Sartwell PE, Diamond EL, Elliott EA: The current mortality rates of radiologists and other physician specialists: Specific causes of death. Am J Epidemiol 1975;101:199–210.

138 Mauch PM, Kalish LA, Marcus KC, Shulman LN, Krill E, Tarbell NJ, Silver B, Weinstein H, Come S, Canellos GP, Coleman CN: Long-term survival in Hodgkin's disease. Relative impact of mortality, second tumors, infection, and cardiovascular disease. Cancer J Sci Am 1995;1:33–42.

139 Mauch PM, Kalish LA, Marcus KC, Coleman CN, Shulman LN, Krill E, Come S, Silver B, Canellos GP, Tarbell NJ: Second malignancies after treatment for laparotomy staged IA–IIIB Hodgkin's disease: Long-term analysis of risk factors and outcome. Blood 1996;87:3625–3632.

140 McCredie JA, Inch WR, Alderson MA: Consecutive primary carcinomas of the breast. Cancer 1975;35:1472–1477.

141 McLaughlin JK, Hrubec Z, Blot WJ, Fraumeni JF Jr: Smoking and cancer mortality among US veterans: A 26-year follow-up. Int J Cancer 1995;60:190–193.

142 Mettler FA Jr, Upton AC: Medical Effects of Ionizing Radiation. Philadelphia, PA, Saunders, 1995.

143 Miller AB, Howe GR, Sherman GJ, Lindsay JP, Yaffe MJ, Dinner PJ, Risch HA, Preston DL: Mortality from breast cancer after irradiation during fluoroscopic examinations in patients being treated for tuberculosis. N Engl J Med 1989;321:1285–1289.

144 Miller JS, Arthur DC, Litz CE, Neglia JP, Miller WJ, Weisdorf DJ: Myelodysplastic syndrome after autologous bone marrow transplantation: An additional late complication of curative cancer therapy. Blood 1994;83:3780–3786.

145 Mitelman F, Brandt L, Nilsson P: Relation among occupational exposure to potential mutagenic/carcinogenic agents, clinical findings, and bone marrow chromosomes in acute nonlymphocytic leukemia. Blood 1978;52:1229–1237.

146 Miura T, Muraoka S, Ogiso T: Effect of ascorbate on Adriamycin-Fe^{3+}-induced lipid peroxidation and DNA damage. Pharmacol Toxicol 1994;74:89–94.

147 Montagnino G, Lorca E, Tarantino A, Bencini P, Aroldi A, Cesana B, Braga M, Lonati F, Ponticelli C: Cancer incidence in 854 kidney transplant recipients from a single institution: Comparison with normal population and with patients under dialytic treatment. Clin Transplant 1996;10:461–469.

148 Morris T, Thacker J: Formation of large deletions by illegitimate recombination in the HPRT gene of primary human fibroblasts. Proc Natl Acad Sci USA 1993;90:1392–1396.

149 Morrison V, Dunn D, Manivel J, Gajl-Peczalska KJ, Peterson BA: Clinical characteristics of post-transplant lymphoproliferative disorders. Am J Med 1994;97:14–24.

150 Mott MG, Boyse J, Hewitt M, Radford M: Do mutations at the glycophorin A locus in patients treated for childhood Hodgkin's disease predict secondary leukaemia? Lancet 1994;343:828–829.

151 Nakagawa I, Nishi E, Naganuma A, Imura N: Effect of preinduction of metallothionein synthesis on clastinogenicity of anticancer drugs in mice. Mutat Res 1995;348:37–43.

152 Nalesnik MA, Randhawa P, Demetris AJ, Casavilla A, Fung JJ, Locker J: Lymphoma resembling Hodgkin disease after posttransplant lymphoproliferative disorder in a liver transplant recipient. Cancer 1993;72:2568–2573.

153 Naoe T, Kudo K, Yoshida H, Horibe K, Ohno R: Molecular analysis of the t(15;17) translocation in de novo and secondary acute promyelocytic leukemia. Leukemia 1997;11(suppl 3):287–288.

154 National Council on Radiation Protection and Measurements (NCRP): The probability that a particular malignancy may have been caused by a specified irradiation. NCRP Statement No 7, Bethesda, 1992.

155 Nayfield SG, Karp JE, Ford LG, Dorr FA, Kramer BS: Potential role of tamoxifen in prevention of breast cancer. J Natl Cancer Inst 1991;83:1450–1459.

156 Neglia JP, Meadows AT, Robison LL, Kim TH, Newton WA, Ruymann FB, Sather HN, Hammond GD: Second neoplasms after acute lymphoblastic leukemia in childhood. N Engl J Med 1991;325:1330–1336.

157 Nelson NJ: Solutions bring new problems: Secondary cancers are a risk for some survivors. News. J Natl Cancer Inst 1997;89:1483–1485.

158 Neugut AI, Murray T, Santos J, Amols H, Hayes MK, Flannery JT, Robinson E: Increased risk of lung cancer after breast cancer radiation therapy in cigarette smokers. Cancer 1994;73:1615–1620.

159 Newstead CG: Assessment of risk of cancer after renal transplantation. Commentary. Lancet 1998;351:610–611.

160 Nichols CR, Breeden ES, Loehrer PJ, Williams SD, Einhorn LH: Secondary leukemia associated with a conventional dose of etoposide: Review of serial germ cell tumor protocols. J Natl Cancer Inst 1993;85:36–40.

161 Nichols CR, Hoffman R, Einhorn LH, Williams SD, Wheeler LA, Garnick MB: Hematologic malignancies associated with primary mediastinal germ-cell tumours. Ann Intern Med 1985;102:603–609.

162 Nichols CR, Loehrer PJ Sr: The story of second cancers in patients cured of testicular cancer: Tarnishing success or burnishing irrelevance? J Natl Cancer Inst 1997;89:1394–1395.

163 Ohe T, Tsuda S, Sakata Y, Taniwaki M, Misawa S, Abe T: Cis-diamminedichloroplatinum(II)-induced sister-chromatid exchanges and chromosome aberration formation in cultured human lymphocytes and their inhibition by sodium thiosulfate. Mutat Res 1990;244:279–285.

164 Olden K: Mutagen hypersensitivity as a biomarker of genetic predisposition to carcinogenesis. J Natl Cancer Inst 1994;86:1660–1661.

165 Opelz G, Schwartz V, Grayson H: Multicenter analysis of posttransplant malignancies; in Touraine JL, Traeger J, Bétuel H, Dubernard JM, Revillard JP, Dupuy C (eds): Cancer in Transplantation; Prevention and Treatment. Dordrecht, Kluwer, 1996, pp 17–23.

166 Osanto S, Thijssen JCP, Woldering VM, van Rijn JL, Natarajan AT, Tates AD: Increased frequency of chromosomal damage in peripheral blood lymphocytes up to nine years following curative chemotherapy of patients with testicular carcinoma. Environ Mol Mutagen 1991;17:71–78.

167 Parker RG, Grimm P, Enstrom JE: Contralateral breast cancers following treatment for initial breast cancers in women. Am J Clin Oncol 1989;12:213–216.

168 Pathak AB, Advani SH, Gopal R, Nadkarni KS, Saikia TK: Urinary bladder cancer following cyclophosphamide therapy for Hodgkin's disease. Leuk Lymphoma 1992;8:503–504.

169 Pedersen-Bjergaard J, Daugaard G, Hansen SW, Philip P, Larsen SO, Rorth M: Increased risk of myelodysplasia and leukaemia after etoposide, cisplatin, and bleomycin for germ-cell tumours. Lancet 1991;338:359–363.

170 Pedersen-Bjergaard J, Ersboll J, Hansen VL, Sorensen BL, Christoffersen K, Hou-Jensen K, Nissen NI, Knudsen JB, Hansen MM: Carcinoma of the urinary bladder after treatment with cyclophosphamide for non-Hodgkin's lymphoma. N Engl J Med 1988;318:1028–1032.

171 Pedersen-Bjergaard J, Larsen S: Incidence of acute nonlymphocytic leukemia, preleukemia, and acute myeloproliferative syndrome up to 10 years after treatment of Hodgkin's disease. N Engl J Med 1982;307:965–971.

172 Pedersen-Bjergaard J, Philip P: Two different classes of therapy-related and de novo acute myeloid leukemia? Cancer Genet Cytogenet 1991;55:119–124.

173 Pedersen-Bjergaard J, Philip P: Balanced translocations involving chromosome bands 11q23 and 21q22 are highly characteristic of myelodysplasia and leukemia following therapy with cytostatic agents targeting at DNA-topoisomerase II. Blood 1991;78:1147–1148.

174 Pedersen-Bjergaard J, Rowley JD: The balanced and the unbalanced chromosome aberrations of acute myeloid leukemia may develop in different ways and may contribute differently to malignant transformation. Blood 1994;83:2780–2786.

175 Pedersen-Bjergaard J, Sigsgaard TC, Nielsen D, Gjedde SB, Philip P, Hansen M, Larsen SO, Rorth M, Mouridsen H, Dombernowsky P: Acute monocytic or myelomonocytic leukemia with balanced chromosome translocations to band 11q23 after therapy with 4-epidoxorubicin and cisplatin or cyclophosphamide for breast cancer. J Clin Oncol 1992;10:1444–1451.

176 Penn I: Cancers complicating organ transplantation. N Engl J Med 1990;323:1767–1768.

177 Perera FP, Motzer RJ, Tang D, Reed E, Parker R, Warburton D, O'Neill P, Albertini R, Bigbee WL, Jensen RH: Multiple biological markers in germ cell tumor patients treated with platinum-based chemotherapy. Cancer Res 1992;52:3558–3565.

178 Pohl H, Reidy JA: Vitamin C intake influences the bleomycin-induced chromosome damage assay: Implications for detection of cancer susceptibility and chromosome breakage syndromes. Mutat Res 1989;224:247–252.

179 Prior P, Pope DJ: Hodgkin's disease: Subsequent primary cancers in relation to treatment. Br J Cancer 1988;58:512–517.

180 Pui CH, Behm FG, Raimondi SC, Dodge RK, George SL, Rivera GK, Mirro J Jr, Kalwinsky DK, Dahl GV, Murphy SB: Secondary acute myeloid leukemia in children treated for acute lymphoid leukemia. N Engl J Med 1989;321:136–142.

181 Pui CH, Ribeiro RC, Hancock ML, Rivera GK, Evans WE, Raimondi SC, Head DR, Behm FG, Mahmoud MH, Sandlund JT: Acute myeloid leukemia in children treated with epipodophyllotoxins for acute lymphoblastic leukemia. N Engl J Med 1991;325:1682–1687.

182 Quesnel B, Kantarjian H, Pedersen-Bjergaard JP, Brault P, Estey E, Lai JL, Tilly H, Stoppa AM, Archimbaud E, Harousseau JL: Therapy-related acute myeloid leukemia with t(8;21), inv(16) and t(8;16): A report on 25 cases and review of the literature. J Clin Oncol 1993; 11:2370–2379.

183 Rabkin CS, Yellin F: Cancer incidence in a population with a high prevalence of infection with human immunodeficiency virus type 1. J Natl Cancer Inst 1994;86:1711–1716.

184 Radis CD, Kahl LE, Baker GL, Wasko MC, Cash JM, Gallatin A, Stolzer BL, Agarwal AK, Medsger TA Jr, Kwoh CK: Effects of cyclophosphamide on the development of malignancy and on long-term survival of patients with rheumatoid arthritis. A 20-year follow-up study. Arthritis Rheum 1995;38:1120–1127.

185 Ratain MJ, Kaminer LS, Bitran JD, Larson RA, Le Beau MM, Skosey C, Purl S, Hoffman PC, Wade J, Vardiman JW: Acute nonlymphocytic leukemia following etoposide and cisplatin combination chemotherapy for advanced non-small-cell carcinoma of the lung. Blood 1987;70:1412–1417.

186 Ratain MJ, Rowley JD: Therapy-related acute myeloid leukemia secondary to inhibitors of to-poisomerase II: From the bedside to the target genes. Ann Oncol 1992;3:107–111.

187 Remick SC: Non-AIDS-defining cancers. Hematol Oncol Clin North Am 1996;10: 1203–1213.

188 Rivas-Olmedo G, Barriga-Arceo SD, Madrigal-Bujaidar E: Inhibition of mitomycin C-induced sister chromatid exchanges by vitamin C in vivo. J Toxicol Environ Health 1992;35: 107–113.

189 Ron E, Lubin JH, Shore RE, Mabuchi K, Modan B, Pottern LM, Schneider AB, Tucker MA, Boice JD Jr: Thyroid cancer after exposure to external radiation: A pooled analysis of seven studies. Radiat Res 1995;141:259–277.

190 Ron E, Modan B, Boice JD Jr, Alfandary E, Stovall M, Chetrit A, Katz L: Tumors of the brain and nervous system after radiotherapy in childhood. N Engl J Med 1988;319:1033–1039.

191 Rosenberg S, Kaplan H: The evolution and summary results of the Stanford randomized clinical trials of the management of Hodgkin's disease: 1962–1984. Int J Radiat Oncol Biol Phys 1985;11:5–22.

192 Rowley J, Golomb H, Vardiman J: Nonrandom chromosomal abnormalities in acute nonlymphocytic leukemia in patients treated for Hodgkin disease and non-Hodgkin lymphomas. Blood 1977;50:759–770.

193 Rubagotti A, Perrotta A, Casella C, Boccardo F: Risk of new primaries after chemotherapy and/or tamoxifen treatment for early breast cancer. Ann Oncol 1996;7:239–244.

194 Salvadori DM, Ribeiro LR, Natarajan AT: Effect of beta-carotene on clastogenic effects of mitomycin C, methyl-methanesulphonate and bleomycin in Chinese hamster ovary cells. Mutagenesis 1994;9:53–57.

195 Samra Y, Hertz M, Lindner A: Urinary bladder tumors following cyclophosphamide therapy: A report of two cases with a review of the literature. Med Pediatr Oncol 1985;13:86–91.

196 Sandoval C, Pui CH, Bowman LC, Heaton D, Hurwitz CA, Raimondi SC, Behm FG, Head DR: Secondary acute myeloid leukemia in children previously treated with alkylating agents, intercalating topoisomerase II inhibitors and irradiation. J Clin Oncol 1993;11:1039–1045.

197 Satoh M, Kondo Y, Mita M, Nakagawa I, Naganuma A, Imura N: Prevention of carcinogenicity of anticancer drugs by metallothionein induction. Cancer Res 1993;53:4767–4768.

198 Seltser R, Sartwell PE: The influence of occupational exposure to radiation on the mortality of radiologists and other specialists. Am J Epidemiol 1965;81:2–22.

199 Shapiro CL, Recht A: Late effects of adjuvant therapy for breast cancer. Monogr Natl Cancer Inst 1994;16:101–112.

200 Shell AG: Development of malignancy following renal transplantation in Australia and New Zealand. Transplant Proc 1992;24:1275–1279.

201 Shirai T: Etiology of bladder cancer. Semin Urol 1993;11:113–126.

202 Sigal SH, Tomaszewski JE, Brooks JJ, Wein A, LiVolsi VA: Carcinosarcoma of bladder following long-term cyclophosphamide therapy. Arch Pathol Lab Med 1991;115:1049–1051.

203 Smith MA, McCaffrey RP, Karp JE: The secondary leukemias: Challenges and research directions. J Natl Cancer Inst 1996;88:407–418.

204 Socié G: Secondary malignancies. Curr Opin Hematol 1996;6:466–470.

205 Sterling W, Wu L, Dowling E, Diethelm AG: Hodgkin's disease in a renal transplant recipient. Transplantation 1974;17:315–317.

206 Storm H, Andersson M, Boice JD Jr, Blettner M, Stovall M, Mouridsen HT, Dombernowsky P, Rose C, Jacobsen A, Pedersen M: Adjuvant radiotherapy and risk of contralateral breast cancer. J Natl Cancer Inst 1992;84:1245–1250.

207 Storm HH, Jensen OM: Risk of contralateral breast cancer in Denmark 1943-80. Br J Cancer 1986;54:483–492.

208 Straus K, Lichter A, Lippman M, Danforth D, Swain S, Cowan K, deMoss E, MacDonald H, Steinberg S, d'Angelo T: Results of the National Cancer Institute early breast cancer trial. Monogr Natl Cancer Inst 1992;11:27–32.

209 Super HJ, McCabe NR, Thirman MJ, Larson RA, Le Beau MM, Pedersen-Bjergaard J, Philip P, Diaz MO, Rowley JD: Rearrangements of the MLL gene in therapy-related acute myeloid leukemia in patients previously treated with agents targeting DNA-topoisomerase II. Blood 1993;82:3705–3711.

210 Swerdlow AJ, Douglas AJ, Hudson GV, Hudson BV, Bennett MH, MacLennan KA: Risk of second primary cancers after Hodgkin's disease by type of treatment: Analysis of 2,846 patients in the British National Lymphoma Investigation. BMJ 1992;304:1137–1143.

211 Tarbell NJ, Gelber RD, Weinstein HJ, Mauch P: Sex differences in risk of second malignant tumors after Hodgkin's disease in childhood. Lancet 1993;341:1428–1432.

212 Tates AD, van Dam FJ, Natarajan AT, Zwinderman AH, Osanto S: Frequencies of HPRT mutants and micronuclei in lymphocytes of cancer patients under chemotherapy: A prospective study. Mutat Res 1994;307:293–306.

213 Tercilla O, Krasin F, Lawn-Tsao L: Comparison of contralateral breast doses from half beam block and isocentric treatment techniques for patients treated with primary breast irradiation with ^{60}Co. Int J Radiat Oncol Biol Phys 1989;17:205–210.

214 Thirman MJ, Gill HJ, Burnett RC, Mbangkollo D, McCabe NR, Kobayashi H, Ziemin-van der Poel S, Kaneko Y, Morgan R, Sandberg AA: Rearrangement of the MLL gene in acute lymphoblastic and acute myeloid leukemias with 11q23 abnormalities. N Engl J Med 1993; 329:958–959.

215 Travis LB, Curtis RE, Bennett WP, Hankey BF, Travis WD, Boice JD Jr: Lung cancer after Hodgkin's disease. J Natl Cancer Inst 1995;87:1324–1327.

216 Travis LB, Curtis RE, Boice JD Jr, Hankey BF, Fraumeni JF Jr: Second cancers following non-Hodgkin's lymphoma. Cancer 1991;67:2002–2009.

217 Travis LB, Curtis RE, Glimelius B, Holowaty EJ, van Leeuwen FE, Lynch CF, Hagenbeek A, Stovall M, Banks PM, Adami J: Bladder and kidney cancer following cyclophosphamide therapy for non-Hodgkin's lymphoma. J Natl Cancer Inst 1995;87:524–530.

218 Travis LB, Curtis RE, Inskip PD, Hankey BF: Lung cancer after treatment for breast cancer (letter). J Natl Cancer Inst 1995;87:60–61.

219 Travis LB, Curtis RE, Storm H, Hall P, Holowaty E, van Leeuwen FE, Kohler BA, Pukkala E, Lynch CF, Andersson M, Bergfeldt K, Clarke EA, Wiklund T, Stoter G, Gospodarowicz M, Sturgeon J, Fraumeni JF Jr, Boice JD Jr: Risk of second malignant neoplasms among long-term survivors of testicular cancer. J Natl Cancer Inst 1997;89:1429–1439.

220 Travis LB, Curtis RE, Stovall M, Holowaty EJ, van Leeuwen FE, Glimelius B, Lynch CF, Hagenbeek A, Li CY, Banks PM: Risk of leukemia following treatment for non-Hodgkin's lymphoma. J Natl Cancer Inst 1994;86:1450–1457.

221 Travis WD, Travis LB, Devesa SS: Lung cancer incidence and survival by histologic type. Cancer 1995;75:191–202.

222 Trizna Z, Hsu TC, Schantz SP: Protective effect of vitamin E against bleomycin-induced genotoxicity in head and neck cancer patients in vitro. Anticancer Res 1992;12:325–327.

223 Trizna Z, Schantz SP, Hsu TC: Effects of N-acetyl-L-cysteine and ascorbic acid on mutagen-induced chromosomal sensitivity in patients with head and neck cancers. Am J Surg 1991; 162:294–298.

224 Trizna Z, Schantz SP, Lee JJ, Spitz MR, Goepfert H, Hsu TC, Hong WK: In vitro protective effects of chemopreventive agents against bleomycin-induced genotoxicity in lymphoblastoid cell lines and peripheral blood lymphocytes of head and neck cancer patients. Cancer Detect Prev 1993;17:575–583.

225 Tucker MA, Coleman CN, Cox RS, Varghese A, Rosenberg SA: Risk of second cancers after treatment for Hodgkin's disease. N Engl J Med 1988;318:76–81.

226 Tucker MA, D'Angio G, Boice JD Jr, Strong LC, Li FP, Stovall M, Stone BJ, Green DM, Lombardi F, Newton W: Bone sarcomas linked to radiotherapy and chemotherapy in children. N Engl J Med 1987;317:588–593.

227 Tucker MA, Jones PH, Boice JD Jr, Robison LL, Stone BJ, Stovall M, Jenkin RD, Lubin JH, Baum ES, Siegel SE: Therapeutic radiation at a young age is linked to secondary thyroid cancer. Cancer Res 1991;51:2885–2888.

228 Tucker MA, Meadows AT, Boice JD Jr, Stovall M, Oberlin O, Stone BJ, Birch J, Voute PA, Hoover RN, Fraumeni JF Jr: Leukemia after therapy with alkylating agents for childhood cancer. J Natl Cancer Inst 1987;78:459–464.

229 Tucker MA, Misfeldt D, Coleman CN, Clark WH Jr, Rosenberg SA: Cutaneous malignant melanoma after Hodgkin's disease. Ann Intern Med 1985;102:37–41.

230 Tucker MA: Solid second cancers following Hodgkin's disease. Hematol Oncol Clin North Am 1993;7:389–400.

231 Uppsala-Örebro Breast Cancer Study Group T: Sector resection with or without postoperative radiotherapy for stage I breast cancer: A randomized trial. J Natl Cancer Inst 1990;82: 277–282.

232 Valagussa P, Moliterni A, Terenziani M, Zambetti M, Bonadonna G: Second malignancies following CMF-based adjuvant chemotherapy in resectable breast cancer. Ann Oncol 1994;5: 803–808.

233 Valagussa P, Santoro A, Fossati-Bellani F, Banfi A, Bonadonna G: Second acute leukemia and other malignancies following treatment for Hodgkin's disease. J Clin Oncol 1986;4:830–837.

234 Veronesi U, Luini A, Del Vecchio M, Greco M, Galimberti V, Merson M, Rilke F, Sacchini V, Saccozzi R, Savio T: Radiotherapy after breast-preserving surgery in women with localized cancer of the breast. N Engl J Med 1993;328:1587–1591.

235 Vittorio CC, Schiffman MH, Weinstock MA: Epidemiology of human papillomaviruses. Dermatol Clin 1995;13:561–574.

236 Vose JM, Kennedy BC, Bierman PJ, Kessinger A, Armitage JO: Long-term sequelae of autologous bone marrow or peripheral stem cell transplantation for lymphoid malignancies. Cancer 1992;69:784–789.

237 Wakabayashi T, Kato H, Ikeda T, Schull WJ: Studies of the mortality of A-bomb survivors, report 7. Part III. Incidence of cancer in 1959–1978, based on tumor registry. Nagasaki Radiat Res 1983;93:112–146.

238 Webster EW: On the question of cancer induction by small x-ray doses: Garland Lecture. AJR 1981;137:647–666.

239 Weijl NI, Cleton FJ, Osanto S: Free radicals and antioxidants in chemotherapy-induced toxicity. Cancer Treat Rev 1997;23:209–240.

240 Whitlock JA, Greer JP, Lukens JN: Epipodophyllotoxin-related leukemia. Identification of a new subset of secondary leukemia. Cancer 1991;68:600–604.

241 Winick NJ, McKenna RW, Shuster JJ, Schneider NR, Borowitz MJ, Bowman WP, Jacaruso D, Kamen BA, Buchanan GR: Secondary acute myeloid leukemia in children with acute lymphoblastic leukemia treated with etoposide. J Clin Oncol 1993;11:209–217.

242 Witherspoon RP, Deeg HJ, Storb R: Secondary malignancies after marrow transplantation for leukemia or aplastic anemia. Transplant Sci 1994;4:33–41.

243 Witherspoon RP, Storb R, Pepe M, Longton G, Sullivan KM: Cumulative incidence of secondary solid malignant tumors in aplastic anemia patients given marrow grafts after conditioning with chemotherapy alone. Blood 1992;79:289–291.

244 Worth PH: Cyclophosphamide and the bladder. Br Med J 1971;iii:182.

245 Ziemin-van der Poel S, McCabe NR, Gill HJ, Espinosa R III, Patel Y, Harden A, Rubinelli P, Smith SD, Le Beau MM, Rowley JD: Identification of a gene, MLL, that spans the breakpoint in 11q23 translocations associated with human leukemias [published erratum appears in Proc Natl Acad Sci USA 1992;89:4220]. Proc Natl Acad Sci USA 1991;88:10735–10739.

246 Zulian GB, Bellorno MJ, Cabrol C, Beris P, Mermillod B, Alberto P: Etoposide and secondary haematological malignancies: Coincidence or causality? Ann Oncol 1993;4:559–566.

J.R. Soedirman, MD
Academisch Ziekenhuis der Vrije Universiteit, Polikliniek, Kamer 0 NBU 48, De Boelelaan 1117, NL–1081 HV Amsterdam (The Netherlands)
Tel. +31-20-4440255, Fax +31-20-642 5085, E-mail jsoedirman@azvu.nl

Rüther U, Nunnensiek C, Schmoll H-J (eds): Secondary Neoplasias following Chemotherapy, Radiotherapy, and Immunosuppression. Contrib Oncol. Basel, Karger, 2000, vol 55, pp 203–224

....

Secondary Malignancies after Allogeneic or Autologous Marrow Transplantation

Robert P. Witherspoon, H. Joachim Deeg, Lloyd Fisher, Gary Schoch, Rainer Storb

Clinical Research Division, Fred Hutchinson Cancer Research Center and Departments of Medicine and Biostatistics of the Schools of Medicine and Public Health, University of Washington, Seattle, WA, USA

Introduction

Secondary malignancies developing after marrow or peripheral blood hematopoietic stem cell transplantation may result from treatment of the underlying disease before marrow transplantation and treatment directly associated with the transplantation process. Immunosuppression resulting from T-lymphocyte depletion of donor marrow used to prevent graft-versus-host disease (GVHD) or antithymocyte globulin (ATG) and anti-T-lymphocyte antibodies used to treat it are often associated with Epstein-Barr virus infection and development of a posttransplant lymphoproliferative disorder (PTLD). Total body irradiation (TBI) used to condition the recipient for a marrow graft is associated with solid nonhematopoietic tumors. Histoincompatibility between donor and recipient, and other predisposing host factors – including genetic predisposition – are more rarely associated with secondary malignancy.

A previous report from this center [1] described 35 malignancies (16 lymphomas, 13 solid tumors and 6 leukemias) in 2,246 patients transplanted between 1969 and 1987. At that time, we found that treatment of acute GVHD with ATG or T64.1, a mouse anti-CD3 monoclonal antibody, and TBI conditioning for grafting were associated with increased risk of developing any secondary malignancy. T-lymphocyte depletion of donor marrow, and HLA incompatibility between donor and recipient had additional associations with secondary PTLD. ATG treatment of acute GVHD was associated with secondary solid tumors.

In this chapter, we update data from the Seattle Marrow Transplant Program, and review the data in the context of literature pertaining to secondary malignancies in hematopoeitic stem cell transplant recipients.

Patients, Records and Treatment

Between 1969 and June 30, 1992, 5,056 patients received bone marrow grafts. Follow-up continued to December 31, 1992. Data were missing on 343 subjects, leaving complete records on 4,713 patients. The donor type and underlying diagnoses for the 4,713 patients are listed in table 1.

Conditioning for grafting for patients with hematologic malignancy consisted of a single dose of 9.6 Gy TBI, or fractionated TBI ranging from 12 to 17 Gy in conjunction with chemotherapy consisting of 120 mg/kg cyclophosphamide or miscellaneous other chemotherapy regimens [2, 3]. Busulfan and cyclophosphamide were used for some patients with myeloid leukemia [4], and bis-dichloroethylnitrosourea (BCNU), cyclophosphamide, and etoposide for patients with lymphoid leukemia who could not tolerate TBI [5]. Patients with aplastic anemia with HLA-identical donors received 200 mg/kg cyclophosphamide [6]. Aplastic anemia patients with HLA partially identical donors received 120 mg/kg cyclophosphamide and 12 Gy TBI.

Treatment to prevent acute GVHD consisted of intermittent methotrexate alone for the first 102 days postgrafting [7], ATG [8], cyclosporine [9], methotrexate given on days 1, 3, 6 and 11, with cyclosporine beginning on the day before the conditioning regimen and continuing for 180 days [10], T-lymphocyte depletion of donor marrow [11], or a combination of prednisone and cyclosporine [12].

Treatment of GVHD consisted of ATG [13], adrenocorticosteroids, cyclosporine [14], monoclonal antibody 64.1 (a murine $IgG2_a$ anti-CD3 monoclonal antibody) [15], monoclonal antibody BC3 (a nonmitogenic $IgG2_b$ anti-CD3 monoclonal antibody) [16], or either Xomazyme-CD5 Plus (a ricin A chain immunotoxin linked to a murine IgG1 anti-CD5 monoclonal antibody) or placebo together with prednisone [17]. Patients who developed chronic GVHD were treated with cyclosporine or prednisone or both [18], or azathioprine [19].

Supportive care was given as described. After discharge home, the patients and their physicians were sent questionnaires every 6 months asking for information about clinical follow-up, including questions regarding the presence of a secondary malignancy. The data on these forms were entered into the database for retrieval with this analysis.

Risk factors for the development of a secondary malignancy considered in this analysis included the diagnosis of hematologic malignancy or aplastic anemia; the age and sex of the recipient; conditioning with a regimen containing TBI or no TBI; the irradiation dose in cGy; receipt of HLA partially identical marrow; prevention of GVHD with methotrexate, cyclosporine, the combination of cyclosporine and methotrexate, or T-lymphocyte depletion of donor marrow; presence of grade 2 or greater acute GVHD; treatment of acute GVHD with ATG, the monoclonal antibody 64.1, or the monoclonal antibody BC3, and the presence of chronic GVHD.

Statistical Analysis

The time from transplantation to the occurrence of second cancer was analyzed using time-to-event survival analysis [20]. The risk of an event over different periods was expressed as the number of events per 100 patient-years at risk, with 95% confidence intervals (CI) constructed with the assumption of a Poisson distribution for the number of events. The probabilities of a second cancer

Donor type		*Table 1.* Characteristics of patients transplanted
Syngeneic donors	203	
HLA-identical family members	2,720	
HLA partially identical family members	729	
Unrelated donors	377	
Autologous marrow	684	
Total	4,713	

Diagnoses at time of transplant	
Acute myelogenous leukemia	1,291
Acute lymphocytic leukemia	936
Chronic myelogenous leukemia	1,106
Myelodysplasia	172
Non-Hodgkin's lymphoma	433
Hodgkin's disease	134
Multiple myeloma	75
Aplastic anemia	339
Paroxysmal nocturnal hemoglobinuria	3
Miscellaneous[1]	224
Total	4,713

[1] Breast carcinoma 41, Ewing's sarcoma 9, sarcoma 13, neuroblastoma 38, thalassemia 10, disorders of metabolism 8, histiocytoses 6, germ cell 4, chronic lymphocytic leukemia 5, glioblastoma 3, medulloblastoma 1, sickle cell anemia 1, pure red cell aplasia 2, refractory anemia with ringed sideroblasts 6, myelosclerosis 5, adenocarcinoma 67, immunodeficiency 5.

were compared with the incidence of primary cancers among residents in Washington State, as obtained from the database of the National Cancer Institute Surveillance, Epidemiology, and End Result (NCI SEER) program. The comparisons were adjusted for age, sex, and the exposure time of the patients making up the control population in the same database. The relatively small number of events occurring among the patients who underwent marrow transplantation was modeled by the Poisson distribution; the larger NCI SEER database (with adjustment for the age, sex, and exposure time of the patients) was used to give a 100% $(1-\alpha/2)$ CI for the number of events expected. The upper limit of this CI was used to evaluate the Poisson probability (p) for a number of events equivalent to or higher than the number observed. If $p+\alpha/2 \leq \alpha$, then the distributions of the time to an event among the patients and the control population differ at the α significance level (with use of the Bonferroni inequality).

The Cox proportional-hazards regression model was used to evaluate univariate statistical significance. Multivariate statistical models were obtained with the stepwise step-up Cox proportional-hazards technique and the BMDP software programs [21]. According to this technique, the predictor with the highest level of statistical significance was used to initiate the model; other variables were then evaluated for further predictive information and added in turn, beginning with the variables with the highest level of statistical significance (i.e., the lowest p values) and continuing as long as the p value for the variable added was ≤ 0.05. The complete list of potential predictors entered in this regression model is given above. Chronic GVHD was entered as a time-dependent covariate. The instantaneous relative risk associated with changing a predictive variable by 1 unit was determined with the Cox models; the estimated magnitude of the relative risk is shown along with its 95% CI.

Outcomes

Secondary Malignancy in Marrow Transplant Patients

Secondary malignancies developed in 103 patients (table 2). The number of patients alive and at risk of developing secondary cancer at the beginning, as well as at 5-, 10-, 15- and 20-year time periods was 4,713, 821, 309, 73 and 6, respectively. The Kaplan-Meier probability of any secondary malignancy was 3% at 5 years (95% CI 2.5–3.5%), 6% at 10 years (CI 3–9%), 12% at 15 years (CI 8–16%) and 17% at 20 years (CI 7–27%) (fig. 1).

PTLD occurred in 24 patients and Hodgkin's disease in 1 patient. A new acute leukemia in donor cells occurred in 11 patients, 6 of which were acute myelogenous leukemia (AML)/myelodysplasia (MDS)/myeloproliferative (MPF) disorders, and 5 acute lymphocytic leukemia (ALL). Solid tumors were identified in 67 patients: 17 squamous cell carcinoma; 6 glioblastoma multiforme; 23 basal cell carcinoma; 3 melanoma; 2 bone sarcoma (myxoid chondrosarcoma, chondrosarcoma); 4 papillary carcinoma of the thyroid, and 8 cases of adenocarcinoma, consisting of 3 originating in the breast, 2 in the colon, and 1 each hepatocellular carcinoma and lung carcinoma and 1 in multiple sites. In addition, 1 patient each had mucoepidermoid carcinoma of the parotid, embryonal cell carcinoma of the testis, rhabdomyosarcoma, and neuroblastoma (table 2).

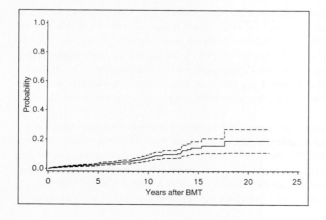

Fig. 1. Kaplan-Meier probability of developing any secondary malignancy after bone marrow transplantation (BMT) (——). Pointwise 95% confidence intervals (-----).

Table 2. Types of
secondary malignancy

Lymphomas	
PTLD	24
HD	1
Acute leukemia	
Lymphoid	5
AML/MDS/MPF	6
Solid tumors	
Squamous cell carcinoma[1]	17
Neurological tumors	6
Basal cell carcinoma	23
Melanoma	3
Bone sarcomas	2
Papillary carcinoma thyroid adenocarcinoma	4
Liver	1
Colon	2
Breast	3
Lung	1
Multiple site	1
Other[2]	4
Total	103

PTLD = Posttransplant lymphoproliferative disorder;
HD = Hodgkin's disease; AML = acute myelogenous leukemia;
MDS = myelodysplasia; MPF = myeloproliferative syndrome.
[1] 14 site-specific carcinomas, and 3 on truncal or extremity
skin.
[2] Neuroblastoma of cranial bone, mucoepidermoid carcinoma
of parotid, embryonal cell carcinoma of testis, rhabdomyosarcoma.

The median time (range) from transplantation to diagnosis of secondary malignancy for the entire group was 4.3 years (1.5 months to 18.2 years). PTLD developed within 4.7 months (1.5 months to 8.31 years); leukemia/MDS occurred within
7.3 months (1.9 months to 2.3 years), and solid tumors developed within 6.6 years
(2.3 months to 18.2 years). Despite treatment, 48 of the 103 patients died of their
secondary malignancy.

*Rates of Secondary Malignancy after Marrow Transplantation Compared to the
General Population*

Table 3 shows the frequencies of secondary malignancy in marrow transplant
recipients compared to the frequencies of the normal population in developing a primary malignancy as reported in the SEER database and as adjusted for transplant

Table 3. Comparison of observed cases to those expected in the general population

Type	Observed (O)	Expected (E)	O/E	One-sided p value
All cancers	103	17.2	5.99	0.0001
PTLD	24	0.6	40.00	0.0001
ALL	5	0.1	50.00	0.0001
AML, MDS	5	0.2	25.00	0.0001
Glioblastoma	6	0.4	15.00	0.0001
Melanoma	3	1.1	2.73	> 0.05
Hodgkin's disease	1	0.4	2.50	> 0.05
Osteosarcoma, chondromyxoid, sarcoma	2	0.1	20.00	0.01
Thyroid, papillary	4	0.5	8.00	0.01
Neuroblastoma, cranium Mucoepidermoid sarcoma, parotid Embryonal, testis Rhabdomyosarcoma	4	0.1	40.00	0.0001
Adenocarcinoma all sites	8	2.1	3.81	0.01
Liver	1	0.0	*	> 0.05
Lung	1	0.4	2.50	> 0.05
Breast	3	1.6	1.88	> 0.05
Colon	2	1.0	2.00	> 0.05
Squamous cell carcinoma				
Oral cavity	3	0.0	*	0.0001
Tongue	6	0.1	60.00	0.0001
Vulva	2	0.0	*	0.001
Cervix	1	0.3	3.33	> 0.05
Penis	1	0.0	*	0.01

PTLD = Posttransplant lymphoproliferative disorder, HD = Hodgkin's disease, AML = acute myelogenous leukemia, MDS = myelodysplasia, MPF = myeloproliferative syndrome.
* The O/E ratio is infinite.

year, sex and age. Transplant recipients were 5.99 times more likely to develop secondary cancer than controls (p = 0.0001). The incidences were elevated in particular for PTLD (p = 0.0001), ALL (p = 0.0001), AML (p = 0.0001), glioblastoma multiforme (p = 0.0001), squamous carcinoma of the tongue (p = 0.0001), and oral mucus membranes other than the tongue (p = 0.0001), vulva (p = 0.001), penis (p = 0.01), osteosarcoma and chondromyxoid carcinoma (p = 0.01), papillary carcinoma of the thyroid (p = 0.01), and the combined group of neuroblastoma, mucoepidermoid carcinoma of the parotid, embryonal cell carcinoma of the testis and rhabdomyosarcoma (p = 0.0001). Overall, the number of adenocarcinomas observed was higher than expected (p = 0.01), but numbers for individual sites of breast, colon, lung and liver were not significantly higher than expected. The incidences of squamous carcinoma of the cervix, Hodgkin's disease and melanoma were not elevated. Because SEER does not track cutaneous squamous carcinoma or basal cell carcinoma, the incidences of cancer for these sites could not be compared with those of the general population.

Factors Associated with Secondary Malignancy
Unifactor Analyses (Data Not Shown)
Development of any secondary malignancy was associated with: treatment of acute GVHD with ATG or monoclonal antibody 64.1 or BC-3; increasing radiation dose; treatment with TBI; acute GVHD of grade II or greater; an HLA partially identical graft, or T-cell depletion of donor marrow to prevent GVHD. Conditioning of aplastic anemia patients with cyclophosphamide alone was associated with fewer secondary malignancies. PTLD was associated with: treatment of acute GVHD with ATG or monoclonal antibodies 64.1 or BC-3; acute GVHD of grade II or greater; partially matched donor marrow or increasing irradiation dose; TBI; methotrexate only as prophylaxis of acute GVHD, or T-cell depletion of donor marrow. Solid tumors occurred less frequently in patients with aplastic anemia. Solid tumors were associated with: increasing dose of irradiation; methotrexate prophylaxis of acute GVHD; presence of TBI, and increasing age. Two of the solid tumor cases occurred in patients who were entered on the Xomazyme-CD5 Plus double-blinded, placebo-controlled trial. One who developed basal cell carcinoma 169 days after transplant for multiple myeloma received Xomazyme-CD5 Plus. The other who developed rhabdomyosarcoma 272 days after transplant for CML received placebo. The power of the analysis to associate Xomazyme-CD5 Plus with secondary malignancy is not sufficient to make a definitive statement about the role of this drug.

No factors were found to be significantly associated with secondary leukemia in donor cells.

Multivariable Analyses
The relative risks (RR) and 95% CI of developing any secondary malignancy derived from the Cox analysis are shown in table 4. Treatment of acute GVHD with the monoclonal antibody 64.1 (RR 9.85 [95% CI 3.02–32.08], p = 0.0001) or ATG (RR 2.57 [1.56–4.24], p = 0.0001) were highly associated with developing a secondary cancer. Patients with aplastic anemia were at reduced risk (RR 0.30 [0.15–0.60], p = 0.0004) of developing any secondary malignancy. The Kaplan-Meier probability of developing a secondary malignancy among patients transplanted for aplastic anemia conditioned with cyclophosphamide alone compared to patients transplanted for malignancy conditioned with chemoradiotherapy is shown in figure 2.

The factors associated with the development of PTLD were treatment of acute GVHD with ATG (RR 9.39 [4.12–21.42], p = 0.0001) or the monoclonal antibodies

Table 4. Factors associated with secondary malignancies – multifactor analyses

Type of secondary malignancy and variable	Step entered	RR	95% CI	Mutivariant p value
All secondary malignancies				
Monoclonal antibody T64.1	1	9.85	3.02 – 32.08	0.0001
ATG	2	2.57	1.56 – 4.24	0.0001
Aplastic anemia	3	0.30	0.15 – 0.60	0.0004
PTLD				
Monoclonal antibody T64.1	1	16.94	4.73 – 60.69	0.0001
ATG	2	9.39	4.12 – 21.42	0.0001
T-cell depletion	3	6.37	1.43 – 28.38	0.0003
Monoclonal antibody BC-3	4	8.01	1.03 – 62.52	0.0182
Radiation dose, cGy	5	1.001	1.000– 1.002	0.0285
Solid tumors				
Aplastic anemia	1	0.29	0.13 – 0.64	0.0005
Age	2	1.02	1.00 – 1.04	0.0212
Squamous cell carcinoma				
Chronic GVHD	1	5.88	2.04 – 16.95	0.0002
Glioblastoma multiforme				
Age, years	1	0.80	0.068 – 0.94	0.0011
Basal cell carcinoma				
Age, years	1	1.07	1.03 – 1.10	0.0001
Aplastic anemia	2	0.10	0.01 – 0.83	0.0139
Adenocarcinoma				
Age, years	1	1.15	1.08 – 1.22	0.0001
ATG	2	9.22	1.61 – 52.86	0.0026

ATG = Antithymocyte globulin; GVHD = graft-versus-host disease. See also table 2 for abbreviations.

64.1 (RR 16.94 [4.73–60.69] p = 0.0001) or BC3 (RR 8.01 [1.03–62.52], p = 0.0182); T-cell depletion of donor marrow, and the incremental dose of irradiation per cGy used for conditioning for grafting (RR 1.001 [1.000–1.002], p = 0.0285) (table 4). The Kaplan-Meier probability of developing PTLD for different radiation doses is shown in figure 3.

For the solid tumors, patients transplanted for aplastic anemia treated with cyclophosphamide alone had a low risk of developing cancer (RR 0.29 [0.13–0.64], p = 0.0003) (table 4). The Kaplan-Meier probability of this relationship is shown in figure 4. Older age was associated with a solid tumor (RR 1.02 [1.00–1.04], p = 0.0212). Chronic GVHD as a time-dependent variable was associated with a significantly elevated risk of developing squamous cell carcinoma (RR 5.88 [2.04–16.95], p = 0.0002). Older patient age was associated with less risk (RR 0.80 [0.68–0.94],

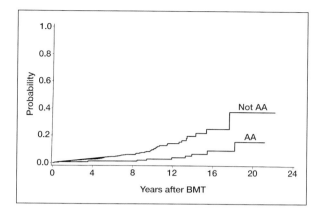

Fig. 2. Kaplan-Meier probability of developing a secondary malignancy among patients transplanted for aplastic anemia (AA) conditioned with cyclophosphamide alone compared to those transplanted for malignancies (not AA) conditioned with chemoradiotherapy.

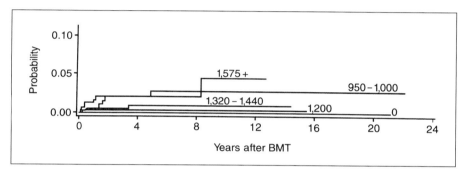

Fig. 3. Kaplan-Meier probability of developing a secondary PTLD after bone marrow transplantation (BMT) with respect to the dose of radiation in cGy. The 0 group received no irradiation. The 950–1,000 cGy group received the dose as a single fraction. The 1,200 cGy group received the dose as 6 fractions of 200 cGy each. The 1,320–1,440 cGy group received 120 cGy fractions 3 times daily to reach the total dose, and the 1,575+ cGy group received 225 cGy daily to reach the total dose. Among the types of irradiation delivered, the delivery of 950–1,000 cGy as a single fraction was associated with higher probability of developing a secondary PTLD than were the 1,200 and 1,320–1,440 cGy fractionated doses.

p = 0.0011) of developing glioblastoma, but with greater risk of developing basal cell carcinoma (RR 1.07 [1.03–1.10], p = 0.0001) or adenocarcinoma (RR 1.15 [1.08–1.22], p = 0.0001). Treatment of acute GVHD with ATG was associated with a greater risk of developing adenocarcinoma (RR 9.22 [1.61–52.86], p = 0.0026). Aplastic anemia was associated with less frequent basal cell carcinoma (RR 0.01 [0.01–0.83], p = 0.0139).

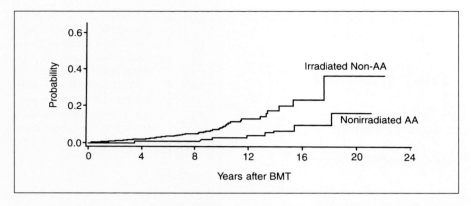

Fig. 4. Kaplan-Meier probability of developing a secondary solid tumor after bone marrow transplantation (BMT). The probability of developing a secondary solid tumor was lower among aplastic anemia (AA) patients who did not receive an irradiation-conditioning regimen (nonirradiated AA) than among those patients transplanted for hematologic malignancy in whom irradiation was used (irradiated non-AA).

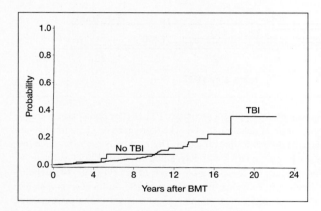

Fig. 5. Kaplan-Meier probability of developing any secondary malignancy after bone marrow transplantation (BMT) among patients transplanted for hematologic malignancy (aplastic anemia patients are excluded) with respect to receiving a conditioning regimen with total body irradiation (TBI) or without TBI.

Additional Aspects of the Effect of Irradiation

By excluding patients transplanted for aplastic anemia, the effect of irradiation-containing conditioning regimens was determined for the remaining patients. Among this group of patients, 673 received chemotherapy conditioning only, consisting mostly of busulfan and cyclophosphamide, and have been followed for 12 years. TBI was used for conditioning in 3,781 patients. For the 12 years of concomitant follow-up, there was no difference in the Kaplan-Meier probability of developing any secondary malignancy with respect to the use or nonuse of irradiation (fig. 5).

Autologous Transplant Recipients

Of 684 autologous transplant patients, 6 (3 transplanted for non-Hodgkin's lymphoma [NHL], 1 ANL, 1 ALL, and 1 adenocarcinoma of the breast) developed secondary cancers (3 basal cell carcinomas, 1 myxoid chondrosarcoma of the mandible, 1 multiple-site adenocarcinoma, 1 squamous carcinoma of the cervix) 410–3,221 (median 1,824) days after transplant. Two patients were conditioned with irradiation-containing regimens and 4 were conditioned with chemotherapy alone.

Review

Risk of Developing Cancer Compared to That of the General Population

The marrow transplant recipients' risk of developing any type of secondary cancer compared to the risk of the general population developing a primary cancer was 5.99 in this group of 4,713 patients. As previously published, PTLD, new leukemia in donor cells, and glioblastoma all continue to be identified as cancers occurring at rates significantly higher than in the general population. In this report, sufficient numbers of new leukemia cases were present to identify the increased risk for both ALL and AML separately, rather than combining them into a single data set of leukemia. In this report, MDS was included with AML. The SEER database does not track MDS. However, these cases of MDS were in the stages of refractory anemia with excess blasts or in transition to acute leukemia. Such cases are likely to have been included in the SEER database previously as AML. Strikingly different from our initial report is the number of patients with squamous cell carcinoma. The sites of oral cavity, tongue, and vulva showed highly significant elevations of risk of squamous cell carcinoma in the marrow transplant population compared to those of the general population.

Tumors occurring less frequently, but at elevated incidence compared to the general population, were also noted: thyroid papillary carcinoma; squamous cell carcinoma of the penis; the combined group of osteosarcoma and chondromyxoid sarcoma, and a group of mesenchymal tumors consisting of rhabdomyosarcoma, embryonal cell carcinoma of the testis, mucoepidermoid carcinoma of the parotid and neuroblastoma of the cranial bone and sinuses. Melanoma and hepatocelluar carcinoma, the incidences of which – compared to the general population – were previously identified as being elevated, were not elevated in this analysis. Furthermore, adenocarcinoma of breast, colon and lung, and squamous cell carcinoma of the cervix occurred with frequencies not significantly elevated compared to the age- and sex-adjusted frequencies seen in the general population.

Transplantation-Related Factors Which Lead to Secondary Cancer

PTLD

Immunosuppression. Clearly, the theme of immunosuppression, permitting uncontrolled Epstein-Barr virus(EBV)-driven B-lymphocyte proliferation, is predominant in the etiology of the lymphomas [22]. As noted previously, treatment of acute GVHD with ATG or the T64.1 monoclonal antibody has profound effects on the immunologic system, which in this study also includes another T-cell monoclonal antibody, BC3. The trials with BC3 ongoing at the time of this study were in dose escalation phases, and it is possible that the higher doses given some of the patients added to immunosuppression, an effect also seen during the initial trials with T64.1. Hodgkin's disease, identified in this group, was also reported in donor cells associated with EBV after transplant for CML [23].

Treatment to eliminate T cells from the graft in order to prevent GVHD was accompanied by a higher incidence of PTLD. The elimination of T cells which regulate EBV-driven B-cell proliferation in vitro [24] and presumably in vivo, appears to give, early after transplant, a window of time when EBV-infected B cells may grow uncontrolled into malignancy. Using tumors from solid-organ transplant patients with PTLD, Liebowitz [25] has recently shown that the in vivo process of B-cell proliferation results from an interaction of the latent membrane protein 1 (LMP1) of EBV-infected B cells and the tumor necrosis factor receptor and its associated proteins. These proteins are capable of linking to nuclear factor κB which is associated with B-cell proliferation. These cellular changes were not seen in tumor tissue which was EBV-negative and LMP1-negative, or in cell lines established from endemic Burkitt's lymphoma which were EBV-positive and LMP1-negative. LMP1, therefore, appears to be critical in the development of EBV-driven PTLD.

The PTLD reported in this study were all monoclonal proliferations linked to EBV. However, in some PTLD, EBV is not identified. T-cell lymphoproliferation has been identified in 3 marrow transplant patients [26], similar to findings in reports after solid-organ transplantation [27]. These reports point out that detailed study will be required to understand the mechanism of expression of types of PTLD other than EBV-associated lymphoproliferations [28].

Irradiation. How irradiation conditioning for grafting affects predisposition to a lymphoma is a bit more puzzling, since the infused donor cells were not irradiated. Nevertheless, those receiving unfractionated TBI were more likely to develop a lymphoma than those not receiving irradiation. In addition, fractionated irradiation in dose levels of 1,200–1,440 cGy reduced the risk from unfractionated TBI, but the risk was again higher among patients who received higher total doses of fractionated irradiation above the 1,440 cGy level (fig. 3). Thus, some type of host effect from irradiation may be important in leading to PTLD. This host effect could be mediated by growth or regulatory cytokines released after irradiation, or by irradiation-induced damage to the lymphoid microenvironment. Another explanation of the effect of irradiation on development of PTLD may be linked to treatment for GVHD. Most patients who received unfractionated TBI had only methotrexate as GVHD prevention and had a higher incidence of severe GVHD than was seen with the combination of methotrexate and cyclosporine used currently for GVHD prophylaxis [29, 30]. In addition, fractionated TBI > 1,200 cGy was associated with more GVHD [31–33]. Patients who received unfractionated TBI or fractionated TBI > 1,200 cGy were more likely to require more treatment for GVHD. This need leads to more immunosuppression, which could then lead to PTLD in patients receiving unfractionated TBI or fractionated TBI > 1,200 cGy.

Treatment for PTLD. PTLD therapy utilizing antiviral drugs such as acyclovir or ganciclovir has not provided long-term survival [34]. Immunotherapeutic approaches have shown some beneficial results. Infusion of lymphocytes from EBV-seropositive donors has resulted in regression of disease, but regrettably, chronic GVHD developed later [35], resulting in mortality [36]. A promising strategy to control chronic GVHD uses EBV-positive donor T lymphocytes into which the HSV-TK gene has been inserted. Treatment of recipients with ganciclovir has the potential to destroy these T cells if chronic GVHD becomes too aggressive [37]. This approach requires sophisticated laboratory facilities and time to create the desired cellular product for infusion. It may have limited application in patients whose rapidly growing tumors necessitate treatment shortly after the diagnosis is made.

Solid Tumors

Immunosuppression. Immunosuppression was an important factor which increased the risk of squamous cell carcinoma and adenocarcinoma. The squamous carcinoma sites were in the oral cavity and extremities where there was extensive involvement with chronic GVHD. Reports from other centers have shown squamous cell cancer being localized to sites of chronic GVHD, which suggests a local effect of GVHD in addition to generalized immunosuppression [38, 39]. Immunosuppressive treatment of chronic GVHD and its correlation with squamous cell carcinoma was shown in a study which combined our data on aplastic anemia patients with those of Hospital St. Louis [40]. In this study, there was a large number of Fanconi anemia patients, who have an elevated risk of developing squamous cancer. Because of their greater risk of developing a malignancy apart from transplantation, the analysis was done with and without their inclusion. Where the Fanconi anemia patients were eliminated from consideration, azathioprine treatment of chronic GVHD was the most important factor which led to squamous cell carcinoma. A similar association between prolonged immunosuppression and squamous cell carcinoma has been described for recipients of renal allografts [41]. Immunosuppressive treatment of GVHD with ATG was identified as a factor predisposing to the 8 cases of adenocarcinoma. This finding was associated with a relative risk of 9.2 (95% CI 1.61–52.86). However, it is difficult to think of a mechanism operating through immunosuppression which could lead to adenocarcinoma, for adenocarcinoma is generally not reported in conjunction with immunosuppression.

Irradiation. TBI increased the risk of solid tumors. Aplastic anemia patients receiving marrow from HLA-identical family members are conditioned in this center with regimens which do not include TBI. The data showed that patients transplanted for aplastic anemia were at a lower risk of developing secondary solid tumors than patients given irradiation-conditioning regimens for malignancies. This effect can be seen especially in the occurrence of basal cell carcinoma which comprised 17 of the 67 cases of solid tumors. Basal cell carcinoma was seen at an RR of only 0.1 in aplastic anemia marrow recipients compared to its occurrence among patients treated for other diseases in whom TBI was used as conditioning (p = 0.0139). TBI is likely to have resulted in the bone sarcomas seen here at elevated risk compared to the general population, similar to reports of bone sarcoma developing after radiotherapy for malignancies in childhood [42].

The combination of Seattle and International Bone Marrow Transplant Registry (IBMTR) data for solid tumors resulted in 80 cases for evaluation among 19,229 patients [43]. When all solid tumors were combined, irradiation dose directly correlated to an elevated risk of developing a secondary solid tumor. When single-fraction TBI was used, the RR of solid tumors developing in patients treated with ≥ 1,000 cGy was 2.7 times that of patients receiving no irradiation (p = 0.0006). This effect was also seen in fractionated irradiation when higher doses were used. The relative risks were 1.2, 1.8, 4.1 and 4.4 for fractionated irradiation < 1,200, 1,200–1,299, 1,300–1,399 and ≥ 1,400 cGy, respectively (p = 0.001). Buccal irradiation to a limited field, especially among males, was associated with the risk of 16.1 to develop oral squamous cancer compared to individuals not irradiated. This treatment consisted of thoracoabdominal irradiation given to patients with aplastic anemia as conditioning therapy for grafting [44, 45].

Melanoma was associated with high-dose TBI in the combined report (RR 8.2, p = 0.01), but was not observed more frequently than in the general population in the Seattle data. In the combined data, the RR of melanoma tended to be higher among recipients of T-lymphocyte-depleted grafts (RR 4.5) compared to those not receiving T-lymphocyte-depleted marrow. Melanoma has been associated with immunosuppressed recipients of renal allografts [46] and in patients with chronic lymphocytic leukemia [47]. Immunosuppression, therefore, may be an important cofactor with irradiation in the development of melanoma in patients after hematopoietic stem cell transplantation.

Age. Younger age correlated with an increased incidence of glioblastoma multiforme. Five of the 6 glioblastoma patients were transplanted for ALL, and 1 for AML. These patients had craniospinal irradiation to prevent or treat central nervous system leukemia before transplant [48]. We did not formally analyze pretransplant craniospinal irradiation. The combined Seattle and IBMTR data show a correlation between glioblastoma and high-dose TBI, defined as ≥ 1,000 cGy single-fraction or ≥ 1,300 cGy from fractionated doses, compared to no or low-dose irradiation. These findings suggest that glioblastoma was accounted for partly by irradiation and not by age alone. In the combined Seattle IBMTR data, the greatest risk of solid-tumor development was seen in patients who were < 10 years of age at the time of transplantation. The observed:expected ratio was 36.6 (95% CI 22.9–55.4) for this group. This risk declined to 1.2 (95% CI 0.7–1.9) among patients ≥ 40 years of age. Although we did not evaluate thyroid cancer by age, the 4 cases occurred in patients who were 5 to 15 years at transplant and 10–23 when they developed papillary carcinoma of the thyroid, which is consistent with thyroid cancer developing later in life after exposure to irradiation at a young age [49, 50]. That brain tumors were associated with younger age at the time of transplant is also consistent with reports of elevated brain and nervous system cancer risk after children were treated with cranial irradiation for tinea capitis [51].

Older patient age (by decade) was associated with an elevated risk of developing adenocarcinoma. However, site-specific adenocarcinoma occurrences were not seen at an elevated risk compared to the age-adjusted incidence of site-specific adenocarcinoma in the general population. Basal cell carcinoma occurred in older patients. One would expect a similar increase in basal cell carcinoma with increasing age in the general population, but since the SEER database does not track basal cell carcinoma, it was not possible to compare the incidence of basal cell carcinoma in older patients with that of the general population.

Donor Leukemias and Myelodysplasia

None of the factors was identified as predisposing to the development of a secondary leukemia, myelodysplasia or a secondary myeloproliferative disorder. We initially hypothesized that transplantation in relapse might lead to a secondary leukemia in donor cells, similar to the in vitro process of transfection of a dominant oncogene from a malignant cell to a normal cell. However, there was no correlation between transplantation in relapse and the subsequent development of new leukemia in donor cells. The tools of molecular biology now available may allow us to study whether an oncogene can be transferred from host to donor tissue.

Tumors after Autologous Transplantation

In this report, 6 of 684 patients given autologous marrow developed secondary solid tumors a median 1,824 days (60.3 months) after transplant. The median follow-up of our autologous patients who did not develop a solid tumor was 208 days. None of the autologous patients developed MDS during this follow-up period. In contrast, secondary MDS occurred after transplantation with autologous hematopoietic stem cells for lymphoma in 20/262 patients reported by Stone et al. [52], in 12/511 reported by Darrington et al. [53], and in 9/206 reported by Miller et al. [54].

Since the median time of follow-up of our autologous patients was 211 days (7.0 months), and the MDS was identified between 31 and 44 months in the other reports, it is possible that our follow-up is too short to identify MDS in autologous transplant patients. Similarly, since the median time to development of a secondary solid tumor in our autologous patients was 60.3 months, the follow-up of the patients in the other reports may not have been long enough to identify solid tumors. In these patients, the pretransplant treatment likely plays a more important role in leading to myelodysplasia or secondary leukemia than does the specific transplantation process [55]. Irradiation and chemotherapy conditioning for marrow grafting are expected to be important in the development of solid tumors [56, 57].

Can the Risk Be Predicted?

As our understanding of the molecular basis for neoplasia grows, some questions arise about secondary cancers in hematopoietic stem-cell transplant patients. In families with the Li-Fraumeni syndrome, individuals develop multiple tumors early in life. The increased frequency of malignancy in these patients has been traced to mutations in the p53 tumor suppressor gene and a defect in the germline DNA. Tumor samples taken from squamous cell carcinoma not associated with the Li-Fraumeni syndrome have also shown mutations in p53 [58, 59]. Similar mutations have been described in malignancies of thyroid [60], parotid [61], colon, breast, lung, and tumor tissue taken from 4 of 59 children and young adults with second primary cancer [62]. It is reasonable to hypothesize that irradiation has the potential to result in mutations in the p53 tumor suppressor gene complex.

Viral infection with EBV and human papilloma virus (HPV) may interact with p53 as well. EBNA5, an EBV nucleoprotein, has been shown to combine with p53 and the retinoblastoma tumor suppressor genes and can potentially affect p53 pathways [63]. HPV type 16, E6 has been demonstrated to bind with p53 and result in its degradation [64]. Patients with epidermodysplasia verruciformis are not capable of containing infection with HPV. Epidermodysplasia verruciformis is very frequent in squamous cell cancers of patients receiving immunosuppression for renal allografts. Acquired mutations in p53 may result from irradiation and/or interaction with EBV and HPV proteins in stem-cell transplant recipients. Study of tumor and normal tissue in these patients will be important to establish these potential links in the pathogenesis of secondary neoplasia and to distinguish those who may undergo transplant treatment with a predisposition for developing cancer.

Conclusion

The risk of developing secondary cancer after marrow transplantation is higher than that of the general population for developing a primary cancer. It is highest in the first year for PTLD and leukemia, and extends beyond 6 years for solid tumors. The risk of secondary malignancy is highest for patients receiving irradiation conditioning and for those being treated with immunosuppressive medications for acute or chronic GVHD. The long risk period for appearance of solid tumors means that lifelong surveillance is vital.

Acknowledgements

The authors wish to thank Keith Sullivan, MD, Mary Flowers, MD, and the long-term follow-up staff of the Clinical Research Division for maintaining the database for these patients; Charles Swartz, Marry Potts, Diane Guay, and Paul Maier of the Cancer Surveillance Statistics Department of the Public Health Sciences Division for preparing the files for comparison with the SEER data, and Kathy Knox for expert technical assistance in preparing the manuscript.

Supported in part by grants CA 18221, CA 18029, CA 15704 and CP 21103 of the National Cancer Institute and HL 36444 of the National Heart, Lung, and Blood Institute of the National Institutes of Health, DHHS, Bethesda, Md., USA.

References

1   Witherspoon RP, Fisher LD, Schoch G, Martin P, Sullivan KM, Sanders J, Deeg HJ, Doney K, Thomas D, Storb R, Thomas ED: Secondary cancers after bone marrow transplantation for leukemia or aplastic anemia. N Engl J Med 1989;321:784–789.
2   Thomas ED, Clift RA, Hersman J, Sanders JE, Stewart P, Buckner CD, Fefer A, McGuffin R, Smith JW, Storb R: Marrow transplantation for acute nonlymphoblastic leukemia in first remission using fractionated or single-dose irradiation. Int J Radiat Oncol Biol Phys 1982;8:817–821.
3   Badger C, Buckner CD, Thomas ED, Clift RA, Sanders JE, Stewart PS, Storb R, Sullivan KM, Shulman H, Flournoy N: Allogeneic marrow transplantation for acute leukemia in relapse. Leuk Res 1982;6:383–387.
4   Santos GW, Tutschka PJ, Brookmeyer R, Saral R, Beschorner WE, Bias WB, Braine HG, Burns WH, Elfenbein GJ, Kaizer H, Mellits D, Sensenbrenner LL, Stuart RK, Yeager AM: Marrow transplantation for acute nonlymphocytic leukemia after treatment with busulfan and cyclophosphamide. N Engl J Med 1983;309:1347–1353.
5   Radich JP, Sanders JE, Buckner CD, Martin PJ, Peterson FB, Bensinger W, McDonald GB, Mori M, Schoch G, Hansen JA: Second allogeneic marrow transplantation for patients with recurrent leukemia after initial transplant with total-body irradiation-containing regimens. J Clin Oncol 1993;11:304–313.
6   Storb R, Thomas ED, Weiden PL, Buckner CD, Clift RA, Fefer A, Fernando LP, Giblett ER, Goodell BW, Johnson FL, Lerner KG, Neiman PE, Sanders JE: Aplastic anemia treated by allogeneic bone marrow transplantation: A report on 49 new cases from Seattle. Blood 1976;48:817–841.
7   Thomas ED, Storb R, Clift RA, Fefer A, Johnson FL, Neiman PE, Lerner KG, Glucksberg H, Buckner CD: Bone-marrow transplantation. N Engl J Med 1975;292:832–843, 895–902.

8   Doney KC, Weiden PL, Storb R, Thomas ED: Failure of early administration of antithymocyte globulin to lessen graft-versus-host disease in human allogeneic marrow transplant recipients. Transplantation 1981;31:141–143.

9   Deeg HJ, Storb R, Thomas ED, Flournoy N, Kennedy MS, Banaji M, Appelbaum FR, Bensinger WI, Buckner CD, Clift RA, Doney K, Fefer A, McGuffin R, Sanders JE, Singer J, Stewart P, Sullivan KM, Witherspoon RP: Cyclosporine as prophylaxis for graft-versus-host disease: A randomized study in patients undergoing marrow transplantation for acute nonlymphoblastic leukemia. Blood 1985;65:1325–1334.

10 Storb R, Deeg HJ, Whitehead J, Appelbaum F, Beatty P, Bensinger W, Buckner CD, Clift R, Doney K, Farewell V, Hansen J, Hill R, Lum L, Martin P, McGuffin R, Sanders J, Stewart P, Sullivan K, Witherspoon R, Yee G, Thomas ED: Methotrexate and cyclosporine compared with cyclosporine alone for prophylaxis of acute graft-versus-host disease after marrow transplantation for leukemia. N Engl J Med 1986;314:729–735.

11 Martin PJ, Hansen JA, Buckner CD, Sanders JE, Deeg HJ, Stewart P, Appelbaum FR, Clift R, Fefer A, Witherspoon RP, Kennedy MS, Sullivan KM, Flournoy N, Storb R, Thomas ED: Effects of in vitro depletion of T cells in HLA-identical allogeneic marrow grafts. Blood 1985;66:664–672.

12 Deeg HJ, Lin D, Leisenring W, Boeckh M, Anasetti C, Appelbaum FR, Chauncey TR, Doney K, Flowers M, Martin P, Nash R, Schoch G, Sullivan KM, Witherspoon RP, Storb R: Cyclosporine or cyclosporine plus methylprednisolone for prophylaxis of graft-versus-host disease: A prospective, randomized trial. Blood 1997;89:3880–3887.

13 Doney KC, Weiden PL, Storb R, Thomas ED: Treatment of graft-versus-host disease in human allogeneic marrow graft recipients: A randomized trial comparing antithymocyte globulin and corticosteroids. Am J Hematol 1981;11:1–8.

14 Kennedy MS, Deeg HJ, Storb R, Doney K, Sullivan KM, Witherspoon RP, Appelbaum FR, Stewart P, Sanders J, Buckner CD, Martin P, Weiden P, Thomas ED: Treatment of acute graft-versus-host disease after allogeneic marrow transplantation: Randomized study comparing corticosteroids and cyclosporine. Am J Med 1985;78:978–983.

15 Martin PJ, Shulman HM, Schubach WH, Hansen JA, Fefer A, Miller G, Thomas ED: Fatal Epstein-Barr-virus-associated proliferation of donor B cells after treatment of acute graft-versus-host disease with a murine monoclonal anti-T-cell antibody. Ann Intern Med 1984;101:310–315.

16 Anasetti C, Martin PJ, Storb R, Appelbaum FR, Beatty PG, Davis J, Doney K, Hill HF, Stewart P, Sullivan KM, Witherspoon RP, Thomas ED, Hansen JA: Treatment of acute graft-versus-host disease with a nonmitogenic anti-CD3 monoclonal antibody. Transplantation 1992;54:844–851.

17 Martin PJ, Nelson BJ, Appelbaum FR, Anasetti C, Deeg HJ, Hansen JA, McDonald GB, Nash RA, Sullivan KM, Witherspoon RP, Scannon PJ, Friedmann N, Storb R: Evaluation of a CD5-specific immunotoxin for treatment of acute graft-versus-host disease after allogeneic marrow transplantation. Blood 1996;88:824–830.

18 Sullivan KM, Witherspoon RP, Storb R, Deeg HJ, Dahlberg S, Sanders JE, Appelbaum FR, Doney KC, Weiden P, Anasetti C, Loughran TP, Hill R, Shields A, Yee G, Shulman H, Nims J, Strom S, Thomas ED: Alternating-day cyclosporine and prednisone for treatment of high-risk chronic graft-versus-host disease. Blood 1988;72:555–561.

19 Sullivan KM, Witherspoon RP, Storb R, Weiden P, Flournoy N, Dahlberg S, Deeg HJ, Sanders JE, Doney KC, Appelbaum FR, McGuffin R, McDonald GB, Meyers J, Schubert MM, Gauvreau J, Shulman HM, Sale GE, Anasetti C, Loughran TP, Strom S, Nims J, Thomas ED:

Prednisone and azathioprine compared with prednisone and placebo for treatment of chronic graft-versus-host disease: Prognostic influence of prolonged thrombocytopenia after allogeneic marrow transplantation. Blood 1988;72:546–554.

20 Kalbfleisch JD, Prentice RL: The Statistical Analysis of Failure Time Data, 1980.

21 Anonymous: BMDP Statistical Software, 1985.

22 Thorley-Lawson DA, Chess L, Strominger JL: Suppression of in vitro Epstein-Barr virus infection. A new role for adult human T lymphocytes. J Exp Med 1977;146:495–508.

23 Meignin V, Devergie A, Brice P, Brison O, Parquet N, Ribaud P, Cojean I, Gaulard P, Gluckman E, Socie G, Janin A: Hodgkin's disease of donor origin after allogeneic bone marrow transplantation for myelogenous chronic leukemia (review). Transplantation 1998;65:595–597.

24 Okos AJ, Lum LG, Storb R: Epstein-Barr virus (EBV) induced immunoglobulin production and suppression by EBV immune T-cells in bone marrow transplant recipients. Blood 1983;62:227A.

25 Liebowitz D: Epstein-Barr virus and a cellular signaling pathway in lymphomas from immunosuppressed patients. N Engl J Med 1998;338:1413–1421.

26 Zutter MM, Durnam DM, Hackman RC, Loughran TP Jr, Kidd PG, Hanke D, Ashley RL, Petersdorf EW, Martin PJ, Thomas ED: Secondary T-cell lymphoproliferation after marrow transplantation. Am J Clin Pathol 1990;94:714–721.

27 Hanson MN, Morrison VA, Peterson BA, Stieglbauer KT, Kubic VL, McCormick SR, McGlennen RC, Manivel JC, Brunning RD, Litz CE: Posttransplant T-cell lymphoproliferative disorders – an aggressive, late complication of solid-organ transplantation. Blood 1996;88:3626–3633.

28 Leblond V, Davi F, Charlotte F, Dorent R, Bitker MO, Sutton L, Gandjbakhch I, Binet JL, Raphael M: Posttransplant lymphoproliferative disorders not associated with Epstein-Barr virus: A distinct entity? J Clin Oncol 1998;16:2052–2059.

29 Storb R, Deeg HJ, Thomas ED, Appelbaum FR, Buckner CD, Cheever MA, Clift RA, Doney KC, Flournoy N, Kennedy MS, Loughran TP, McGuffin RW, Sale GE, Sanders JE, Singer JW, Stewart PS, Sullivan KM, Witherspoon RP: Marrow transplantation for chronic myelocytic leukemia: A controlled trial of cyclosporine versus methotrexate for prophylaxis of graft-versus-host disease. Blood 1985;66:698–702.

30 Storb R, Deeg HJ, Farewell V, Doney K, Appelbaum F, Beatty P, Bensinger W, Buckner CD, Clift R, Hansen J, Hill R, Longton G, Lum L, Martin P, McGuffin R, Sanders J, Singer J, Stewart P, Sullivan K, Witherspoon R, Thomas ED: Marrow transplantation for severe aplastic anemia: Methotrexate alone compared with a combination of methotrexate and cyclosporine for prevention of acute graft-versus-host disease. Blood 1986;68:119–125.

31 Nash RA, Pepe MS, Storb R, Longton G, Pettinger M, Anasetti C, Appelbaum FR, Bowden R, Deeg HJ, Doney K, Martin PJ, Sullivan KM, Sanders J, Witherspoon RP: Acute graft-versus-host disease: Analysis of risk factors after allogeneic marrow transplantation and prophylaxis with cyclosporine and methotrexate. Blood 1992;80:1838–1845.

32 Clift RA, Buckner CD, Appelbaum FR, Bryant E, Bearman SI, Petersen FB, Fisher LD, Anasetti C, Beatty P, Bensinger WI, Doney K, Hill RS, McDonald GB, Martin P, Meyers J, Sanders J, Singer J, Stewart P, Sullivan KM, Witherspoon R, Storb R, Hansen JA, Thomas ED: Allogeneic marrow transplantation in patients with chronic myeloid leukemia in the chronic phase: A randomized trial of two irradiation regimens. Blood 1991;77:1660–1665.

33 Clift RA, Buckner CD, Appelbaum FR, Bearman SI, Petersen FB, Fisher LD, Anasetti C, Beatty P, Bensinger WI, Doney K, Hill R, McDonald G, Martin P, Sanders J, Singer J, Stewart P,

Sullivan KM, Witherspoon R, Storb R, Hansen J, Thomas ED: Allogeneic marrow transplantation in patients with acute myeloid leukemia in first remission: A randomized trial of two irradiation regimens. Blood 1990;76:1867–1871.

34   Sullivan JL, Medveczky P, Forman SJ, Baker SM, Monroe JE, Mulder C: Epstein-Barr-virus induced lymphoproliferation. Implications for antiviral chemotherapy. N Engl J Med 1984;311:1163–1167.

35   Rooney CM, Smith CA, Ng CY, Loftin S, Li C, Krance RA, Brenner MK, Heslop HE: Use of gene-modified virus-specific T lymphocytes to control Epstein-Barr-virus-related lymphoproliferation. Lancet 1995;345:9–13.

36   Papadopoulos EB, Ladanyi M, Emanuel D, Mackinnon S, Boulad F, Carabasi MH, Castro-Malaspina H, Childs BH, Gillio AP, Small TN, Young JW, Kernan NA, O'Reilly RJ: Infusions of donor leukocytes to treat Epstein-Barr virus-associated lymphoproliferative disorders after allogeneic bone marrow transplantation. N Engl J Med 1994;330: 1185–1191.

37   Bonini C, Ferrari G, Verzeletti S, Servida P, Zappone E, Ruggieri L, Ponzoni M, Rossini S, Mavilio F, Traversari C, Bordignon C: HSV-TK gene transfer into donor lymphocytes for control of allogeneic graft-versus-leukemia. Science 1997;276:1719–1724.

38   Lishner M, Patterson B, Kandel R, Fyles G, Curtis JE, Meharchand J, Minden MD, Messner HA: Cutaneous and mucosal neoplasms in bone marrow transplant recipients. Cancer 1990;65:473–476.

39   Lowsky R, Lipton J, Fyles G, Minden M, Meharchand J, Tejpar I, Atkins H, Sutcliffe S, Messner H: Secondary malignancies after bone marrow transplantation in adults. J Clin Oncol 1994;12:2187–2192.

40   Deeg HJ, Socié G, Schoch G, Henry-Amar M, Witherspoon RP, Devergie A, Sullivan KM, Gluckman E, Storb R: Malignancies after marrow transplantation for aplastic anemia and Fanconi anemia: A joint Seattle and Paris analysis of results in 700 patients. Blood 1996;87:386–392.

41   Gupta AK, Cardella CJ, Haberman HF: Cutaneous malignant neoplasms in patients with renal transplants. Arch Dermatol 1986;122:1288–1293.

42   Tucker MA, D'Angio GJ, Boice JD Jr, Strong LC, Li FP, Stovall M, Stone BJ, Green DM, Lombardi F, Newton W, Hoover RN, Fraumeni JF Jr: Bone sarcomas linked to radiotherapy and chemotherapy in children. N Engl J Med 1987;317:588–593.

43   Curtis RE, Rowlings PA, Deeg HJ, Shriner DA, Socié G, Travis LB, Horowitz MM, Witherspoon RP, Hoover RN, Sobocinski KA, Fraumeni JF Jr, Boice JD Jr, Schoch HG, Sale GE, Storb R, Travis WD, Kolb HJ, Gale RP, Passweg JR: Solid cancers after bone marrow transplantation. N Engl J Med 1997;336:897–904.

44   Socié G, Henry-Amar M, Cosset JM, Devergie A, Girinsky T, Gluckman E: Increased incidence of solid malignant tumors after bone marrow transplantation for severe aplastic anemia. Blood 1991;78:277–279.

45   Socié G, Henry-Amar M, Bacigalupo A, Hows J, Tichelli A, Ljungman P, McCann SR, Frickhofen N, Van't Veer-Korthof E, Gluckman E, for the European Bone Marrow Transplantation-Severe Aplastic Anaemia Working Party: Malignant tumors occurring after treatment of aplastic anemia. N Engl J Med 1993;329:1152–1157.

46   Greene MH, Young TI, Clark WH Jr: Malignant melanoma in renal transplant recipients. Lancet 1981;i:1196–1199.

47   Manusow D, Weiberman BH: Subsequent neoplasia in chronic lymphocytic leukemia. JAMA 1975;232:267–269.

48   Sanders J, Sale GE, Ramberg R, Clift R, Buckner CD, Thomas ED: Glioblastoma multiforme in a patient with acute lymphoblastic leukemia who received a marrow transplant. Transplant Proc 1982;14:770–774.

49   Ron E, Modan B, Preston D, Alfandary E, Stovall M, Boice JD Jr: Thyroid neoplasia following low-dose radiation in childhood. Radiat Res 1989;120:516–531.

50   Shore RE, Hildreth N, Dvoretsky P, Andresen E, Moseson M, Pasternack B: Thyroid cancer among persons given X-ray treatment in infancy for an enlarged thymus gland. Am J Epidemiol 1993;137:1068–1080.

51   Ron E, Modan B, Boice JD Jr, Alfandary E, Stovall M, Chetrit A, Katz L: Tumors of the brain and nervous system after radiotherapy in childhood. N Engl J Med 1988;319:1033–1039.

52   Stone RM, Neuberg D, Soiffer R, Takvorian T, Whelan M, Rabinowe SN, Aster JC, Leavitt P, Mauch P, Freedman AS, Nadler LM: Myelodysplastic syndrome as a late complication following autologous bone marrow transplantation for non-Hodgkin's lymphoma. J Clin Oncol 1994;12:2535–2542.

53   Darrington DL, Vose JM, Anderson JR, Bierman PJ, Bishop MR, Chan WC, Morris ME, Reed EC, Sanger WG, Tarantolo SR, Weisenburger DD, Kessinger A, Armitage JO: Incidence and characterization of secondary myelodysplastic syndrome and acute myelogenous leukemia following high-dose chemoradiotherapy and autologous stem-cell transplantation for lymphoid malignancies. J Clin Oncol 1994;12:2527–2534.

54   Miller JS, Arthur DC, Litz CE, Neglia JP, Miller WJ, Weisdorf DJ: Myelodysplastic syndrome after autologous bone marrow transplantation: An additional late complication of curative cancer therapy. Blood 1994;83:3780–3786.

55   Govindarajan R, Jagannath S, Flick JT, Vesole DH, Sawyer J, Barlogie B, Tricot G: Preceding standard therapy is the likely cause of MDS after autotransplants for multiple myeloma. Br J Haematol 1996;95:349–353.

56   Andre M, Henry-Amar M, Blaise D, Colombat P, Fleury J, Milpied N, Cahn JY, Pico JL, Bastion Y, Kuentz M, Biron P, Ferme C, Gisselbrecht C: Incidence of second cancers and causes of death after autologous stem cell transplantation for Hodgkin's disease. Blood 1995;86:460a, abstract 1826.

57   Bhatia S, Ramsay NK, Steinbuch M, Dusenbery KE, Shapiro RS, Weisdorf DJ, Robison LL, Miller JS, Neglia JP: Malignant neoplasms following bone marrow transplantation. Blood 1996;87:3633–3639.

58   Nylander K, Nilsson P, Mehle C, Roos G: p53 mutations, protein expression and cell proliferation in squamous cell carcinomas of the head and neck. Br J Cancer 1995;71:826–830.

59   Nylander K, Schildt EB, Eriksson M, Magnusson A, Mehle C, Roos G: A non-random deletion in the p53 gene in oral squamous cell carcinoma. Br J Cancer 1996;73:1381–1386.

60   Fogelfeld L, Bauer TK, Schneider AB, Swartz JE, Zitman R: p53 gene mutations in radiation-induced thyroid cancer. J Clin Endocrinol Metab 1996;81:3039–3044.

61   Gallo O, Franchi A, Bianchi S, Boddi V, Giannelli E, Alajmo E: p53 oncoprotein expression in parotid gland carcinoma is associated with clinical outcome. Cancer 1995;75:2037–2044.

62   Malkin D, Jolly KW, Barbier N, Look AT, Friend SH, Gebhardt MC, Andersen TI, Borresen AL, Li FP, Garber J, Strong LC: Germline mutations of the p53 tumor-suppressor gene in children and young adults with second malignant neoplasms. N Engl J Med 1992; 326:1309–1315.

63   Szekely L, Selivanova G, Magnusson KP, Klein G, Wiman KG: EBNA-5, an Epstein-Barr virus-encoded nuclear antigen, binds to the retinoblastoma and p53 proteins. Proc Natl Acad Sci USA 1993;90:5455–5459.

64   Werness BA, Levine AJ, Howley PM: Association of human papillomavirus types 16 and 18
      E6 proteins with p53. Science 1990;248:76–79.

Robert P. Witherspoon, MD, Fred Hutchinson Cancer Research Center, Clinical Research
Division, 1100 Fairview Ave N, PO Box 19024, Seattle, WA 98109-1024 (USA)
Fax +1 206 667 7693

Rüther U, Nunnensiek C, Schmoll H-J (eds): Secondary Neoplasias following Chemotherapy, Radiotherapy, and Immunosuppression. Contrib Oncol. Basel, Karger, 2000, vol 55, pp 225–241

Malignancy following Kidney Transplantation

Christoph J. Olbricht

Transplantationszentrum Stuttgart, Katharinenhospital, Stuttgart, Deutschland

Introduction

Compared with an age-matched control population, postrenal transplantation patients have a higher risk of developing malignancies. The first indication that immunosuppressed transplant patients were susceptible to cancer came with the transplantation of apparently normal kidneys removed from donors dying of cancer. It was soon recognized that such organs could harbor malignant cells that could proliferate in the recipient [1, 2]. A few years later, the first reports of cancer arising de novo in transplant recipients appeared [3, 4]. Given the predisposition of immunosuppressed transplant recipients to malignant disease, we must ask whether it is safe for patients who have had malignancies to undergo transplantation.

In an early review of patients with preexisting cancer who went on to renal transplantation, an increased recurrence rate of malignancies was demonstrated [5]. Three different mechanisms may contribute to this increased risk of malignancy following renal transplantation: recurrence of previous malignancies, transferred malignancies, and de novo malignancies. While the risk of malignancies is increased following renal transplantation in comparison to an age-matched control population, one must ask whether the risk is also increased compared to that of patients undergoing dialysis. Therefore, this chapter will also review the occurrence of malignancies in dialysis patients.

Malignancies in Dialysis Patients

The incidence of malignancies in patients undergoing dialysis is increased [6–13]. However, this correlation does not prove a causal relationship between chronic uremia and the pathogenesis of malignancy. Nor is it surprising that cancers affecting renal function are much more common in patients on dialysis than in the general population. For instance, renal failure may be the consequence of having removed all functioning renal tissue to cure renal or ureteral malignancies. Or, multiple myeloma may cause terminal renal failure in a substantial number of affected patients. In yet other cases, patients have conditions which cause renal failure and which are also associated with a high incidence of malignancy; for instance, analgesic nephropathy or long-term treatment with cyclosporine for extrarenal indications.

There is controversy over whether dialysis patients are more susceptible to malignancy other than that affecting the renal tract. Most authors conclude that there is an increased incidence of malignancy in chronic renal failure [6–10, 12]. Others find no increase [11], or an increase in skin and colon cancer only [13]. The most detailed and reliable information concerning cancer in dialysis patients comes from the Australia and New Zealand Combined Dialysis and Transplant Registry. The 1991 Registry Report included 13,524 patients on dialysis. Of these, 380 (3%) developed malignancies involving the skin, and an additional 337 (2%) developed malignancies of other organs [12]. All malignancies were diagnosed for the first time while patients were on dialysis, and in no case did a patient need dialysis because of malignancy. Almost one third of malignancies other than skin involved the kidney, bladder and ureter (122 patients). The reasons for this surprisingly high incidence include the presence of analgesic nephropathy with the associated increased risk of urothelial carcinoma, and the development of secondary renal cysts in approximately 80% of patients with terminal renal failure, which is associated with a 6–7% risk of renal cancer [14–17]. If the group with renal and urothelial malignancies is not considered, the rate of cancer development is still approximately twice that expected in the age-matched general population. Taken together, there is considerable evidence indicating increased risk of developing malignancy during renal replacement therapy with dialysis. Periodic careful cancer screening, including of the native kidneys, is therefore recommended.

Recurrence of Malignancy following Renal Transplantation

It is generally accepted that immunosuppressive therapy favors the growth of existing cancer cells. Therefore, a current malignancy excludes transplantation. Only patients with curative cancer treatment are candidates for renal transplantation. However, the recurrence of cancer after transplantation is a considerable risk in these patients also, so that a prudent waiting period extending from the time of malignancy therapy to the time of transplantation will exclude patients who would otherwise develop recurrence. The best available data on this topic were collected by the Cincinnati Transplant Tumor Registry (CTTR), an international registry for malignancies in solid organ transplantation [18]. The CTTR data show that 87% of recurrences occur within 5 years following kidney transplantation. However, such a long waiting time prior to registration on the transplant waiting list is not practical, particularly in the many elderly individuals requiring a kidney graft. Overall, a 2-year waiting period would eliminate about 53% of recurrences and seems to be an acceptable hiatus for most, but not all, types of malignancy. Tumor screening of all patients should be performed prior to acceptance for renal transplantation. Even so, it is not uncommon for some malignancies, including prostate, stomach and multiple myeloma, to be missed prior to transplantation or to develop during an extended waiting time before transplantation. Hence, older patients who have been on the transplant waiting list for an extended period of time should be evaluated periodically for occult tumors.

Multiple Myeloma

Approximately 40% of patients with myeloma may have recurrent plasmocytic bone marrow infiltration. Furthermore, 75% of patients with monoclonal gammopathy progress to multiple myeloma after transplantation, a number considerably higher than that observed in patients without immunosuppression. Many patients with a history of multiple myeloma who undergo transplantation succumb to systemic bacterial or fungal infection [19, 20].

Urogenital Tumors

According to the CTTR data, asymptomatic *renal cell carcinomas* discovered incidentally before or at the time of transplantation did not recur [18]. This is probably because of the discovery of the tumor at an early stage. In these patients, a 1-year waiting period prior to transplantation may be appropriate. However, if the incidental tumor is large or has infiltrated beyond the confines of the kidney, a longer waiting period is mandatory. In patients with a symptomatic renal tumor, a 30% recurrence rate was observed following solid organ transplantation. 61% of the cases occurred during the first 2 years after transplantation; 33% within 2–5 years, and 6% beyond 5 years. Therefore, a waiting time of at least 2 years should eliminate 61% of the recurrences. Likewise, the recommended waiting time for *Wilm's tumor* is at least 2 years following therapy. Shorter waiting times were associated with high mortality following transplantation (79%) [18, 21].

Patients with *in situ bladder cancer* or noninvasive papilloma tumors have a low risk of recurrence, and in general do not require a waiting period [18]. Invasive bladder cancer necessitates a waiting time of 2 years to eliminate recurrence in almost two thirds of the cases.

In the CTTR data, the vast majority of patients with *in situ cervical cancers* did not develop recurrence. This is partially explained by the fact that most patients had a 2- to 5-year hiatus between treatment and transplantation. Given the very small number of published cases, it is difficult to make a definitive recommendation for the management of patients with a history of invasive cervical cancer. Cervical cytology screening should probably be routinely performed every 1–3 years in women aged 20–65 years, as recommended for the adult general population [22]. In patients with *uterine body cancer,* a recurrence rate of 11% has been described, with a time lag of up to 60 months [18].

Testicular cancers, including seminomas, teratomas, embryomas, choriocarcinomas and unclassified tumors, have a low recurrence rate of 3%, attributed to the generally longer interval between treatment and transplantation. In fact, 26% have a 2- to 5-year waiting period, and 52% have a waiting period of more than 5 years. In summary, a waiting period of 2 years and testicular examination regularly are recommended [18, 22]. In patients with *prostate cancer,* the recurrence rate was 24%, and 40% of the recurrences developed in patients treated less than 2 years before transplantation. The average time of recurrence following transplantation in the remaining 60% was 44 months. The recommended waiting time is 2 years [18].

Sarcomas

The CTTR included 16 patients with osteosarcoma, Ewing's sarcoma, fibrosarcoma, Kaposi's sarcoma, leiomyosarcoma, and angioleiomyosarcoma. Recurrence was noted in 4 patients at 2, 3.5 and 20 years after transplantation. Patients who did not develop recurrence were treated more than 2–5 years before transplantation. Hence, it is difficult to make a recommendation. It seems prudent to allow a waiting time of more than 2 years.

Thyroid Carcinoma

The different forms of thyroid carcinoma – including papillary, follicular, mixed, medullary and unclassified tumors – were noted in 39 patients of the CTTR database. Three recurrences occurred in patients treated variably from 1 week to 96 months before transplantation. Those without recurrence either had low-grade papillary tumors or had been treated more than 2–5 years before transplantation. Therefore, it is reasonable to wait for 2 years before permitting patients with thyroid cancer to undergo renal transplantation [18].

Breast Cancer

The recurrence rate was 25% in a time frame of between less than 5 years and more than 15 years. This time span makes it difficult to give a recommendation. Risk factors for recurrence included regional lymph node involvement, bilateral disease and inflammatory histopathology. Patients with in situ lobular carcinoma may have a relatively favorable prognosis, so that a prolonged waiting time may not be warranted. However, for many patients it may be prudent to wait at least 2 and possibly more than 5 years [18]. Breast examination should be performed yearly in women over 40, and yearly after the age of 35 if breast cancer occurred before menopause in a first-degree relative [22].

Colorectal Cancers

Recurrence of colorectal cancer was noted in 8 (21%) of 38 patients in the CTTR data [18]. Only 1 patient was treated 2 years before transplantation. Of the patients without recurrence, 20 (57%) were treated more than 2–5 years before transplantation. Patients with in situ Duke's A carcinoma may have a relatively favorable prognosis, so that a prolonged waiting time may not be necessary. For all other patients with previous colorectal cancer, a waiting time of 5 years is mandatory. Routine testing for occult blood in the stool in individuals over 50 should be performed yearly; in individuals over 40 with a history of colon cancer in a first-degree relative or a history of inflammatory bowel disease, testing for occult blood in the stool and periodic sigmoidoscopy may be warranted [23]. Colonoscopy may be considered in individuals with more than 1 first-degree relative with colon cancer or a history of ulcerative colitis for at least 10 years, adenomatous polyps, or familial polyposis [22, 23].

Lymphoma and Skin Cancers

Recurrence was observed in approximately 10% of patients with *non-Hodgkin's lymphoma,* but not in patients with Hodgkin's lymphoma [18]. At least a 2-year waiting period is recommended. The recurrence rate in *melanoma* patients was 30%. Fifty percent of the patients were treated less than 2 years before transplantation; 33% were treated between 2 and 5 years, and 17% were treated 10 years before transplantation. It seems prudent that patients with melanoma should wait 5 years before undergoing transplantation. In patients with *nonmelanoma skin cancer,* 62% developed recurrence and/or new lesions. Most recurrences (61%) were observed within 2 years following transplantation. It is therefore recommended that patients with *squamous cell carcinomas* wait for 2 years before transplantation. *Basal cell cancers* have a lesser tendency to invade and metastasize and may thus not require a waiting period [18].

In summary, for most malignancies, patients should have been free of recurrence for 2 years before transplantation. However, a longer waiting period may be advisable for most malignant melanomas, breast cancer and colorectal carcinomas. No waiting period may be necessary for some malignancies such as incidentally discovered renal cell carcinomas, in situ carcinomas, and basal cell skin cancer [18].

Transferred Malignancies in Renal Transplant Recipients

A large proportion of patients who receive organ grafts from cancer-affected donors develop cancer both in the organ transplanted and systemically [24]. In rare cases, cessation of immunosuppressive therapy and removal of the allograft result in rejection of the cancer with apparent cure [25, 26]. However, most patients with transferred cancer go on to die of malignancy [27]. Potential organ donors with malignancies, therefore, should be excluded from further consideration as donors. Because of the severe shortage of donor organs, exceptions are made for donors with primary intracerebral malignancy or those with low-grade cancer of the skin, because such tumors rarely metastasize. However, most transplant centers may not use organs from patients with a recurrence of cerebral malignancy, since prior surgery may increase the risk of metastasis considerably. Transmission of the cerebral cancer with a transplanted organ has been observed. Furthermore, transmission of metastases with liver grafts has been observed from donors with glioblastoma. Hence, patients dying of intracerebral glioblastoma should probably not be considered as organ donors, irrespective of prior brain surgery [28–31].

De novo Malignancies after Renal Transplantation

Compared to an age-matched control population, the risk of de novo malignancies is increased following renal transplantation [13, 32–41]. In addition, in renal transplantation it is appropriate to compare the risk of de novo cancer following transplantation with the risk of patients with renal replacement therapy by dialysis. Unfortunately, there are no prospective data available, although in a retrospective analysis of a comparatively small number of patients from California, no significant difference between cancer risks in dialysis patients (3%) and after transplantation (4.9%) was present [9]. The registry of the European Dialysis and Transplant Society showed a slightly higher incidence of all malignancies following renal transplantation – compared with dialysis patients – in men over 45 and in women aged

65–74. Malignancies with significantly higher incidence included colon cancer in males, cervical cancer in females, lymphoma and skin malignancies [13].

The data should be interpreted with great caution since reporting to this registry has recently been consistently low (44–67%). It is therefore conceivable that the data included are biased [42]. However, all reports taken together showed clear evidence of an increased rate of skin malignancies and lymphomas in patients after renal transplantation, compared with patients undergoing dialysis.

Reports on the incidence of cancer in transplant recipients vary considerably. Transplant centers from Germany, Denmark and Japan reported a cancer incidence following renal transplantation of 2.8, 4.4 and 4.1%, respectively [32, 35, 39, 41]. Series from Great Britain and the US with a longer observation period showed an incidence of malignancies after transplantation of between 7 and 19.7%. The Australia and New Zealand Combined Dialysis and Transplant Registry demonstrated a cancer incidence of 26% [12, 36, 40]. In part, these differences are related to the different length of follow-up. Taking time after transplantation into consideration, the risk of malignancy 10 years after transplantation is between 14 and 30%, and amounts to 40–60% at 20 years [12, 37, 38]. A good deal of the variation is due to the high incidence of skin malignancies in high-risk areas (ultraviolet radiation from sunshine) for the development of these cancers.

Considerable differences in the type of cancer are reported. In most countries, skin cancer is the leading malignancy following renal transplantation, accounting for 40–75% of all cancers [33, 36–38, 43]. The rate of skin cancer was only 6% in a report from Japan [41]. This difference is most likely related to different exposure to the sun, although a racial difference cannot be excluded. Lymphoma and urogenital cancer are the two second-most common malignancies after transplantation, accounting for approximately 10–15% of all malignancies, respectively [12, 33, 36–38, 43]. The incidence of Kaposi's sarcoma, hepatobiliary carcinomas, and a variety of sarcomas seems to be increased as well. In contrast, the incidence of many of the most common tumors in the general population – lung, prostate, colon and invasive uterine carcinomas – is not increased in comparison to an age-matched population according to the large databases of the CTTR and the Collaborative Transplant Study (CTS) [33, 34, 43]. Furthermore, according to the CTS including 23,729 female first cadaver kidney recipients, the incidence of breast cancer in women after renal transplantation appears to be reduced by 25–30% [43].

All major series consistently report no difference in the rate of malignancies between immunosuppression with azathioprine and cyclosporine [36–39]. Antilymphocyte therapy, as with OKT3 or antilymphocyte serum, specifically predisposes to posttransplant lymphoproliferative disorders which are induced by Epstein-Barr virus. With this exception, there is no evidence that a particular immunosuppressive agent causes a specific type of malignancy. Rather, it is the overall level of immunosuppression that the patient has received and continues to receive that increases the risk of posttransplant malignancy. This relationship explains why lymphoproliferative disorders, for example, are more common in recipients of solid nonrenal organs such as the heart. These patients receive more aggressive antirejection therapy – since loss of such organs would result in death – while renal transplant recipients can return to dialysis [44, 45]. This may also explain some of the differences observed between American and European registries. The lower incidence of posttransplant malignancies in Europe may be related – in part – to the usually lower overall dose of immunosuppression and the avoidance of induction therapy by OKT3 or antilymphocyte serum following renal transplantation in many transplant centers in Europe [32–40, 43].

When all cancers are considered, the average patient age is 41 years and the average time of appearance is approximately 5 years after transplantation. The average onset of certain neoplasms occurs at distinct time intervals after transplantation; for instance, Kaposi's sarcoma at 21 months; lymphomas at 32 months (although the incidence is highest during the first year, which is the time of the most intense immunosuppression); epithelial cancers at 69 months, and cancer of the vulva and perineum at 112 months [43].

General Outline of Treatment

Treatment for specific malignancies is described in the respective sections. An approach to treatment of posttransplant malignancies should begin with preventive measures. In particular, excess immunosuppression or repeated exposure to antilymphocytic drugs should be avoided. With regard to skin cancers, sun exposure should be limited by either avoidance or protective sunscreens and clothing. Patients should be examined regularly and any premalignant lesion should be treated. There are two malignancies in which reduction in, or cessation of, immunosuppressive therapy may result in regression of the tumor: lymphoma and Kaposi's sarcoma. Here, reducing exposure to cyclosporine may be particularly important. This approach is useful primarily in renal transplantation, since loss of the graft due to rejection is not a final event (see below). Solid tumors not affecting the skin are treated by standard surgical, radiotherapeutic or chemotherapeutic modalities. If chemotherapy is needed, azathioprine should be discontinued to avoid added bone marrow toxicity. Not surprisingly, the course of these malignancies appears to be more aggressive in transplant recipients, and tumor stage at detection is a critical factor in outcome.

Skin Cancer

The most common posttransplant cancers are those involving the skin and the lips. In the CTTR of more than 5,000 patients, these malignancies developed in 37%

of cases [33, 34]. The rate of occurrence corresponded with the amount of sun exposure. That is, the lower incidence of 6% in Japan [41] and 20% in Germany [35, 39], versus the higher incidence of 75% in Australia [36], may be best explained by differences in sun exposure. Premalignant and malignant skin conditions that occur in transplant recipients include keratoacanthomas, Bowen's disease, basal cell carcinoma (BCC), squamous cell carcinoma (SCC), malignant melanoma and Merkel cell carcinoma.

Skin cancer in transplant recipients differs in a number of ways from similar lesions in the general population. For example, SCC is more common than BCC [34, 36], which is the reverse of what occurs in the general population. The lesions develop at a younger age (30 vs. 60 years), and occur in multiple sites on the skin [36, 46]. In high-risk areas with strong sun exposure, the frequency of SCC is calculated to be at least 20 times that expected in a comparable population [36, 40]. Although SCC occurs mostly in parts of the body exposed to the sun, this is by no means always the case. Some patients develop almost generalized SCCs of the skin and require repeated operations for removal of lesions. In some patients, SCC involving the vulva, vagina and anus occur. There is a tendency for lesions to be multiple and aggressive and prone to recurrence and metastasis [36, 40]. SCCs can also develop from warts, although rarely. Approximately 40% of transplant recipients develop these lesions. In nearly every affected patient, there is a history of warts as a child, suggesting that development after transplantation is the result of reactivation of latent viruses rather than primary infection [47, 48]. It is still not clear whether BCC is increased in transplant recipients compared to the general population [46].

Skin cancers following renal transplantation are often characterized by a rapid course and the frequency of recurrences. These features justify immediate excision with clinical follow-up. Node metastases are more frequent than in the general population, ranging between 5 and 10% in the different studies [46]. Treatment of SCC and BCC quite often involves surgery, followed by histological control to ensure that the excision has been complete both laterally and in depth. The frequent recurrence of these cancers in transplant patients requires that systematic clinical follow-up be carried out after surgery. Treatment of multiple recurrences or progressive and extensive development of a carcinoma may benefit from concomitant radiotherapy or chemotherapy with surgery. Moreover, the recurrence and multiple lesions or a rapidly spreading carcinoma may require a reduction or discontinuation of immunosuppression. Two immunomodulatory treatments are available: oral retinoids and interferon-α. Acitretin and isoretinoin have been used at doses of between 0.5 and 1 mg/kg. Partial and complete remissions have been reported in studies with a limited number of subjects that do not allow the true value of these substances to be evaluated [49–51]. These substances may have a potential for the prevention of recurrences. Interferon-α has proved effective in treating viral cutaneous lesions and skin cancers. It can be injected intralesionally in smaller lesions or subcutaneously in larger lesions. However, we do not recommend this type of treatment since interferon may induce graft rejection [46]. Bleomycin has been proposed for intralesional treatment. Cisplatin and 5-fluorouracil are used either in association with surgery in highly progressive forms of carcinoma or in cases with more than two recurrences.

It is likely that malignant melanoma occurs with increased frequency after solid-organ transplantation [12, 46, 52]. The reported incidence in transplant recipients is 4 times that expected in the normal population. Prevention plays an essential role in reducing the risk of melanoma. Patients should be advised to avoid exposure to the sun and to use sun creams with high protection (UV index > 20). Any suspected melanocytic nevi should be removed.

Although rare, Merkel cell carcinoma deserves mention because of its grave prognosis. This tumor derives from the Merkel cell, a neuroendocrine cell present in the skin. In transplant recipients, this tumor is characterized by rapid development, frequent locoregional recurrence, and a high nodal and visceral metastatic power. A thorough excision of these tumors should be performed immediately, associated with radiotherapy at the excision site and possibly on adjacent nodal areas. Immunosuppressive treatment should be reduced or stopped, given the risk of disease progression and the fact that chemotherapy is relatively ineffective at the metastatic stage [46, 53–55].

Kaposi's Sarcoma

The occurrence of Kaposi's sarcoma (KS) in transplant patients is increased, with reported prevalence between 0.06 and 4.1%. The higher percentage was observed in populations also affected by sporadic and endemic KS, such as in subjects from black African countries and the Caribbean and Mediterranean areas. The magnitude of the increase of risk of KS conferred by transplantation was evaluated in several studies. It ranged from 25- to 400-fold [56–59]. No genetic predisposition has been identified. There is a male preponderance from 2 to 40 in different studies [summarized in 59]. The average interval between organ transplantation and onset of KS is 20 months, ranging from a few weeks to 18 years. Skin lesions are seen in >90% of all cases with KS. Leg edema often predates the skin lesions. In this situation, serological tests for human herpesvirus-8 (HHV-8) may be useful to make an early diagnosis, since HHV-8 is clearly associated with the development of KS. Oral lesions consist of purple stains on the palate and gingival hyperplasia. Extracutaneous KS most frequently involves the lymph nodes, the gastrointestinal tract and the lungs [58]. The gastrointestinal lesions rarely cause clinical symptoms, and instead usually are detected by chance.

Pulmonary involvement appears to be at a more advanced stage of the disease; it may cause dyspnea, hypoxemia, and hypercapnia due to diffuse interstitial infiltrates, pulmonary nodules and pleural effusion. Many other localizations have been reported. Regardless of the localization, the diagnosis of KS can be confirmed on the basis of its histologic features. The treatment of KS varies greatly between different transplant centers. In general, immunosuppression should be reduced to the lowest possible margin. KS may disappear in 16–17% of patients after reduction of immunosuppression [58, 59]. In renal transplant recipients with more advanced stages of KS, immunosuppression can be removed completely. Other therapeutic options include cryotherapy, cryosurgery, laser or surgical removal in cases with spreading KS, functional or aesthetic discomfort, or life-threatening risks. Intralesional chemotherapy has also been recommended, but is less popular because it is painful.

Lesions regress more rapidly after radiotherapy, but this modality poses the long-term risk of skin cancer. Different regimens of chemotherapy have been recommended, including vinblastine, bleomycin, adriamycin and doxorubicin in patients with multivisceral involvement. Mortality from KS after renal transplantation is approximately 20% [59].

Kidney and Urinary Tract Cancer

Renal transplant recipients may also be at increased risk of developing carcinoma of the native kidney, the ureter and the bladder. For instance, one study used ultrasonography to screen for masses in the native kidneys of 129 consecutive renal transplant recipients. Five patients had kidney cancer, an incidence approximately 100 times greater than that observed in the general population [60]. Other studies confirm these findings [61, 62]. Likewise, the incidence of urothelial carcinomas seems to be increased. The reasons for this much higher than expected incidence include (1) the presence of analgesic nephropathy, with the associated increased risk of urothelial carcinoma, and (2) the development of secondary renal cysts in approximately 80% of patients with terminal renal failure, which is associated with a 6–7% risk of renal cancer [14–17]. Therefore, meticulous screening for renal cell carcinoma and urothelial carcinoma prior to transplantation and during follow-up is of prime importance. Some transplant centers recommend ureteronephrectomy prior to renal transplantation in patients with analgesic nephropathy to prevent the development of urothelial carcinoma [63].

Lymphoproliferative Disorders

Lymphoproliferative disorders are some of the most serious and potentially fatal complications of chronic immunosuppression in organ transplant recipients. They account for about 20% of all malignancies following renal transplantation, versus 5% of malignancies in the general population [33, 43]. The incidence of lymphoproliferative disease in renal transplant recipients is approximately 1%, or 30–50 times higher than in the general population, with a recent trend towards increased frequency. The degree of overall immunosuppression is a major determinant of the development of a lymphoproliferative disorder [33, 45, 64].

Transplant patients who are at increased risk for lymphoproliferative disorders are those treated with both cyclosporine and azathioprine or with polyclonal or monoclonal (OKT3) antilymphocyte antibodies. In OKT3-treated patients, both the dose and the duration of therapy are important [65, 66]. The role of immunosuppression was illustrated in the CTS with the following observations: The incidence of lymphoproliferative disease was highest in the first year, the time of the most intensive immunosuppression, and fell about 80% thereafter. The incidence was much greater in heart transplant recipients in whom a greater degree of immunosuppression is required because of the more serious consequences of transplant rejection. Among patients who develop lymphoproliferative disease, renal transplant recipients were much more likely to have renal lymphoma (14.2 vs. 0.7% in heart transplant recipients), while heart transplant recipients were more likely to develop lymphoma in the heart and the lungs (17.9 vs. 6.8% in renal transplant recipients). These findings suggest that the local immune reaction against the graft may be one of the factors promoting malignant transformation [65].

The pathogenesis of posttransplant lymphoproliferative disease appears to be related to B-cell proliferation induced by infection with Epstein-Barr virus (EBV) in the setting of chronic immunosuppression [67–69]. Studies of liver transplant recipients, for example, have demonstrated EBV mRNA in hepatic tissue in most patients before overt lymphoproliferative disease was documented; this finding was generally absent in controls who did not go on to develop lymphoproliferative disease [69]. Three types of EBV-related lymphoproliferative disease occur in transplant recipients:

(1) Benign polyclonal lymphoproliferation is an infectious mononucleosis-type acute illness which develops 2–8 weeks after induction or antirejection therapy. This disorder is characterized by polyclonal B-cell proliferation with normal cytogenetics and no evidence of immunoglobulin gene rearrangements to suggest malignant transformation. It accounts for approximately 55% of cases [70].

(2) The second EBV-induced disorder is similar to the first in its clinical presentation, but is characterized by polyclonal B-cell proliferation with evidence of early malignant transformation, such as clonal cytogenetic abnormalities and immunoglobulin gene rearrangements. It accounts for approximately 30% of cases.

(3) The last disorder, accounting for about 15% of cases, is usually an extranodal condition presenting with localized solid tumors characterized by monoclonal B-cell proliferation with malignant cytogenic abnormalities and immunoglobulin gene rearrangements [70].

Not all posttransplant lymphoproliferative tumors are directly associated with EBV. Lymphomas not due to EBV appear to differ clinically from EBV-related tumors. For instance, tumors not related to EBV present much later (2,324 vs. 546 days posttransplant), and were much more virulent, with a mean survival of only 1 month as compared to 37 months in EBV-associated disease [71]. Although uncommon, posttransplant lymphoproliferative disease may also originate from T cells. Among 24 cases at one center, for example, 3 (12.5%) were T-cell lymphomas [73].

Lymphoproliferative disorders occurring after transplantation differ from those occurring in the general population [33, 72]. Non-Hodgkin's lymphoma accounts for 65% of lymphomas in the general population, as compared to 93% in transplant recipients. These tumors are mostly large-cell lymphomas, the vast majority of which are of the B-cell type. Extranodal involvement is common, occurring in approximately 70% of the cases. Twenty to 25% have central nervous system disease, which is rare in the general population, and a similar proportion have infiltrative lesions in the allograft itself.

The first two polyclonal EBV-induced diseases are generally treated by antiviral therapy and by reducing immunosuppressive medications [74, 75]. The majority of these lesions either resolve completely (44%) or improve significantly (23%) with reduced immunosuppression [74]. On the other hand, there is as yet no convincing evidence of the efficacy of antiviral therapy, nor consensus on whether acyclovir or gancyclovir is preferred.

The third condition is monoclonal malignant lymphoma. Patients with this disorder, and those with polyclonal disease that does not respond to reduced immunosuppression, are treated with radiation, chemotherapy, and occasionally surgical resection [76]. Mortality from monoclonal malignancies is reported to be approximately 80%. Information on mortality of patients with posttransplant lymphoproliferative disease is largely based upon case reports and retrospective studies. Although the prognosis varies with clonality, published series suggest overall survival rates of 25–35% [77]. T-cell lymphomas have an extremely poor prognosis.

References

1   Martin DC, Rubini M, Rosen VJ: Cadaveric renal homotransplantation with inadvertent transplantation of carcinoma. JAMA 1965;192:752.
2   McPhaul JJ, McIntosh DA, Hall W: Tissue transplantation still vexes. N Engl J Med 1965;272:105.
3   Doak PB, Montgomerie JL, North JDK, Smith F: Reticulum cell sarcoma after renal homotransplantation and azathioprine and prednisone therapy. Br Med J 1968;iv:746.
4   Penn I, Hammond W, Brettschneider L, Starzl TE: Malignant lymphomas in transplantation patients. Transplant Proc 1969;1:106.

5 Penn I: Renal transplantation in patients with preexisting malignancies. Transplant Proc 1983;15:1079.

6 Matas AJ, Simmons RL, Kjellstrand CM, Buselmeier TJ, Najarian JS: Increased incidence of malignancy during chronic renal failure. Lancet 1975;i:883.

7 Miach PJ, Dawborn JK, Xipell J: Neoplasia in patients with chronic renal failure on long-term dialysis. Clin Nephrol 1976;5:101.

8 Sutherland GA, Glass J, Gabriel R: Increased incidence of malignancy in chronic renal failure. Nephron 1977;18:182.

9 Herr HW, Engen DE, Hostetler J: Malignancy in uremia: Dialysis versus transplantation. J Urol 1979;121:584.

10 Lidner A, Farewell VT, Sherrard DJ: High incidence of neoplasia in uremic patients receiving long-term dialysis. Nephron 1981;27:292.

11 Slifkin RF, Goldberg J, Neff MS, Baez A, Mattoo N, Gupta S: Malignancy in end-stage renal disease. ASAIO Trans 1977;23:34.

12 Sheil AGR; in Disney APS (ed): XIVth Report of the Australia and New Zealand Combined Dialysis and Transplant Registry. Woodville/SA, The Queen Elizabeth Hospital, 1991, p 100.

13 Brunner FP, Landais P, Selwood NH: Malignancies after renal transplantation: The EDTA-ERA Registry experience. Nephrol Dial Transplant 1995;10:74–80.

14 Ishikawa I, Saito Y, Shikura N, Kitada H, Shinoda A, Suzuki S: Ten-year prospective study on the development of renal cell carcinoma in dialysis patients. Am J Kidney Dis 1990;16: 452–458.

15 MacDougall ML, Welling LW, Wiegmann TB: Prediction of carcinoma in acquired cystic disease as a function of kidney weight. J Am Soc Nephrol 1990;1:828–831.

16 Levine E, Slusher SL, Grantham JJ, Wetzel LH: Natural history of acquired renal cystic disease patients: A prospective longitudinal CT study. AJR 1991;156:501–506.

17 Truong LD, Krishnan B, Cao JT, Barrios R, Suki WN: Renal neoplasm in acquired cystic kidney disease. Am J Kidney Dis 1995;26:1–12.

18 Penn I: The effect of immunosuppression on preexisting cancers. Transplantation 1993;55: 742–747.

19 Bumgardner GL, Matas AJ, Payne WD, Dunn DL, Sutherland DER, Najarian JS: Renal transplantation in patients with paraproteinemias. Clin Transplant 1990;4:399–405.

20 De Lima JJ, Kourilsky O, Meyrier A, Morel-Maroger L, Sraer JD: Kidney transplant in multiple myeloma. Early recurrence in the graft with sustained normal renal function. Transplantation 1981;31:223–224.

21 Pais E, Pirson Y, Squifflet JP, Ninane J, Cornu G, Alexandre GP, van Ypersele de Strihou C: Kidney transplantation in patients with Wilms' tumor. Transplantation 1992;53:782–785.

22 Sox HC Jr: Preventive health services in adults. N Engl J Med 1994;330:1589–1595.

23 Toribara NW, Sleisenger MH: Screening for colorectal cancer. N Engl J Med 1995;332: 861–867.

24 Penn I: Development of cancer as a complication of clinical transplantation. Transplant Proc 1977;9:1121.

25 Wilson RE, Hager EB, Hampers CL, Corson JM, Merrill JP, Murray JE: Immunologic rejection of human cancer transplanted with renal allograft. N Engl J Med 1968;278:479.

26 Zukoski CF, Killen DA, Ginn E, Matter B, Lucas DO, Seigler HF: Transplanted carcinoma in an immunosuppressed patient. Transplantation 1970;9:71.

27 Penn I: Some contributions of transplantation to our knowledge of cancer. Transplant Proc 1980;12:676.

28 Morse JH, Turcotte JG, Merion RM, Campbell DA Jr, Burtch GD, Lucey MR: Development of a malignant tumor in a liver transplant graft procured from a donor with a cerebral neoplasm. Transplantation 1990;50:875–877.

29 Jonas S, Bechstein WO, Lemmens HP, Neuhaus R, Thalmann U, Neuhaus P: Liver graft-transmitted glioblastoma multiforme. A case report and experience with 13 multiorgan donors suffering from primary cerebral neoplasia. Transplant Int 1996;9:426–429.

30 Fecteau AH, Penn I, Hanto DW: Peritoneal metastasis of intracranial glioblastoma via a ventriculoperitoneal shunt preventing organ retrieval: Case report an review of the literature. Clin Transplant 1998;12:348–350.

31 Frank S, Muller J, Bonk C, Haroske G, Schackert HK, Schackert G: Transmission of glioblastoma multiforme through liver transplantation. Lancet 1998;352:31.

32 Birkeland SA: Malignant tumors in renal transplant patients. Cancer 1983;51:1571–1575.

33 Penn I: Cancers complicating organ transplantation. N Engl J Med 1990;323:1767.

34 Penn I: The changing patterns of posttransplant malignancies. Transplant Proc 1991;23:1101.

35 Walz MK, Albrecht KH, Niebel W, Eigler FW: De-novo-Malignome unter medikamentöser Immunsuppression. Dtsch Med Wochenschr 1992;117:927–934.

36 Sheil AGR, Disney APS, Mathew TH, Amiss N: De novo malignancy emerges as a major cause of morbidity and late failure in renal transplantation. Transplant Proc 1993;25: 1383–1384.

37 Gaya SBM, Rees AJ, Lechler RI, Williams G, Mason PD: Malignant disease in patients with long-term renal transplants. Transplantation 1995;59:1705–1709.

38 London NJ, Farmery SM, Will EJ, Davison AM, Lodge JPA: Risk of neoplasia in renal transplant patients. Lancet 1995;346:403.

39 Fahlenkamp D, Reinke P, Kirchner S, Schnorr D, Lindeke A, Loening SA: Malignant tumours after renal transplantation. Scand J Urol Nephrol 1996;30:357–362.

40 Sheil AGR: Cancer in immune-suppressed organ transplant recipients: Aetiology and evolution. Transplant Proc 1998;30:2055–2057.

41 Akiyama T, Imanishi M, Matsuda H, Nishioka T, Kunikata S, Kurita T: Difference among races in posttransplant malignancies: Report from an oriental country. Transplant Proc 1998; 30:2058–2059.

42 Tsakiris D, Simpson HKL, Jones HP, Briggs JD, Elinder CG, Mendel S, Piccoli G, dos Santos JP, Tognoni G, Vanrenterghem Y, Valderrabano F: Rare diseases in renal replacement therapy in the ERA-EDTA Registry. Nephrol Dial Transplant 1996;11:4–20.

43 Stewart T, Tsai SCJ, Grayson H, Henderson R, Opelz G: Incidence of de-novo breast cancer in women chronically immunosuppressed after organ transplantation. Lancet 1995;346:796–798.

44 Penn I: Solid tumors in cardiac allograft recipients. Ann Thorac Surg 1995;60:1559.

45 Swinnen LJ, Costanzo-Nordin MR, Fisher SG, O'Sullivan EJ, Johnson MR, Heroux AL, Dizikes GJ, Pifarre R, Fisher RI: Increased incidence of lymphoproliferative disorder after immunosuppression with the monoclonal antibody OKT3 in cardiac transplant recipients. N Engl J Med 1990;323:1723–1728.

46 Dreno B, Mansat E, Legoux B, Litoux P: Skin cancers in transplant patients. Nephrol Dial Transplant 1998;13:1374–1379.

47 Spencer ES, Anderson HK: Clinically evident, nonterminal infections with herpesviruses and the wart virus in immunosuppressed renal allograft recipients. Br Med J 1970;iii:251.

48 Koranda FC, Dehmel EM, Kahn G, Penn I: Cutaneous complications in immunosuppressed renal homograft recipients. JAMA 1974;229:419.

49   Bavinck JNB, Tieben LM, Van Der Woude FJ, Tegzess AM, Hermans J, Schegget JT, Vermeer BJ: Prevention of skin cancer and reduction of keratotic skin lesions during acitretin therapy in renal transplant recipients: A double-blind, placebo-controlled study. J Clin Oncol 1995; 13:1933–1938.

50   Rook AH, Jaworsky C, Nguyen T, Grossman RA, Wolfe JT, Witmer WK, Kligman AM: Beneficial effect of low-dose systemic retinoid in combination with topical tretinoin for the malignant skin lesions in renal transplant recipients. Transplantation 1995;59:714–719.

51   Bellman BA, Eaglstein WH, Miller J: Low-dose isotretinoin in the prophylaxis of skin cancer in renal transplant patients. Transplantation 1996;61:173.

52   Penn I: Malignant melanoma in organ allograft recipients. Transplantation 1996;61:274–278.

53   Douds AC, Mellotte GJ, Morgan SH: Fatal Merkel-cell tumour (cutaneous neuroendocrine carcinoma) complicating renal transplantation. Nephrol Dial Transplant 1995;10:2346–2348.

54   Gooptu C, Woollons A, Ross J, Price M, Wojnarowska F, Morris PJ, Wall S, Bunker CB: Merkel-cell carcinoma arising after therapeutic immunosuppression. Br J Dermatol 1997; 137:637–641.

55   Williams RH, Morgan MB, Mathieson IM, Rabb H: Merkel-cell carcinoma in a renal transplant patient: Increased incidence? Transplantation 1998;65:1396–1397.

56   Shepherd FA, Maher E, Cardella C, Cole E, Greig P, Wade JA, Levy G: Treatment of Kaposi's sarcoma after solid organ transplantation. J Clin Oncol 1997;15:2371–2377.

57   Harwood AR, Osoba D, Hofstader SL, Goldstein MB, Cardella CJ, Holecek M, Kunynetz O, Gammarco JA: Kaposi's sarcoma in recipients of renal transplants. Am J Med 1979; 67:759–765.

58   Penn I: Kaposi's sarcoma in transplant recipients. Transplantation 1997;64:669–673.

59   Frances C: Kaposi's sarcoma after renal transplantation. Nephrol Dial Transplant 1998;13: 2768–2773.

60   Doublet JD, Peraldi MN, Gattegno B, Thibault P, Sraer JD: Renal cell carcinoma of native kidneys: Prospective study of 129 renal transplant patients. J Urol 1997;158:42–44.

61   Kliem V, Kolditz M, Behrend M, Ehlerding G, Pichlmayr R, Koch KM, Brunkhorst R: Risk of renal cell carcinoma after kidney transplantation. Clin Transplant 1997;11:255–258.

62   Avinash CG, Daily PP, Kilambi NK, Hamrick-Turner JE, Butkus DE: Prospective pretransplant ultrasound screening in 206 patients for acquired renal cysts and renal cell carcinoma. Transplantation 1998;66:1669–1672.

63   Kliem V, Thon W, Krautzig S, Kolditz M, Behrend M, Pichlmayr R, Koch KM, Frei U, Brunkhorst R: High mortality from urothelial carcinoma despite regular tumor screening in patients with analgesic nephropathy after renal transplantation. Transplant Int 1996;9:231–235.

64   Gifford RR, Wofford JE, Edwards WG Jr: Carcinoma of the bladder in renal transplant patients. A case report and collective review of cases. Clin Transplant 1998;12:65–69.

65   Opelz G, Henderson R for the Collaborative Transplant Study: Incidence of non-Hodgkin's lymphoma in kidney and heart transplant recipients. Lancet 1993;342:1514.

66   Cockfield SM, Preiksaitis JK, Jewell LD, Parfrey NA: Post-transplant lymphoproliferative disorder in renal allograft recipients. Clinical experience and risk factor analysis in a single center. Transplantation 1993;56:88.

67   Patton DF, Wilkowski CW, Hanson CA, Shapiro R: Epstein-Barr virus determines clonality in post-transplant lymphoproliferative disorders. Transplantation 1990;49:1080.

68   Hanto DW, Frizzera G, Gajl-Peczalska KJ: Epstein-Barr-virus induced B-cell lymphoma after renal transplantation: Acyclovir therapy and transition from polyclonal to monoclonal B-cell proliferation. N Engl J Med 1992;306:913.

69   Randhawa PS, Jaffe R, Demetris AJ, Nalesnik M, Starzl TE, Chen YY, Weiss LM: Expression of Epstein-Barr virus-encoded small RNA (by the EBER-1 gene) in liver specimens from transplant recipients with posttransplantation lymphoproliferative disease. N Engl J Med 1992;327:1710–1714.

70   Nalesnik MA, Jaffe R, Starzl TS, Demetris AJ, Porter K, Burnham JA, Makowka L, Ho M, Locker J: The pathology of posttransplant lymphoproliferative disorders occurring in the setting of cyclosporine A-prednisone immunosuppression. Am J Pathol 1988;133:173–192.

71   Leblond V, Davi F, Charlotte F, Dorent R, Bitker MO, Sutton L, Gandjbakhch I, Binet JL, Raphael M: Posttransplant lymphoproliferative disorders not associated with Epstein-Barr virus: A distinct entity? J Clin Oncol 1998;16:2052–2059.

72   Nalesnik MA, Makowka L, Starzl TE: The diagnosis and treatment of posttransplant lympho-proliferative disorders. Curr Probl Surg 1988;25:367.

73   Leblond V, Sutton L, Dorent R, Davi F, Bitker MO, Gabarre J, Charlotte F, Ghoussoub, JJ, Fourcade C, Fischer A, Gandjbakhch I, Binet JL, Raphael M: Lymphoproliferative disorders after organ transplantation: A report of 24 cases observed in a single center. J Clin Oncol 1995;13:961–968.

74   Flinner RL: Neoplasms occurring in solid organ transplant recipients; in Hammond EH (ed): Solid Organ Transplantation Pathology. Philadelphia, PA, Saunders, 1994, pp 262–273.

75   Starzl TE, Nalesnik MA, Porter KA, Ho M, Iwatsuki S, Griffith BP, Rosenthal JT, Hakala TR, Shaw BW Jr, Hardesty RL, Atchison RW, Jaffe R: Reversibility of lymphomas and lympho-proliferative lesions developing under cyclosporin-steroid therapy. Lancet 1984;i:583–587.

76   De Mario MD, Liebowitz DN: Lymphomas in the immunocompromised patient. Semin Oncol 1998;25:492.

77   Savage P, Waxman J: Post-transplant lymphoproliferative disease. Q J Med 1997;90:497.

Prof. Dr. Christoph J. Olbricht, Transplantationszentrum Stuttgart, Katharinenhospital, Kriegsbergstraße 60, D–70174 Stuttgart (Germany)
Tel. + 49 711 278-5300, Fax -5309, E-mail olbricht.nep@katharinenhospital.de

Rüther U, Nunnensiek C, Schmoll H-J (eds): Secondary Neoplasias following Chemotherapy, Radiotherapy, and Immunosuppression. Contrib Oncol. Basel, Karger, 2000, vol 55, pp 242–255

Malignancy after Heart and Lung Transplantation

Olaf Wendler, Hans-Joachim Schäfers

Department of Thoracic and Cardiovascular Surgery,
University Hospitals, Homburg/Saar, Germany

Compared to the transplantation of kidney or liver, the history of heart transplantation is relatively short. The first clinical heart transplant in 1967 was followed by early enthusiasm, and then disappointment due to poor results. It is primarily the Stanford group which deserves credit for their perseverance in this field. They continued with their clinical program of heart transplantation and were able to improve clinical management, so that 1-year survival continuously increased from 20 to 40% during the first decade [43, 59].

The introduction of endomyocardial biopsy and the advent of cyclosporine revolutionized heart transplantation. The early and highly specific diagnosis of rejection provided the basis for more accurate adjustment of immunosuppression to minimize unwanted immunologic or toxic effects [6]. Using cyclosporine-based immunosuppression, the clinical appearance of graft rejection was altered from a very dramatic course, with rapid development of heart failure and potential death, to a gradual process that could be reversed much more easily and safely [70].

Results improved, with 1-year survival rates of up to 90% in the early 1980s, and heart transplantation rapidly evolved into a standardized treatment option for terminal heart failure. Currently, approximately 4,000 heart transplants are performed worldwide on an annual basis, as reported by the registry of the International Society for Heart and Lung Transplantation. This registry contains data on more than 50,000 heart transplants performed. One-year survival is currently approximately 85%, and 10-year survival rates of approximately 40% are being reported [32].

Lung and heart-lung transplantation have an even more recent history than cardiac transplantation. The transplants performed during the 1960s and 1970s must in retrospect be considered as clinical experiments that ultimately failed [68]. Lessons learned from other fields of organ transplantation, primarily heart transplantation, led to the first successful heart-lung transplant in 1981 by Reitz et al. [56] in Stanford, and the first isolated lung transplant by Cooper et al. [66] in Toronto.

Despite the initial success, many aspects of donor criteria, organ preservation and postoperative patient management were still undefined. Maintaining patient stability and graft function after transplantation proved to be more difficult in lung than in heart transplantation. A major problem arose from the fact that the lung is the only internal organ in constant contact with the environment, and thus the most susceptible to infection. In addition, common phenomena such as rejection, infection, reperfusion injury, and even certain types of malignant disease, result in similar clinical and radiologic manifestations.

With increasing experience, however, results improved, and from 1990 on, lung transplantation evolved into a globally accepted form of treatment for patients with end-stage pulmonary disease [64]. Given this development, combined heart-lung transplantation played a significant role only in the 1980s. With improved results of isolated lung transplantation and an increasing number of active transplant centers, the scarcity of donor organs led to a general preference for isolated lung transplantation for pulmonary disease. Currently, heart-lung transplantation is reserved for those patients suffering from a combination of pulmonary and irreversible cardiac pathology [64].

The registry of the International Society for Heart and Lung Transplantation currently reports approximately 1,000 pulmonary transplant procedures performed worldwide each year. The total number of lung and heart-lung transplants is approximately 10,000. One-year survival rates range around 70% in the world registry, while survival rates of up to 85% have been reported by individual centers. Five-year survival is approximately 45% in the world registry, compared to more than 60% in selected single centers [32, 64].

Specific Aspects of Thoracic Organ Transplantation

Compared to renal transplantation, both cardiac and lung transplantation differ with respect to the inherent prognostic consequences. Despite the development of uni- or biventricular cardiac assist devices, replacement of cardiac function or mechanical circulatory support is still in the experimental stages and far from being a true alternative to adequate function of the native or transplanted heart [18, 37]. For terminal pulmonary disease, there is not even a medium-term substitute for the biologic function of the natural organ. By definition, heart and lung transplant candidates have a poor spontaneous prognosis (life expectancy of less than 24 months). Compared to renal and hepatic transplantation patients, they have a lesser chance of survival in the face of restricted postoperative graft function. Likewise, they have only a limited possibility of functional recovery from significant graft dysfunction [35].

Thus, for both heart and lung transplants, recipients and transplant physicians are faced with the choice of having either (a) a well-functioning graft transplanted within a reasonable time from the moment of initial decision, and maintaining adequate graft function throughout the posttransplant period, or (b) death from native organ or graft failure. These facts generate pressure to maintain good posttransplant graft function which is considerably higher than for renal or hepatic transplantation. Consequently, the degree of immunosuppression – either due to the dose of individual agents or the choice of specific and highly effective immunosuppressants – is generally higher than in renal and liver transplantation. This can significantly impact aspects that would already preoccupy a competent immune system, such as the incidence and natural course of malignancies [10].

The Role of Malignant Disorders in Thoracic Organ Transplantation

As cardiac and lung transplantation evolved, malignant disorders in the postoperative course became more and more relevant beginning in the 1980s. With improved posttransplant survival and increased numbers, the first reports on posttransplant lymphoproliferative disease appeared in 1982 [69]. At that time, the Cincinnati Transplant Tumor Registry, for example, contained data on less than 60 patients with malignant disease following cardiac replacement [50].

Further research has disclosed the full spectrum of malignant disorders in cardiac and, recently, in pulmonary transplantation. In addition, many similarities have been found between the range of neoplastic disorders in thoracic and abdominal organ transplantation [53]. Malignant complications have evolved into a relevant cause of morbidity and mortality during the long-term follow-up of patients after thoracic organ transplantation [16, 43].

Depending on the origin of the malignant disease, neoplastic disorders after thoracic organ transplantation can be divided into three categories: (*1*) *Transplanted malignancy:* Transplantation of an organ carrying malignant cells from the donor. (*2*) *Preexisting malignancy:* Transplantation where the recipient has a previous history of a malignant disorder. This includes transplantation to treat malignancy in either heart or lung that is not amenable to conventional resection; and transplantation without knowledge of existing neoplasm. (*3*) *De-novo malignancy:* Malignant disease which occurs after transplantation and without a history of transplanted or preexistent malignancy.

Transplanted Malignancy

The possibility of transferring malignant cells with the graft has been under consideration for 20 years. While such malignant cells of foreign origin would normally be rejected, the situation is naturally different in organ transplantation: Normal immunosuppression that prevents a relevant immune response which could result in functional impairment of the graft will automatically also prevent immune response to malignant cells [51]. For this reason, careful screening of the potential cadaver donor in order to rule out malignancy has been conducted in the past two decades [14, 34].

There is limited information on organ donors who suffered from unsuspected malignancy despite careful screening. In renal transplantation, some reports have demonstrated a 40% probability for recipients to develop malignancies identical to those in the original donor if the donor suffered from malignancy up to 5 years before transplantation [48–50]. For this reason, avoidance of donors with a history of cancer has also been recommended for thoracic organ transplantation [34]. It is probably thanks to strict adherence to this policy that transmission of malignant donor cells to the recipient has been observed only anecdotally in cardiac transplantation [42].

In light of the available evidence, avoidance of donors with bronchogenic carcinoma, renal cell carcinoma and malignant melanoma appears mandatory both in heart and lung transplantation. However, since cardiac metastases in other tumors are very rare, and transmission of malignant cells by cardiac allograft transplantation is rare, the use of such donor hearts may be considered in selected cases. This approach may be justified where primary neoplasms of the brain are involved, as they rarely metastasize outside the central nervous system. In lung transplantation, however, it is generally inadvisable. The possibility of pulmonary metastases in most malignancies of donor origin is sufficiently high to warrant exclusion of lung donation if the donor has a history or current clinical evidence of any malignant disease.

Preexisting Malignancy

It has long been suspected that with positive tumor history before transplantation, subsequent immunosuppressive therapy may impair the ability of the host immune defense to control any residual malignant cells. This aspect has been most thoroughly researched in renal and hepatic transplantation. In renal transplantation, a series of 823 malignancies treated at varying intervals before transplantation resulted in an overall recurrence rate of 22% posttransplantation [55]. An even higher recurrence rate has been observed in hepatic transplantation to treat primary or metastatic liver neoplasm [52].

Only limited information is available on heart transplantation, in part because most centers have considered a history of malignancy as a contraindication to heart transplantation [41, 46]. Arico et al. [1] and Goenen et al. [24] reported individual cases of successful cardiac transplantation in patients with doxorubicin cardiomyopathy. After a follow-up of less than 12 months, both patients appeared free of recurrence. Armitage et al. [2] reported preliminary results in 10 patients who had undergone transplantation after previous treatment for neoplastic disease. During the follow-up, no evidence of recurrent neoplastic disease was found. Ueberfuhr et al. [67] made similar observations. Edwards et al. [20] reported on a series of 9 patients with preexisting neoplasm who underwent heart transplantation. Of these, 1 patient with previous adenocarcinoma of the colon died 16 months after transplantation and almost 5 years following colectomy performed for diffuse metastatic disease. All the other patients, who had been treated for lymphoma, did not exhibit any evidence of recurrence during a mean follow-up of approximately 3 years. Of concern was that 2 patients recently treated for lymphoma died of sepsis during the early postoperative phase.

Apart from these individual center reports, little data is available on larger collectives of heart transplant patients. A thorough analysis of more than 5,000 patients who had undergone cardiac transplantation between 1990 and 1997 documented that a history of malignancy prior to transplantation increased the probability of posttransplantation death due to malignancy (12% vs. 2% in 3 years, $p = 0.001$) [19].

Even more interesting is the question of transplantation as treatment for a cardiac tumor which is otherwise nonresectable. Ueberfuhr et al. [67] recently reported on 4 patients who underwent heart transplantation for angiosarcoma (n = 2), hemangiopericytoma (n = 1) and leiomyosarcoma (n = 1). Three of these 4 patients died within 18 months after heart transplantation due to recurrence of the tumor. The fourth patient had a follow-up of less than 12 months at the time of the report. This contrasted sharply with 10 other patients in this group who presented noncardiac tumors with a mean time gap of approximately 5 years between treatment of the neoplasm and heart transplantation. Of these 10 patients, 1 developed local recurrence following thyroid carcinoma; all others were tumor-free at a mean follow-up of more than 4 years [67].

Because lung transplantation has not been as well researched or developed, a history of preexistent or current neoplasm remains a contraindication – even despite the great scarcity of donor organs. Accordingly, there are no comparable data on preexisting malignancies and their consequences for transplantation of this organ. The only publication, which is by Santamauro et al. [58], reports successful transplantation in a young man with induced fibrosis 9 years after chemotherapy for acute lymphoblastic leukemia.

Current knowledge in cardiopulmonary transplantation with preexistent neoplasm justifies taking the conservative approach. Every decision in favor of cardiac or pulmonary transplantation despite a history of malignant disease must consider the individual's tumor history, organ availability, and the possibility of death if action is not taken. If transplantation is seriously considered, at least 3 years should have passed without evidence of local recurrence or distant metastases between initial treatment of malignancy and transplantation.

De novo Malignancy

The bulk of neoplasms occurring after solid-organ transplantation is classified as de novo malignancy. While this may be true, a small proportion of cases may involve transplanted tumors not diagnosed correctly or preexistent tumor that simply was not diagnosed before transplantation.

The incidence reported in cardiac patients varies from around 2.7% at 1 year to 25% at 5 years. Several reports from Australia and the Southern US give higher figures, which may be due to specific climate conditions [8, 25, 38]. The risk of death due to neoplasms is substantial in thoracic organ transplantation. Approximately 8–10% of deaths are due to malignant disorder.

Lanza et al. [40] compared the incidence of cancer in cardiac transplant recipients with that of renal allograft patients. They found a 2-fold increase of all neoplasms in cardiac patients, with a nearly 6-fold increase in the incidence of visceral malignancy. The higher incidence of malignancy is also confirmed by an analysis from the Pittsburgh group, which demonstrated an overall incidence of lymphoma in heart transplantation of 3.4% and lung transplantation of 7.9%, compared to an incidence of only 1% in renal transplantation [2]. Thus, even though figures vary quite significantly between different centers and reports, there tends to be a higher risk of malignancy in heart and particularly lung transplantation [44].

The reasons are unclear at this time. Initially, cyclosporine A was held responsible for the increased incidence [55]. More recent observations, however, show no difference between conventional immunosuppression (azathioprine and corticosteroids) and cyclosporine-based immunosuppression [47, 60]. It is currently felt that the general degree of immunosuppression and possibly the use of antilymphocyte antibodies may contribute to this relationship [15, 39, 65].

A group in Brazil reported an elevated incidence of malignancies (37.5% at a mean follow-up time of 25 months) after cardiac transplantation in 16 patients with Chagas' disease [7]. The authors hypothesized that these findings are due to drug toxicity or to chronic infection with an immunomodulator protozoan.

After heart transplantation, the most common tumors involve skin and lips [54]. Carcinomas of breast, prostate, colon and uterus are observed with an incidence similar to that seen in the general population [54]. Carcinomas of the lung have recently been reported to occur somewhat more often than in the general population [17, 19, 23]. Tumors with a significantly elevated probability are lymphoma, Kaposi's sarcoma, and sarcoma in general [54]. While lymphoma and Kaposi's sarcoma appear at an earlier stage (average 32 and 22 months), carcinomas of vulva and perineum present rather late after transplantation (average 110 months). Epithelial malignancies appear on an average of 70 months following transplantation [54].

Cancer of Skin and Lips

The most common tumors following thoracic organ transplantation involve skin and lips. Their incidence apparently depends on the amount of sun exposure [45, 54]. In regions with limited exposure, incidence is 4–7 times higher than in the general population. In areas with increased sunshine exposure, an almost 21-fold increase over that seen in the local population was observed, primarily due to an increase in squamous cell carcinoma [21]. This mechanism could certainly explain the relatively high incidence observed in Australia and the Southern US [8, 60]. An increased incidence is also reported in areas with little sunshine, such as Canada, Norway and Scotland [36]. In these regions, the increased incidence of squamous cell carcinomas may be related to malignant change in papillomavirus-induced cutaneous warts under the influence of immunosuppression [4, 61].

Among the different skin cancer types, squamous cell carcinoma predominates over basal cell carcinoma. The incidence appears to increase with older age, male sex, and fair skin of the patient [11, 39, 57]. As in renal transplantation, squamous cell carcinomas are more aggressive in cardiac transplant recipients than in the general population. Higher incidences of metastases to lymph nodes as well as distant metastases have been observed [22, 54].

Lymphoproliferative Disorders

Lymphomas are the second most frequent malignant disorder in thoracic as well as other organ transplant patients. The vast majority of lymphomas (94%) after transplantation are non-Hodgkin's lymphomas (NHL). There is a 30- to 50-fold increase in allograft recipients over that seen in age-matched controls [13, 54].

Morphologically, most NHLs have been classified as immunoblastic sarcomas, reticular cell sarcomas, microgliomas or large-cell lymphomas. The majority of these lymphomas is apparently of B-lymphocyte origin; only 13% arise from T cells. Whereas extranodal involvement occurs in only a minority of patients with NHL in the general population, it is present in more than 70% of NHLs in transplant patients [54]. Interestingly, in the general population, approximately 1% of NHLs involve the brain; whereas in organ transplant recipients, 24% affect the central nervous system, usually in a multicentric fashion (fig. 1) [29, 54]. The incidence is considerably higher in thoracic transplantation than in renal transplantation patients [3]. In the latter area, a 1% incidence is seen, compared to a 2.3% incidence in cardiac allograft recipients and a 3.8% incidence in recipients of lung transplants [3]. Immunologic and serologic evidence of primary or secondary Epstein-Barr virus infection has been observed in the majority of patients [3, 26–28, 30, 31].

Organ involvement and radiologic manifestations may vary widely. Allografts have shown involvement with lymphoma in a number of thoracic organ recipients. The lungs are frequently affected organs of lymphoma, after both heart and lung transplantation (fig. 2) [3]. In cardiac recipients, the lymphomatous infiltrate may be mistaken for rejection when biopsies, performed because of allograft dysfunction, are studied microscopically [3]. With diffuse involvement of the cardiac allograft, the clinical and hemodynamic picture of restrictive cardiomyopathy may be encountered, which is reversible upon administration of chemotherapy. In lung transplantation, the radiologic manifestations of lymphoproliferative disease resemble those of

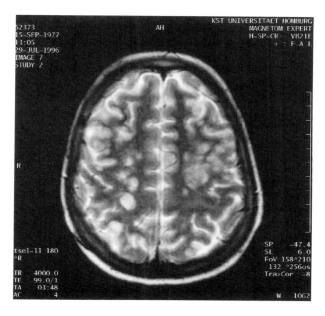

Fig. 1. NHL involving the brain in a patient after lung transplantation.

infectious complications (fig. 3). Lung biopsy is required in order to obtain exact information for diagnosis and treatment.

These lymphomas have a wide variety of causes. Most occur within the first year after transplantation due to the high initial immunosuppressive therapy. In approximately 20–30% of patients, the only treatment used with a subsequent excess was reduction of immunosuppressive therapy [62]. The mortality of early-onset lymphoma is substantial, with more than 30% dying of the disease [3]. By comparison, late-onset lymphoma usually requires specific treatment, such as chemotherapy. In this subset, mortality rates of 70% and higher have been reported [3].

There is speculation on whether some lymphoproliferative lesions in these patients should be regarded as true lymphomas, or as typical B-cell hyperplasia induced by the Epstein-Barr virus, which is frequently seen in immunosuppressed patients. The confusion arises from the variable histologic manifestations of the NHLs, the differences in clonality, and the differences in spontaneous as well as posttherapeutic prognoses. One theory suggests a spectrum of lesions ranging from infectious mononucleosis, like polyclonal B-cell proliferation, to frank monoclonal lymphomas. Between these two extremes lies the stage where some polyclonal proliferations undergo a clonal cytogenetic change evidenced by malignant manifestations [3].

Kaposi's Sarcoma

Kaposi's sarcoma is the classic malignancy of the immunosuppressed patient. The 6% incidence in organ transplant recipients is much higher than in the general

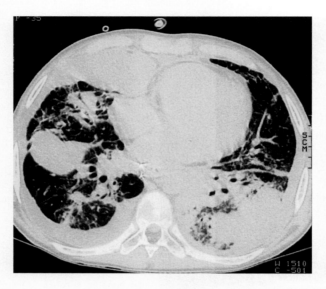

Fig. 2. NHL involving both lungs in a patient after double lung transplantation.

population [54]. It has long been believed that the infectious agent is transmitted by sexual contact or tissue transplantation [33]. Recently, a herpesvirus-like DNA sequence, termed human herpesvirus, was identified in lesions of patients with Kaposi's sarcoma – both in HIV and heart transplant patients, as well as in recipients of other organ transplants [9, 63]. Also hypothesized is an association with the use of OKT3 in postoperative immunosuppression [5, 9, 39]. This is confirmed by reports of Kaposi's sarcoma regressing under conditions of normalized immune response [5, 12].

Carcinoma of the Lung

While large-scale studies do not report any difference between the incidence of bronchogenic carcinoma in cardiac transplant patients and that in the general population [54], an increased risk of lung carcinoma has recently been reported in these patients. The incidence of adenocarcinoma in particular was increased [17, 19, 23]. Here, the risk factors are currently unknown, but it may be significant that more than half of the cardiac transplant recipients suffer from ischemic heart disease and had a positive history of smoking prior to transplantation. At this time, no sufficient numbers exist in lung transplantation to judge the relative importance of bronchogenic carcinoma.

Miscellaneous Epithelial Malignancies

Carcinomas of breast, prostate, colon and kidney have occasionally been observed in thoracic organ transplants, but at the same rate of incidence as in the gen-

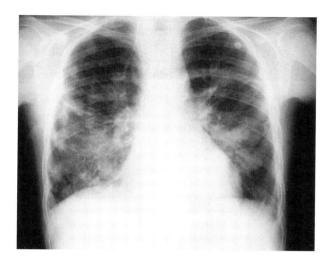

Fig. 3. Bilateral infiltrations due to NHL in a patient after double lung transplantation.

eral population [54]. Experience in cardiac transplantation is still insufficient to determine whether thoracic organ recipients have higher incidences of carcinomas of vulva and perineum, as is the case for renal transplantation. Papillomavirus infections, however, appear to increase the risk for immunosuppressed women to contract lower genital intraepithelial neoplasms [61].

Conclusion

Over the last 15 years, cardiac and pulmonary transplantation has evolved into an accepted option to treat end-stage heart and lung disease. At the same time, with improved long-term survival, complications like malignant disorders have become more significant. The overall risk of a patient developing cancer after cardiac transplantation is more than 10% within the first 5 postoperative years.

Although the prognosis for malignant disorders after thoracic organ transplantation is generally worse than that for the general population, some forms of lymphoproliferative disease can be treated, with acceptable results, by reducing immunosuppression or administering chemotherapy. In general, the risk of secondary malignancy is higher in thoracic than in abdominal transplantation.

In patients with cardiac or pulmonary failure caused by chemotherapy for malignant disorders, an elevated risk of neoplasm remains; heart or lung transplantation is, however, possible in selected patients. Only further research will show whether more specific immunosuppression will ultimately decrease the probability and clinical impact of this group of sequelae in thoracic organ transplantation.

References

1   Arico M, Pedroni E, Nespoli L, Vigano M, Porta F, Burgio GR: Long-term survival after heart transplantation for doxorubicin-induced cardiomyopathy. Arch Dis Child 1991;66:985–986.

2   Armitage JM, Kormos RL, Griffith BP, Fricker FJ, Hardesty RL: Heart transplantation in patients with malignant disease. J Heart Transplant 1990;9:627–629.

3   Armitage JM, Kormos RL, Stuart RS, Frederick FJ, Griffith BP, Nalesnik M, Hardesty RL, Dummer JS: Posttransplant lymphoproliferative disease in thoracic organ transplant patients: Ten years of cyclosporine-based immunosuppression. J Heart Lung Transplant 1991;10:877–887.

4   Barr BB, Benton EC, McLaren K, Bunney MH, Smith IW, Blessing K, Hunter JA: Human papilloma virus infection and skin cancer in renal allograft recipients. Lancet 1989; i:124–129.

5   Bhoopchand A, Cooper DKC, Novitzky D, Rose AG, Path MRC, Reichart B: Regression of Kaposi's sarcoma after reduction of immunosuppressive therapy in a heart transplant patient. J Heart Transplant 1986;5:461–464.

6   Billingham ME: Diagnosis of cardiac rejection by endomyocardial biopsy. J Heart Transplant 1981;1:25–30.

7   Bocchi EA, Higuchi ML, Vieira MLC, Stolf N, Bellotti G, Fiorelli A, Uip D, Jatene A, Pileggi F: Higher incidence of malignant neoplasms after heart transplantation for treatment of chronic Chagas' heart disease. J Heart Lung Transplant 1998;17:399–405.

8   Bouwes Bavinck JN, Robertson I, Wainwright RW, Green A: Excessive numbers of skin cancers and pre-malignant skin lesions in an Australian heart transplant recipient. Br Heart J 1995;74:468–470.

9   Briz M, Alonso-Pulpon L, Crespo-Leiro MG, Exposito C, Almagro M, Busto MJ, Fernandez MN: Detection of herpesvirus-like sequences in Kaposi's sarcoma from heart transplant recipients. J Heart Lung Transplant 1998;17:288–293.

10 Brumbaugh J, Baldwin JC, Stinson E, Oyer PE, Jamieson SW, Bieber CP, Henle W, Shumway NE: Quantitative analysis of immunosuppression in cyclosoporine-treated heart transplant patients with lymphoma. J Heart Transplant 1985;4:307–311.

11 Bull DA, Karwande SV, Hawkins JA, Neumayer LA, Taylor DO, Jones KW, Renlund DG, Putnam CW: Long-term results of cardiac transplantation in patients older than sixty years. J Thorac Cardiovasc Surg 1996;111:423–428.

12 Carmeli Y, Mevorach D, Kaminski N, Raz E: Regression of Kaposi's sarcoma after intravenous immunoglobulin treatment for polymyositis. Cancer 1994;73:2859–2861.

13 Clearly ML, Sklar J: Lymphoproliferative disorders in cardiac transplant recipients are multiclonal lymphomas. Lancet 1984;ii:489–493.

14 Copeland JG, Emery RW, Levinson MM, Icenogle TB, Carrier M, Ott RA, Copeland JA, McAleer-Rhenman MJ, Nicholson SM: Selection of patients for cardiac transplantation. Circulation 1987;75:2–9.

15 Cotton JR, Searl AG, Remmers AR, Lindley JD, Beathard GA, Cottom DL, Fish JC, Townsend CM Jr, Ritzmann SE: The appearance of reticulum cell sarcoma at the site of anti-lymphocyte globulin injection. Transplantation 1973;16:154–157.

16 Couetil JP, McGoldrick JP, Wallwork J, English TAH: Malignant tumors after heart transplantation. J Heart Lung Transplant 1990;9:622–626.

17 Curtil A, Schjöth B, Billès MA, Trochu JN, Tronc F, Villemot JP, Laborde N, Despins P, Champsaur G: Do heart transplant recipients present an unusual incidence of lung neoplasms? J Heart Lung Transplant 1998;1:70.

18   DeRose JJ, Argenziano M, Sun BC, Reemtsma K, Oz M, Rose EA: Implantable left ventri-cular assist devices: An evolving long-term cardiac replacement therapy. Ann Surg 1997;226:461–470.

19   DeSalvo TG, Naftel DC, Kasper EK, Rayburn BK, Leier CV, Massin EK, Cintron GB, Yancy CW, Keck S, Aaronson K, Kirklin JK: The differing hazard of lymphoma vs. other malig-nancies in the current era – A multiinstitutional study. J Heart Lung Transplant 1998;1:70.

20   Edwards BS, Hunt SA, Fowler MB, Valentine HA, Stinson EB, Schroeder JS: Cardiac trans-plantation in patients with preexisting neoplastic diseases. Am J Cardiol 1990;65:501–504.

21   Espana A, Redondo P, Fernandez A, Jabala M, Herreros J, Llorens R, Quintanilla E: Skin can-cer in heart transplant recipients. J Am Acad Dermatol 1995;32:458–465.

22   Euvrard S, Kanitakis J, Pouteil-Noble C, Dureau G, Touraine JL, Faure M, Claudy A, Thivolet J: Comparative epidemiological study of premalignant epithelial cutaneous lesions developing after kidney and heart transplantation. J Am Acad Dermatol 1995;33:222–229.

23   Gallo P, Agozzino L, Angelini A, Arbustini E, Bartolini G, Bernucci P, Bonacina E, Bosman C, Catani G, diGioia C, Giordana C, Leone O, Motta T, Pucci A, Rocco M: Causes of late failure after heart transplantation: A ten-year survey. J Heart Lung Transplant 1997; 16:1113–1121.

24   Goenen M, Baele P, Lintermans J, Lecomte C, Col J, Ponlot R,Schoevardts JC, Chalant C: Orthotopic heart transplantation eleven years after left pneumonectomy. J Heart Transplant 1988;7:309–311.

25   Goldstein DJ, Williams DL, Oz MC, Weinberg AD, Rose EA, Mitchler RE: De novo solid malignancies after cardiac transplantation. Ann Thorac Surg 1995;60:1783–1789.

26   Hanto DW, Sakamoto K, Purtilo DT, Simmons RL, Najarian JS: The Epstein-Barr virus in the pathogenesis of posttransplant lymphoproliferative disorders. Surgery 1981;90:204–213.

27   Hanto DW, Frizzera G, Gail-Peczalska K, Sakamoto K, Purtilo DT, Balfour HH Jr, Simmons RL, Najarian JS: Epstein-Barr virus-induced B-cell lymphoma after renal transplantation. N Engl J Med 1982;306:913–918.

28   Hanto DW, Simmons RL, Narjarian JS: Epstein-Barr virus-induced lymphoproliferative diseases in renal allograft recipients. J Heart Transplant 1984;3:121–130.

29   Harris KM, Schwarz ML, Slasky BS, Nalesnik M, Makowka L: Posttransplantation cyclo-sporine-induced lymphoproliferative disorders: Clinical and radiologic manifestation. Radiology 1987;162:697–700.

30   Ho M, Miller G, Atchison W, Breinig MK, Dummer JS, Andiman W, Starzl TE, Eastman R, Griffith BP, Hardesty RL: Epstein-Barr virus infections and DNA hybridization studies in posttransplantation lymphoma and lymphoproliferative lesions: The role of primary infection. J Infect Dis 1985;152:876–886.

31   Ho M, Jaffe R, Miller G, Breinig MK, Dummer JS, Makowka L, Atchison RW, Karrer F, Nalesnik MA, Starzl TE: The frequency of Epstein-Barr virus infection and associated lym-phoproliferative syndrome after transplantation and its manifestations in children. Transplantation 1988;45:719–727.

32   Hosenpud JD, Bennet LE, Keck BM, Daily P: The Registry of the International Society for Heart and Lung Transplantation: 15th official report – 1998. J Heart Lung Transplant 1998;17:656–668.

33   Huang YQ, Li JJ, Kaplan MH, Poiesz B, Katabira E, Zhang WC, Feiner D, Friedman-Kien AE: Human herpesvirus-like nucleic acid in various forms of Kaposi's sarcoma. Lancet 1995;345:759–761.

34   Hunt SA, Stinson EB: Cardiac transplantation. Annu Rev Med 1981;32:213–220.

35   Hunt SA: Complications of heart transplantation. Heart Transplant 1983;11:70–74.

36   Jensen P, Clausen OPF, Geiran O, Simonsen S, Relbo A, Hansen S, Langeland T: Cutaneous complications in heart transplant recipients in Norway 1983–1993. Acta Derm Venereol 1995;75:400–403.

37   Koul B, Solem JO, Steen S, Casimir AH, Granfeldt H, Lohn UJ: HeartMate left ventricular assist device as bridge to heart transplantation. Ann Thorac Surg 1998;65:1625–1630.

38   Krikorian JG, Anderson JL, Bieber CP, Penn I, Stinson EB: Malignant neoplasms following cardiac transplantation. JAMA 1978;240:639–643.

39   Lampros TD, Cobanoglu A, Parker F, Ratkovec R, Norman DJ, Hershberger R: Squamous and basal cell carcinoma in heart transplant recipients. J Heart Lung Transplant 1998;17:586–591.

40   Lanza RP, Cooper DKC, Cassidy MJD, Barnard CN: Malignant neoplasms occurring after cardiac transplantation. JAMA 1983;249:1746–1748.

41   Levitt G, Bunch K, Rogers CA, Whitehead B: Cardiac transplantation in childhood cancer survivors in Great Britain. Eur J Cancer 1996;32A:826–830.

42   Loh E, Couch FJ, Hendrichsen C, Farid L, Kelly PF, Acker MA, Tomaszewski JE, Malkowicz SB, Weber BL: Development of donor-derived prostate cancer in a recipient following orthotopic heart transplantation. JAMA 1997;277:133–137.

43   McGiffin DC, Kirklin JK, Naftel DC, Bourge RC: Competing outcomes after heart transplantation: A comparison of eras and outcomes. J Heart Lung Transplant 1997;16:190–198.

44   Mihalov ML, Gattuso P, Abraham K, Holmes EW, Reddy V: Incidence of post-transplant malignancy among 674 solid-organ-transplant recipients at a single center. Clin Transplant 1996;10:248–255.

45   O'Connell BM, Abel EA, Nickoloff BJ, Bell BJ, Hunt SA, Theodore J, Shumway NE, Jacobs PH: Dermatologic complications following heart transplantation. J Heart Transplant 1986;5:430–436.

46   Oechslin E, Kiowski W, Schneider J, Follath F, Turina M, Gallino A: Pretransplant malignancy in candidates and posttransplant malignancy in recipients of cardiac transplantation. Ann Oncol 1996;7:1059–1063.

47   Olivari MT, Diekmann RA, Spencer HK, Braunlin E, Jamieson SW, Ring WS: Low incidence of neoplasia in heart and heart-lung transplant recipients receiving triple-drug immunosuppression. J Heart Transplant 1990;9:618–621.

48   Penn I: Tumors arising in organ transplant recipients; in Klein G, Weinhouse S (eds): Advances in Cancer Research. New York, New York Academic Press, 1978, vol 28, pp 31–61.

49   Penn I: The price of immunotherapy. Curr Probl Surg 1981;18:682–751.

50   Penn I: Problems of cancer in organ transplantation. J Heart Transplant 1982;2:71–77.

51   Penn I: Why do immunosuppressed patients develop cancer?; in Pimenkel E (ed): CRC Critical Reviews in Oncogenesis. Boca Raton, FL, CRC Press, 1989, pp 27–52.

52   Penn I: Hepatic transplantation for primary and metastatic cancers of the liver. Surgery 1991;110:726–734.

53   Penn I: Tumors after renal and cardiac transplantation. Hematol Oncol Clin North Am 1993;7:431–445.

54   Penn I: Incidence and treatment of neoplasia after transplantation. J Heart Lung Transplant 1993;12:328–336.

55   Penn I: Neoplasia: An example of plasticity of the immune response. Transplant Proc 1996;28:2089–2093.

56   Reitz BA, Pennock JL, Shumway NE: Simplified method of heart and lung transplantation. J Surg Res 1981;31:1–5.

57   Rickenbacher PR, Lewis NP, Valantine HA, Luikart H, Stinson EB, Hunt SA: Heart transplantation in patients over 54 years of age. Eur Heart J 1997;18:870–878.

58   Santamauro JT, Stover DE, Jules-Elysee K, Maurer JR: Lung transplantation for chemotherapy-induced pulmonary fibrosis. Chest 1994;105:310–312.

59   Sarris GE, Moore KA, Schroeder JS, Hunt SA, Fowler MB, Valantine HB, Vagelos RH, Billingham ME, Oyer PE, Stinson EB, Reitz BA, Shumway NE: Cardiac transplantation: The Stanford experience in the cyclosporine era. J Thorac Cardiovasc Surg 1994;108:240–252.

60   Sheil AGR, Disney APS, Mathew TH, Livingston BER, Keogh AM: Lymphoma incidence, cyclosporine, and the evolution and major impact of malignancy following organ transplantation. Transplant Proc 1997;29:825–827.

61   Sillman F, Stanek A, Sedlis A, Rosenthal J, Lanks KW, Buchhagen D; Nicrasti A, Boyce J: The relationship between human papillomavirus and lower genital intraepithelial neoplasia in immunosuppressed women. Am J Obstet Gynecol 1984;150:300–308.

62   Starzl TE, Nalesnik MA, Porter KA, Ho M, Iwatsuki S, Griffith BP, Rosenthal JT, Hakala TR, Shaw BW, Hardesty RL: Reversibility of lymphomas and lymphoproliferative lesions developing under cyclosporine-steroid therapy. Lancet 1984;i:583–587.

63   Su IJ, Hsu YS, Chang YC, Wang IW: Herpesvirus-like DNA sequence in Kaposi's sarcoma from AIDS and non-AIDS patients in Taiwan. Lancet 1995;345:722–723.

64   Sundaresan S, Cooper JD: Lung transplantation. Ann Thorac Surg 1998;65:293–294.

65   Swinnen LJ, Costanzo-Nordin MR, Fisher SG, O'Sullivan EJ, Johnson MR, Heroux AL, Dizikes GJ, Pifarre R, Fisher RI: Increased incidence of lymphoproliferative disorder after immunosuppression with the monoclonal antibody OKT3 in cardiac-transplant recipients. N Engl J Med 1990;323:1723–1728.

66   Toronto Transplant Group: Unilateral lung transplantation for pulmonary fibrosis. N Engl J Med 1986;314:1140–1145.

67   Ueberfuhr P, Meiser B, Kraatz M, Schmidt D, Schirmer J, Issels R, Stempfle U, Reichart B: Is there an increased risk for patients with a tumor history after HTx? J Heart Lung Transplant 1998;1:70.

68   Veith FJ, Koerner SK, Hagstrom JW, Attai L, Bloomberg A, Jacobson E, Nagashima H, Boley SJ, Gliedman ML: Experience in clinical lung transplantation. JAMA 1972;222:779–782.

69   Weintraub J, Warnke RA: Lymphoma in cardiac allograft recipients. Clinical histological features and immunological phenotye. Transplantation 1982;33:347–351.

70   White DJ, Calne RY: The use of cyclosporin A immunosuppression in organ grafting. Immunol Rev 1982;65:115–131.

Olaf Wendler, MD, Chirurgische Klinik, Abteilung für Thorax- und Herz-Gefäßchirurgie, Universitätskliniken des Saarlandes, D–66421 Homburg/Saar (Germany)
Tel. +49 6841-16 2501, Fax -16 2788, E-mail chowen@med-rz.uni-sb.de

Rüther U, Nunnensiek C, Schmoll H-J (eds): Secondary Neoplasias following Chemotherapy,
Radiotherapy, and Immunosuppression. Contrib Oncol. Basel, Karger, 2000, vol 55, pp 256–263

Secondary Neoplasms following Liver and Pancreas Transplantation

B. Nashan

Klinik für Viszeral- und Transplantationschirurgie, Medizinische Hochschule
Hannover, Deutschland

Increased incidence of de novo malignancies of lymphoid and nonlymphoid
origin is observed in immunosuppressed patients [14–19, 21]. The pattern of these
malignancies varies according to the origin of impairment. Thus, patients with primary immunodeficiency disorders have an increased risk for leukemia, non-
Hodgkin's and Hodgkin's lymphomas, and gastric cancer [17]. Patients with acquired immunodeficiency syndrome (AIDS) suffer in particular from Kaposi's
sarcoma, malignancies of the oral and anal tract, as well as non-Hodgkin's lymphomas [20]. On the other hand, patients on immunosuppressive medication following organ transplantation demonstrate a variety of different malignancies without a
given pattern. Depending on several factors, this population in particular demonstrates considerable modulation of the risk of developing cancer.

Cumulative knowledge, especially in the kidney recipient population, has
demonstrated that cancer risk is determined by several factors, of which none is assumed to act in isolation. These factors are: (1) Replication of oncogenic viruses
(EBV, CMV, HSV1 and 2, human papillomavirus, HBV, HCV) [5]. (2) Immunosuppressive agents (azathioprine, cyclosporine, tacrolimus, polyclonal and monoclonal
antibody preparations directed against lymphocytes) [5, 6, 9]. (3) Time of immunosuppressive medication [21]. (4) Age of the patient [19, 21]. (5) Genetic background
of the individual [21]. These same factors could be also classified as local (immunosuppression, viral infections, pre-existing diseases) or general (age, sex, genetic diversity, time after transplantation).

While there is considerable knowledge on renal transplant recipients (reaching
back more than 20 and, in some registries, even 30 years), information is sparse on
liver transplant recipients, and nearly nonexistent for pancreas transplantees. Long-
term observation (20–30 years) of renal transplant recipients has been based on pa-

	Ref. 4 (n = 1,657)	Ref. 8 (n = 888)	Ref. 7 (n = 458)	Ref. 12 (n = 1,416)
De novo nonlymphoid malignancies	64/50 (3.9%)	42/38 (1.6%)	27/26 (5.6%)	12/12 (0.9%)
Immunosuppression	CyA, steroids (Aza) FK, steroids	CyA, steroids Aza FK, steroids	ATG or BT563, CyA, steroids Aza FK, steroids	CyA, steroids FK, steroids

tients receiving azathioprine as maintenance immunosuppression. It is thus difficult to extrapolate our knowledge from the renal transplant population to other types, since they differ as to observation time, type of maintenance immunosuppression and total numbers of patients. This is not a problem of *reporting,* but of the *number* of events. Especially in the early years of transplantation medicine, fewer patients received liver transplants, and even fewer pancreas grafts, compared to renal transplants. As a result, insufficient means of immunosuppression led to unfavorable outcomes. Therefore, liver and pancreas were not transplanted in large numbers until the early 1980s, when the introduction of cyclosporine improved patient and graft survival and made both organs eligible for transplantation in great numbers. Our report will focus on data of liver transplant patients as reported from four centers [4, 7, 8, 12].

Incidence

The numbers of de novo nonlymphoid malignancies reported vary from center to center. Those numbers observed at The Recanati/Miller Transplantation Institute, Mount Sinai Hospital, New York [8]; the Pittsburgh Transplantation Institute [4]; the Department of Visceral and Transplantation Surgery at the Medizinische Hochschule Hannover [12], and at the Department of Surgery and Transplantation Medicine, Charité, Humboldt University, Berlin [7] (table 1), concur with those of J.Penn [18, 19] and others [22] observed in renal transplantation. They do not indicate that patients after liver transplantation have an increased risk of contracting commonly observed malignancies (i.e., carcinomas of the colon and rectum, lung, breast and prostate). The incidences and diagnoses are given in detail in table 2.

On the other hand, more skin carcinomas are observed in the liver transplantee population, as is a shift from basal cell to squamous cell carcinomas, an inverse relation which is likewise noted in renal transplant recipients [19, 21]. One center re-

Table 2. Incidences and diagnoses reported from four centers (see text)

De novo nonlymphoid malignancy	Ref. 4 (n = 1,657)	Ref. 8 (n = 888)	Ref. 7 (n = 458)	Ref. 12 (n = 1,416)
Skin carcinoma	37 (2.2%)	15 (1.7%)	6 (1.2%)	3 (0.2%)
Basiloma	16	3	3	1
Squamous	13	12	3	2
Melanoma	4	0	0	0
Bowen	4	0	0	0
Skin sarcoma	2 (0.1%)	5 (0.6%)	1 (0.2%)	0
Kaposi's	2	4	1	0
Ewing	0	1		0
Skin (other)	2 (0.1%)	0	2 (0.4%)	0
Prostate carcinoma	1 (0.05%)	4 (0.5%)		0
Uterine cervical dysplasia	2 (0.1%)	4 (0.5%)	7 (1.5%)	0
Uterus	2 (0.1%)	1 (0.1%)	0	0
Colorectal	6 (0.3%)	3 (0.3%)	0	1 (0.05%)
Breast	3 (0.2%)	2 (0.2%)	3 (0.6%)	
Ovary	2 (0.1%)			1 (0.05%)
Oropharyngeal		2 (0.2%)	2 (0.4%)	
Laryngeal	2 (0.1%)			
Lungs	2 (0.1%)	2 (0.2%)	3 (0.6%)	1 (0.05%)
Gastric	2 (0.1%)	0	1 (0.2%)	
Esophageal	0	0	0	1 (0.05%)
Hepatocellular	0	0	0	1 (0.05%)
Pancreatic	0	1 (0.1%)		1 (0.05%)
Thyroid	0	0	1 (0.2%)	
Embryonal testicular	0	0	1 (0.2%)	0
Neural	0	0	0	2 (0.1%)
Bone	1 (0.05%)	0	0	
Bladder	0	1 (0.1%)	0	0
Craniopharyngeoma	0	1 (0.1%)	0	0
Total	64	41	27	12

ports an increased incidence of uterine cervical dysplasia [7]. EBV-associated leiomyosarcomas, which are mesenchymal malignancies with smooth muscle cell differentiation and which are extremely rare in children, have been found in pediatric liver recipients [11, 23]. EBV may be a possible mechanism for neoplastic smooth muscle proliferation analogous to the posttransplantation lymphoproliferative syndrome, and is more often reported in patients receiving increased amounts of cumulative immunosuppression.

Despite these particular findings, long-term follow-up (10–20 years) [1, 12] in liver-transplanted children showed no evidence of increased incidence of de novo nonlymphoid malignancies. Out of 202 children [1], only 1 developed cancer, and none of the 214 children of the Hannover center showed evidence of a tumor. Rates of 0.9–5.6% for de novo nonlymphoid malignancies in the adult liver transplant recipient group [4, 7, 8, 12] are comparable to those observed in the renal transplant group (average of 6%) [3, 14]. The total incidence of tumorigenesis after liver transplantation was much lower than that of the nonliver-transplanted population [13].

Types of Neoplasms

De novo nonlymphoid malignancies after liver transplantation make up the set of carcinomas and sarcomas found in the general population [4, 7, 8, 12, 13]. A list is given in table 2. Concerning the different types, no specific pattern of malignancy was detected. Differences between the centers may be due to local or general factors, like type of immunosuppression (table 1), age of recipient, or time of follow-up. Skin cancer outscores all other malignancies, which clearly makes it the most common tumor in the liver- transplanted population, a result similar to that in kidney recipients [14, 18, 21].

Recipient Age

A comparison of patients receiving a transplant and concomitant immunosuppression did not suggest that de novo nonlymphoid malignancies tended to occur at an earlier age in them than in the general population [4, 7, 8, 12, 13]. The gross number of tumors appeared at ages 50–60 years. Though the numbers of the studies are small, incidence and distribution of tumors did not differ.

Follow-Up Time after Transplantation

Few liver transplantations were conducted before the early 1980s. Over time, incidence of de novo nonlymphoid malignancies reported has increased, although no estimate on the further development could be made here. In renal transplant patients, an increase from 34–50% after 20 years to 80% after 30 years in patients with carcinoma was observed [21]. Data from large series in centers performing liver transplantations indicate that (1) the primary disease indication for liver transplantation does not correlate with the time at which the de novo nonlymphoid malignancies were observed; nor (2) was an increase over time observed correlating to that of renal transplant patients [4, 7, 8, 12].

Comorbidity

Patients undergoing liver transplantation in particular bear an increased risk of developing malignancies. Indications prone to this development are HBV and HCV cirrhosis, inflammatory bowel disease or alcoholic cirrhosis. The New York group (with 58 inflammatory bowel disease patients) reported 1 patient with primary sclerosing cholangitis. This patient underwent transplantation and later developed a colorectal carcinoma. A different group, however, reported an increased risk for this setting [2].

In Hannover, 12 years after liver transplantation to treat HBV, 1 patient developed reinfection of the graft and hepatocellular carcinoma there [12]. One patient with alcoholic liver cirrhosis developed pancreatic carcinoma, and 1 patient with alcoholic liver cirrhosis developed esophageal carcinoma. Both carcinomas are frequently seen in patients with alcoholism. The Pittsburgh and Berlin groups observed that lung carcinomas and tongue carcinomas were ascribable to smoking and drinking [4, 7]. Although no significant correlation between de novo nonlymphoid malignancies and etiology of liver cirrhosis was proven, the data indicate that social history is an important modulator in the incidence of some tumors, as in the general population, despite transplantation and immunosuppression. Out of 58 inflammatory bowel disease patients of the New York series, only 1 developed a colorectal malignancy [8]. Other authors describe subsets of patients with inflammatory bowel disease and primary sclerosing cholangitis who had an increased risk of developing colorectal cancer [2]. An association between primary biliary cirrhosis and breast cancer has been reported [25]; here, 2 patients (1 in the Berlin group and 1 in the New York group) had this combination.

Immunosuppression

Immunosuppressive therapy has advanced considerably in the last 30 years. The use of certain immunosuppressive substances like azathioprine, cyclosporine, tacrolimus or ATG preparations may alter the incidence and types of tumors observed. Increasingly, attention is also focusing on the cumulative amount of immunosuppression as an indicator of the pattern of posttransplant malignancies. Since the introduction of calcineurin inhibitors, the incidence of lymphomas and Kaposi's sarcomas has risen, while the incidence of skin and cervical carcinomas has fallen [16]. It is unclear if the latter is due to the switch from azathioprine to cyclosporine as the basic immunosuppressant in the early 1980s. Unfortunately, numbers are not large enough to substantiate these observations. Nevertheless, post-liver transplant groups using azathioprine for maintenance immunosuppression tend to evince greater incidence of either skin carcinomas or cervical dysplasia [7].

Immunosuppression itself may change host immune defense capabilities. Jonas et al. [7] reported a significantly decreased CD4/CD8 lymphocyte ratio in patients who developed de novo nonlymphoid malignancies. This finding is typical for induction therapy with antilymphocytic or antithymocytic globulins, and may be observed even 5 years after renal transplantation in patients with ATG induction [10]. Decreased CD4/CD8 ratios are typical of HIV-positive patients, who are prone to certain types of malignancies, such as oral and anal carcinomas, Kaposi's sarcoma and non-Hodgkin's lymphomas. Via a dose-dependent mechanism, cyclosporine and tacrolimus have been found to increase the release of TGF-ß. TGF-ß is a cytokine with a variety of functions, including carcinogenesis [6, 9]. Whether these in vitro observations apply to clinical findings is debatable, because the concentrations required in in vitro conditions are 2–10 times higher than the therapeutic levels in patients. Reports from liver transplant centers using tacrolimus as maintenance immunosuppression stress that they see fewer de novo nonlymphoid malignancies than in their groups administered cyclosporine [4, 7]. In contrast to cyclosporine, which was part of a triple therapy including azathioprine [8], or part of a quadruple therapy including antilymphocytic induction [7], tacrolimus was given in combination with steroids. Other reports do not provide detailed information [4, 24] for baseline immunosuppression. Hence, comparison is difficult, and may be biased in favor of the transplant population receiving tacrolimus. This population received its grafts 6–10 years later, and thus has had a shorter observation period. Moreover, the numbers in each of these retrospective analyses are too low to make comparisons meaningful.

Conclusions

Liver transplant patients evince a lower incidence of de novo nonlymphoid malignancies compared to other transplant populations. In particular, there is no evidence that liver-transplanted children are at greater risk of developing cancer. What is more, compared to renal transplant patients, the entire liver transplant population is 'younger' in terms of posttransplantation survival time. Therefore, this lower rate may be due to the shorter follow-up time here. As in renal transplant patients, skin carcinomas are the leading group of tumors found in liver transplant recipients. Because this higher incidence is well documented in all transplant recipients, prolonged and unprotected sun exposure should be avoided. However, none of these retrospective analyses has irrefutably demonstrated that liver transplant patients have a greater than normal risk of developing de novo nonlymphoid solid-organ tumors.

References

1 Andrews W, Sommerauer J, Roden J, Andersen J, Conlin C, Moore P: Ten years of pediatric liver transplantation. J Pediatr Surg 1996;31:619–624.

2 Bleday R, Lee E, Jessurun J, Heine J, Wong D: Increased risk of early colorectal neoplasms after hepatic transplant in patients with inflammatory bowel disease. Dis Colon Rectum 1993;36:908–912.

3 Blohme I, Brynger H: Malignant disease in renal transplant patients. Transplantation 1985;39:23–25.

4 Frezza EF, Fung JJ, Van Thiel DH: Non-lymphoid cancer after liver transplantation. Hepato-gastroenterology 1997;44:1172-1181.

5 Gruber S, Matas AG: Etiology and pathogenesis of tumors occurring after organ transplantation. Transplant Sci 1994;4:87-104.

6 Hojo M, Morimoto T, Maluccio M, Asano T, Morimoto K, Lagman M, Shimbo T, Suthanthiran M: Cyclosporine induces cancer progression by a cell-autonomous mechanism. Nature 1999;397:530-534.

7 Jonas S, Rayes N, Neumann U, Neuhaus R, Bechstein WO, Guckelberger O, Tullius SG, Serke S, Neuhaus P: De novo malignancies after liver transplantation using tacrolimus-based protocols or cyclosporine-based quadruple immunosuppression with an interleukin-2 receptor antibody or antithymocyte globulin. Cancer 1997;80:1141–1150.

8 Kelly DM, Emre S, Guy SR, Miller CM, Schwartz ME, Sheiner PA: Liver transplant recipients are not at increased risk for nonlymphoid solid organ tumors. Cancer 1998;83:1237–1243.

9 Khanna A, Cairns V, Hosenpud JD: Tacrolimus induces increased expression of transforming growth factor-ß$_1$ in mammalian lymphoid as well as nonlymphoid cells. Transplantation 1999;67:614–619.

10 Lange H, Müller TF, Ebel H, Kuhlsmann U, Grebe SO, Heymanns J, Feiber H, Riedmiller H: Immediate and long-term results of ATG induction therapy for delayed graft function compared to conventional therapy for immediate graft function. Transplant Int 1992;12:2–9.

11 Lee ES, Locker J, Nalesnik M, Reyes J, Jaffe R, Alashari M, Nour B, Tzakis A, Dickman PS: The association of Epstein-Barr virus with smooth-muscle tumors occurring after organ transplantation. N Engl J Med 1995;332:19–25.

12 Medizinische Hochschule Hannover, Klinik für Viszeral- und Transplantationschirurgie, Liver Transplant Registrar, unpubl data.

13 Parker SL, Tong T, Bolden S, Wings PA: Cancer statistics 1996. CA Cancer J Clin 1996;65:5–27.

14 Penn I: Why do immunosuppressed patients develop cancer? Crit Rev Oncol Hematol 1989;1:27–52.

15 Penn I: Cancer in the immunosuppressed organ recipient. Transplant Proc 1991;23:1771–1772.

16 Penn I: The changing pattern of post-transplant malignancies. Transplant Proc 1991;23:1101–1103.

17 Penn I: Depressed immunity and the development of cancer. Cancer Detect Prev 1994;18:241–252.

18 Penn I: The problem of cancer in organ transplant recipients. Transplant Sci 1994;4:23–32.

19 Penn I: Posttransplant malignancies. Transplant Proc 1999;31:1260–1262.

20 Selik R, Starcher ET, Curran JW: Opportunistic diseases reported in AIDS patients: Frequencies, association and trends. AIDS 1987;1:125.

21 Sheil AGR: Patterns of malignancies following renal transplantation. Transplant Proc 1999; 31:1263–1265.

22 Tan-Shalaby J, Tempero M: Malignancies after liver transplantation. A comparative review. Semin Liver Dis 1995;15:156–164.

23 Timmons CF, Dawson DB, Richards CS, Andrews WS, Katz JA: Epstein-Barr virus-associated leiomyosarcomas in liver transplantation recipients. Cancer 1995;76:1481–1489.

24 Todo S, Fung JJ, Starzl TE, Tzakis A, Doyle H, Abu-Elmaghd K, Jain A, Selby R, Bronsther O, Marsh W, et al: Single-center experience with primary orthotopic liver transplantation with FK-506 immunosuppression. Ann Surg 1994;220:297–308.

25 Wolke AM, Schaffner F, Kapelman B, Sacks HS: Malignancy in primary biliary cirrhosis. High incidence of breast cancer in affected women. Am J Med 1984;76:1075–1078.

Prof. Dr. med. Björn Nashan, Medizinische Hochschule Hannover, Viszeral- und Transplantationschirurgie, D–30623 Hannover (Germany)
Tel. +49 511-532 6534/2267, Fax -532 2265

Rüther U, Nunnensiek C, Schmoll H-J (eds): Secondary Neoplasias following Chemotherapy, Radiotherapy, and Immunosuppression. Contrib Oncol. Basel, Karger, 2000, vol 55, pp 264–274

....

Therapy of Secondary Acute Myeloid Leukemia and Secondary Myelodysplastic Syndrome

U. Rüther[a], B. Rothe[a], C. Nunnensiek[b]

[a] Stuttgart
[b] Ärztliche Praxis, Reutlingen, Deutschland

Introduction

Secondary or therapy-related myelodysplastic syndrome (t-MDS) leading to acute myeloid leukemia (t-AML) is increasing due to the vast amount of cytotoxic drugs available, dose-escalated therapeutic regimens, prolonged survival rates, and better cure rates for many malignant diseases. Bone marrow and peripheral stem cell transplantation following intense induction chemotherapy is the gold standard today for many malignant hematologic and for some nonmalignant diseases, and such therapies themselves increase the risk of therapy-related malignancy.

t-MDS and t-AML are late complications following chemotherapeutic treatment of malignant disease, particularly with alkylating agents or topoisomerase inhibitors. Radiotherapy, on the other hand, is more commonly associated with secondary solid tumors. Especially in younger patients with increased long-term survival rates, t-MDS and t-AML have become two of the most serious and feared complications of current cancer chemotherapy.

MDS is an acquired clonal expansion of the hematopoietic stem cell. It is characterized by ineffective hematopoiesis and progressive peripheral cytopenias. MDS increases the risk of transformation to AML. Infections due to neutropenia and thrombocytopenic bleeding are the most frequent causes of death. Ten to 40% of these patients proceed to AML [Ganser and Hoelzer, 1992]. MDS has been classified by the French-American-British (FAB) Group into five subcategories: refractory anemia (RA); refractory anemia with ring sideroblasts (RARS); refractory anemia with excess of blasts (RAEB); refractory anemia with excess of blasts in transformation (RAEBt), and chronic myelomonocytic leukemia (CMML). The clinical course of MDS varies from an indolent form to a rapidly fatal disease. The distinction between MDS and AML, however, is not always clear, and some conditions of MDS may be indistinguishable from acute leukemia.

Risk of t-AML and t-MDS

The risk of t-AML and t-MDS correlates to the cumulative dose of chemotherapeutic drugs, rather than to particular treatment protocols, and generally peaks 5–10 years following therapy. Older patients (> 50 years) have a higher risk of developing t-AML than younger patients. Ten years after chemotherapy, the incidence for all patients equals that of the general population [Miller et al., 1988].

Drugs that may induce t-MDS / t-AML are: (a) alkylating agents: nitrogen mustard and its derivatives: chlormethine, chlorambucil, busulfan, melphalan; (b) oxazaphosphorines: cyclophosphamide, ifosfamide, trophosfamide; (c) nitrosourea derivatives: nimustine, carmustine, lomustine, bendamustine; (d) aziridine/ethylenimine derivatives: thiotepa; (e) others: treosulfan; (f) alkaloids, podophyllin and podophyllotoxin derivatives: etoposide, teniposide, and (g) platinum derivatives: cisplatin, carboplatin.

Patients treated for non-Hodgkin's lymphoma are reported to have a 20- to 105-fold greater risk of contracting t-AML than does the general population. This risk increases with the number of cycles containing mechlorethamine [Ellis and Lishner, 1993, Kollmannsberger et al., 1998] during primary treatment. The incidence of t-AML peaks 4–8 years after chemotherapy. Splenectomy or radiation of the spleen appears to increase the risk of t-AML.

Patients with NHL, breast or testicular cancer experience a 2- to 15-fold risk of t-AML. Epipodophyllotoxins are apparently a predisposing factor for t-AML in patients with testicular cancer, just as mechlorethamine and prednimustine are for patients with NHL.

The exposure of stem cells to alkylating agents used particularly in myeloablative transplant conditioning also seems to be a major risk factor. A 9% cumulative risk of developing t-AML at 5 years has been observed for NHL patients who have undergone allogenic bone marrow transplantation or peripheral stem cell transplantation [Kollmannsberger et al., 1998, Traweek et al., 1994]. However, most of these patients have also been treated with alkylating agents before bone marrow transplantation, making it unclear whether the high-dose conditioning regimen adds significantly to the risk of secondary MDS/AML. The risk of developing t-MDS or t-AML appears to be even higher if this dose-escalated conditioning therapy, which is necessary prior to transplantation, is administered as second-line therapy after many courses of chemotherapeutic regimens that include alkylating agents. Therefore, high-dose chemotherapy followed by autologous stem cell therapy is now recommended as first-line chemotherapy for patients with malignant lymphomas.

Different alkylating agents have different propensities for inducing secondary AML. For example, higher rates are reported for melphalan and busulfan, or for the combination of nitrogen mustard and procarbazine; and lower rates for cyclophosphamide-based regimens [Kollmannsberger et al., 1998]. Because of the risk of secondary MDS and AML, the use of alkylating agents has been markedly reduced for benign diseases such as rheumatoid arthritis, nephritis and systemic lupus erythematosus disease. Secondary leukemias, however, are also being diagnosed more frequently as autologous stem cell transplantation is increasingly conducted to treat solid tumors.

Pathology and Prognosis

The onset of t-AML is usually 3–5 years after chemotherapy, with a preceding myelodysplastic phase [Rege et al., 1998]. Long-term follow-up of patients has shown that risk increases in proportion to the cumulative dose of chemotherapy received, the age of the patient, and whether total-body irradiation or local radiotherapy was administered [Miller et al., 1994]. Secondary leukemias following therapy with alkylating agents usually occur after 5–7 years, and are often preceded by a preleukemic period of myelodysplasia. Secondary leukemias associated with topoisomerase II inhibitors have a shorter latency period and are rarely preceded by a myelodysplastic prephase [Kollmannsberger et al., 1998; Smith et al., 1999; Karp and Smith, 1997].

The principal reason for the fact that secondary AML/MDS has a worse prognosis than primary AML/MDS is its association with chromosomal abnormalities, such as deletions or monosomies involving chromosomes 5 and/or 7. These are often accompanied by other, complex changes [Karp and Smith, 1997]. Recently, secondary MDS and AML with balanced translocations to chromosome bands 11q23 and 21q22 have demonstrated significant association with previous therapy with DNA topoisomerase II inhibitors. On the other hand, in 60–90% of cases, alkylating agents cause aberrations in chromosomes 5 and 7 [Pedersen-Bjergaard and Philip, 1991; Larson et al., 1992]. Patients with double or complex cytogenetic abnormalities have the worst prognosis [Kantarjian et al., 1986; Yunis et al., 1986; Geddes et al., 1990; Greenberg et al., 1997].

Greenberg et al. [1997] postulate that once bone marrow blast percentage, number of cytopenias, and cytogenetic subgroup are considered as risk variables determining outcome (International Prognostic Scoring System [IPSS]), it no longer makes a difference whether the patient presents with de novo MDS/AML or with t-MDS / t-AML. There is no evidence of a difference in outcome between primary and secondary MDS/AML patients within a given IPSS category [Estey, 1998].

Therapy of t-MDS and t-AML

Supportive Therapy

There are no satisfactory therapeutic options for patients with secondary MDS. The majority should therefore participate in clinical trials, since most of the patients with secondary MDS today are not expected to live more than 2 years. For patients with a median predicted survival time in excess of 2 years (IPSS category low or INT-1), principal therapies are supportive, such as transfusions only, the use of erythropoietin (EPO) ± granulocyte colony-stimulating factor (G-CSF), or granulocyte-macrophage colony-stimulating factor (GM-CSF). Therapy for MDS using growth factors (EPO, G-CSF and GM-CSF) aims for differentiation induction, and can prolong survival and improve the quality of life in some patients. A significant reduction in infection risk has been retrospectively demonstrated in responding patients compared to pretreatment episodes. However, the general benefit is very limited.

Therapy with the iron chelator desferrioxamine should be considered after 10–20 red cell transfusions in order to prevent organ damage and to prolong survival [Cohen et al., 1984]. Patients with inappropriately low levels of EPO may respond to recombinant human EPO therapy, in contrast to the majority of patients with normal or elevated levels of EPO. Estey [1998] suggests a 3-month trial of EPO. Successful treatment is reflected by stable hemoglobin and a serum EPO level > 200. Another option is the combination treatment of EPO and G-CSF/GM-CSF. A synergistic effect on hemoglobin levels in anemic patients with MDS can be observed when G-CSF is combined with EPO. Overall hemoglobin values are less likely to fall in the G-CSF/GM-CSF+EPO group, so that transfusion requirements are decreased [Estey, 1998].

Differentative therapy, such as non-AML-type chemotherapy with low-dose cytostatic agents like 5-azacytidine and amifostine, may be considered in the context of a clinical trial. Patients under 60 years with poor-risk features might profit from this combination chemotherapy [List et al., 1996]. In t-AML, complete remissions in 10–15% of patients have been reported, with improved blood counts in another 25–30% [Estey, 1998].

For patients with a better prognosis, Estey [1998] also suggests a trial of antithymocyte globulin (ATG) ± cyclosporine. This is an accepted therapy for aplastic anemia, and may restore pancytopenia in cases of hypoplastic MDS without changing the course of the leukemic clone. Complete remission with this therapy was reported in 18% and partial remission in 23% of 22 patients in low or INT-1 categories of IPSS [Moldrem et al.,1996].

Low-intensity therapies *not* recommended are G-CSF or GM-CSF alone; low-dose cytosine arabinoside; androgens; and vitamin A and vitamin D analogs. In pilot studies, those therapies have failed to induce a substantial percentage of complete remissions or better survival than in the control group treated with supportive care only [De Witte et al., 1995]. Nor are there any reports of reduced infection rates. Miller et al. [1988] also compared supportive care to low-dose arabinoside, and reported no difference in survival.

Conventional Chemotherapy

In the early 1980s, conventional multidrug chemotherapy, such as that applied to induce complete remission in de novo AML, was demonstrated to be effective for MDS, with complete remission rates of 15–51% [De Witte, 1994]. Later results obtained with combinations of cytosine arabinoside (ara-C), daunorubicin, thioguanine and vincristine showed complete remissions in 15–64% of the patients [Kantarijian et al., 1986; Anderson et al., 1993]. However, intensive AML-type chemotherapy in the management of high-risk t-MDS / t-AML remains controversial. Although increasing remission rates have been reported, the exact role of high-dose ara-C, idarubicin, fludarabine and growth factors has yet to be demonstrated. Complete remissions can be expected in only about 35% of unselected patients. In view of the treatment-related toxicity, these relatively low and brief complete remission rates (median remission duration and overall survival time are 3–9 months) are disappointing [De Witte et al., 1995, Ganser et al., 1993], and only a few patients are likely to be cured by chemotherapy alone. The high failure rate of remission-induction therapy is partly due to the long-term hypoplasia after chemotherapy and to strong drug resistance of the leukemic clone [De Witte et al., 1995, Greenberg et al., 1995]. Therefore, postremission therapy must also be modified, particularly in patients not suited for transplantation.

In a few patients with a worse overall prognosis (IPSS scores INT-2 or higher), treatment with AML-type chemotherapy regimens may induce complete remissions (15–61%) [Löffler et al., 1992]. However, remission is brief, and survival rate at 3 years is only 7%. About 40% of patients under 60 years with normal karyotype t-MDS can expect a complete remission lasting > 2 years following AML-type chemotherapy with high dosage of ara-C [Anderlini et al., 1996].

Estey [1998], however, suggests that those patients should also receive newer agents such as deoxyazacytidine (DAC), topotecan and *all-trans*-retinoic acid (ATRA) combined with chemotherapy. DAC is a pyrimidine analog able to methylate DNA, and may therefore enhance differentiation. Topotecan interacts with the topoisomerase I enzyme, resulting in cell death. It is useful in patients with cytogenetic abnormalities associated with poor response to standard therapies [Beran et al., 1996]. ATRA is of interest for AML and MDS because it decreases concentrations of proteins such as BCL-2 that interfere with chemotherapy-induced apoptosis.

Compared to the same chemotherapy regimen without ATRA, ATRA combined with fludarabine, ara-C and idarubicin prolonged disease-free survival from the start of treatment and from the time of complete remission [Estey et al., 1997].

Gardin et al. [1997] reported results for 34 patients treated with a combination intensive chemotherapy (12 mg/m^2 of idarubicin on days 1–3 and 100 mg/m^2 of cytarabine on days 1–7 in older patients, or 1 g/m^2 every 12 h on days 1–5 in younger patients) followed by G-CSF. G-CSF appears to reduce the incidence of resistant leukemia and, in some patients, seems to enhance the antileukemic effect of chemotherapy. There is a significant increase in remission *rate* but not in remission *duration* or overall survival [Bernasconi et al., 1998, Büchner et al., 1990]. However, only patients who undergo bone marrow / stem cell transplantation achieve long-term survival. The induction of complete remission prior to transplantation results in an even better outcome [Runde et al., 1995; De Witte, 1994].

Allogenic Bone Marrow Transplantation

Allogenic bone marrow transplantation improves chances for long-term disease-free survival, making it the treatment of choice for younger patients with short disease duration, high leukocyte count and a high hematocrit. Bone marrow transplantation should therefore be considered early on for t-MDS or t-AML patients under 55 years and with an HLA-identical sibling or closely matched unrelated donor [De Witte et al., 1990]. The results depend more on the patients transplanted than on the regimens used. Outcome varies considerably, depending on the stage of the disease at the time of transplantation and on clinical factors such as cytogenetic abnormalities, age, and the percentage of blasts in the bone marrow at the time of transplantation [De Witte et al., 1990].

A study by Arnold et al. [1998] on unrelated bone marrow transplantation in patients with MDS and secondary AML showed, at 2 years, a 28% probability of survival; 28% disease-free survival; a 35% relapse risk, and transplant-related mortality of 58%. Transplant-related mortality is significantly influenced by the age of the recipient, whereas the relapse rate after transplantation correlates to the FAB classification of the underlying disease. As in other allogenic bone marrow transplantations, the relapse rate is directly related to the graft-versus-leukemia effect. Patients treated in Seattle within 1 year of diagnosis had a 3-year survival rate of 65%, versus 30% for patients receiving transplants more than 3 years after diagnosis. Therefore, allogenic bone marrow transplantation is recommended early in the course of MDS [Estey, 1998].

Unfortunately, two thirds of the patients with MDS who may benefit from allogenic bone marrow transplantation lack a suitable family donor. Unrelated bone marrow transplantation cures a certain proportion of patients, but transplant-related mortalities are also high. A graft from an HLA-matched, unrelated donor seems most promising for younger patients (< 35 years) with poor-risk t-MDS or t-AML. Donors should therefore be sought early in the course of the disease. Most transplant centers will only consider allogenic bone marrow transplantation for t-AML after remission-induction therapy. If allogenic bone marrow transplantation is performed during a stage of excess blasts or during overt transformation, a relapse risk of 50–80% may be expected [De Witte et al., 1995]. Remission in patients treated with AML-type remission-induction chemotherapy is usually brief – particularly in patients with cytogenetic abnormalities. Sandler et al. [1994] also report improved survival for children with t-AML after bone marrow transplantation. Disease-free survival was 33% at 5 years, while regimen-related deaths occurred in 30% of the patients. Transplantation for t-MDS showed disease-free survival of 62%, and therapy-related mortality of 8%.

Whether bone marrow transplantation should be preceded by remission-induction chemotherapy is still under discussion. The remission rate is low, the risk of death during induction chemotherapy ranges from 15 to 64%, and it is unclear whether remission at the time of transplantation improves the outcome. Anderson et al. [1993] report a 5-year estimate of 24.4% disease-free survival, and a cumulative probability of 31.3% for relapse mortality and of 44.3% for nonrelapse mortality for patients transplanted without prior therapy. Three factors are associated with improved outcome: young age; short range of time from diagnosis to transplant – resulting in a lower nonrelapse mortality rate, and fewer blasts – leading to a lower relapse rate. This underscores the importance of transplanting as soon as possible after diagnosis of t-AML or before t-MDS progresses into t-AML.

Autologous Transplantation with Peripheral Blood Stem Cells

Autologous stem cell transplantation should be considered for patients without a suitable donor who achieve cytogenetic remission after intense chemotherapy [Bernasconi et al., 1998]. Hindering the more widespread use of autotransplants is the dearth of grafts of progenitor cells that are predominantly or completely disease-free. Carella et al. [1996] reported promising results for mobilization of peripheral blood progenitor cells (PBSC) without chromosomal aberrations and with consecutive autografting in patients with high-risk AML transformed from MDS. It was demonstrated that in this clonal neoplastic disease, progenitor cells lacking the clonal marker can be collected. In 6 out of 9 patients, the leukapheresis product was entirely karyotypically normal and could be used for autologous transplantation, ensuring a short recovery time. Demuynck et al. [1996] reported the same results for patients with high-risk MDS where adequate numbers of PBSC were harvested, enabling rapid and stable engraftment after reinfusion.

The possibility of mobilizing karyotypically normal PBSC into peripheral blood and the consecutive transplantation is therefore a very attractive treatment option – particularly for older patients who cannot risk allogenic bone marrow transplantation.

Conclusions

While debate on allogenic bone marrow transplantation versus AML-type chemotherapy for patients with t-MDS/t-AML is intense, the fact remains that neither therapy is currently satisfactory for these patients. AML-type intensive chemotherapy usually achieves only low and brief complete remission rates, so that its actual benefit for t-AML patients is controversial [Gardin et al., 1997]. Overall, long-term disease-free survival of patients with untreated t-MDS / t-AML or of those undergoing stem cell transplantation is poor, with high relapse and nonrelapse mortality.

Nevertheless, because some patients *are* cured with transplantation and are given a prognosis superior to those treated with chemotherapy, suitable patients should be transplanted as soon as possible. Moreover, since pretransplant remission induction does not benefit every patient, mild myeloablative therapy followed by transplantation of stem cells may be a more appropriate strategy. It is, in any case, an approach that also allows us to transplant older patients with poor performance status. In this manner, long-term remission may be achieved for some patients with otherwise fatal disease. Finally, strategies for the early detection of lethal treatment complications need to be pursued more extensively, particularly in times of reduced health-care budgets.

Acknowledgement

We would like to thank S. Frank (literature) and D. Crawford (translation and editing).

References

Anderlini P, Pierce S, Kantarjian H: AML-type chemotherapy for myelodysplasia. J Clin Oncol 1996;14:1404–1405.

Anderson JE, Appelbaum FR, Fisher LD: Allogenic bone marrow transplantation for 93 patients with myelodysplastic syndrome. Blood 1993;82:677–681.

Anderson JE, Gooley TA, Schoch G, Anasetti C, Bensinger WI, Clift RA, Hansen JA, Sanders JE, Storb R, Appelbaum FR: Stem cell transplantation for secondary acute myeloid leukemia: Evaluation of transplantation as initial therapy for following induction chemotherapy. Blood 1997;89:2578–2585.

Arnold R, De Witte T, Van Biezen A, Hermans J, Jacobsen N, Runde V, Gratwohl A, Apperley JF: Unrelated bone marrow transplantation in patients with myelodysplastic syndromes and secondary acute myeloid leukemia: An ABMT survey. Bone Marrow Transplant 1998;21: 1213–1216.

Beran M, Kantarjian H, O'Brien S: Topotecan, a topoisomerase I inhibitor, is active in the treatment of myelodysplastic syndrome and chronic myelomonocytic leukemia. Blood 1996;88:2473–2479.

Bernasconi C, Alessandrino EP, Bernasconi P, Bonfichi M, Lazzarino M, Canevari A, Catelli G, Brusamolina E, Pagnucco G, Gastagnola C: Randomized clinical study comparing aggressive chemotherapy with or without G-CSF support for high-risk myelodysplastic syndromes or secondary acute myeloid leukaemia evolving from MDS. Br J Haematol 1998;102:678–683.

Büchner T, Hiddemann W, Königsmann M: Recombination human GM-CSF following chemotherapy in high-risk AML. Bone Marrow Transplant 1990;6(suppl 1):131–134.

Carella AM, Dejana D, Lerma E, Podesta M, Benbenuto F, Chimirri F, Parodi C, Sessarego M, Prencipe E, Frassoni F: In vivo mobilization of karyotypically normal peripheral blood progenitor cells in high-risk MDS, secondary or therapy-related acute myelogenous leukemia. Br J Haematol 1996;95:127–130.

Cohen A, Martin M, Schwartz E: Depletion of excessive liver iron stores with desferrioxamine. Br J Haematol 1984;58:369–372.

De Witte T: New treatment approaches for myelodysplastic syndrome and secondary leukaemias. Ann Oncol 1994;5:401–408.

De Witte T, Suciu S, Peetermans M, Fenaux P, Strijckmans P, Hayat M, Jaksic B, Selleslag D, Zittoun R, Dardenne M, Solbu G, Zwierzina H, Muus P: Intensive chemotherapy for poor prognosis myelodysplasia (MDS) and secondary acute myeloid leukemia following MDS of more than 6 months' duration. A pilot study by the Leukemia Cooperative Group of the European Organisation for Research and Treatment in Cancer (EORTC-LCG). Leukemia 1995;9:1805–1811.

De Witte T, Zwaan F, Hermans J, Vernant J, Kolb H, Vossen J, Lönnquist B, Beelen D, Ferrant A, Gmür J, Liu Yin J, Troussard X, Cahn J, Ban Lint M, Gratwohl A: Allogeneic bone marrow transplantation for secondary leukaemia and myelodysplastic syndrome: A survey by the Leukaemia Working Party of the European Bone Marrow Transplantation Group. Br J Haematol 1990;74:151–155.

Demuynck H, Delforge M, Verhoef GEG, Zachee P, Vandenberghe P, Van Den Berghe H, Bougaerts MA: Feasibility of peripheral blood progenitor cell harvest and transplantation in patients with poor-risk myelodysplastic syndromes. Br J Haematol 1996;92:351–359.

Ellis J, Lishner M: Second malignancies following treatment in non-Hodgkin's lymphoma. Leuk Lymphoma 1993;9:337–342.

Estey E: Prognosis and therapy of secondary myelodysplastic syndromes. Haematologica 1998;83: 543–549.

Estey E, Beran M, Pierce S, Kantarjian H, Keating M: ATRA may improve results of chemotherapy in poor prognosis non-APL, AML and MDS: A randomized study. Blood 1997;90: 1221–1223.

Ganser A, Heil G, Kolbe K, Maschmeyer G, Fischer JT, Bergmann L, Mitrou PS, Heit W, Heimpel H, Huber C, Hoelzer D: Aggressive chemotherapy combined with G-CSF and maintenance therapy with interleukin-2 for patients with advanced myelodysplastic syndrome, subacute or secondary acute myeloid leukemia – initial results. Ann Hematol 1993;66:123–125.

Ganser A, Hoelzer D: Clinical course of myelodysplastic syndromes. Hematol Oncol Clin North Am 1992;6:607–618.

Gardin C, Chaibi P, DeRevel T, Rousselot P, Turlure P, Miclea JM, Nedellec G, Dombret H: Intensive chemotherapy with idarubicin, cytosine arabinoside and granulocyte colony-stimulating factor in patients with secondary and therapy-related acute myelogenous leukemia. Leukemia 1997;11:16–21.

Geddes A, Bowen D, Jacobs A: Clonal karyotypic abnormalities and clinical progress in the myelodysplastic syndrome. Br J Haematol 1990;76:194–202.

Greenberg P, Cox D, LeBeau MM, Fenaux P, Morel P, Sanz G, Sanz M, Vallespi T, Hamblin T, Oscler D, Ohyashiki K, Toyama K, Aul C, Mufti G, Bennet J: International scoring system for evaluating prognosis in myelodysplastic syndromes. Blood 1997;99:2079–2088.

Greenberg P, O'Brien S, Goldman J, Sawyers C: Myelodysplastic syndromes and myeloproliferative disorders: Clinical, therapeutic and molecular advances. Hematology. Educational Program ASH, Seattle, Wash. 1995, pp 10–21.

Kantarjian HM, Keating MJ, Walters RS, Smith TL, Cork A, McCredie KB, Freireich EJ: Therapy-related leukemia and myelodysplastic syndrome: Clinical, cytogenetic and prognostic features. J Clin Oncol 1986;4:1748–1757.

Karp JE, Smith MA: The molecular pathogenesis of treatment-induced (secondary) leukemias. Foundations for treatment and prevention. Semin Oncol 1997;24:103–113.

Kollmannsberger C, Harmann JT, Kanz L, Bokemeyer C: Risk of secondary myeloid leukemia and myelodysplastic syndrome following standard-dose chemotherapy or high-dose chemotherapy with stem cell support in patients with potentially curable malignancies. J Cancer Res Clin Oncol 1998;124:207–214.

Larson RA, Le Beau MM, Ratain MJ, Rowley JD: Balanced translocations involving chromosome bands 11q23 and 21q22 in therapy-related leukemia. Blood 1992;79:1892–1893.

List AF, Heaton R, Glinsmann-Gibson B, et al.: Amifostine promotes multilineage hematopoiesis in patients with myelodysplastic syndrome: Results of a phase I/II clinical trial. Blood 1996; 88:453a.

Löffler H, Schmitz N, Gassmann W: Intensive chemotherapy and bone marrow transplantation for myelodysplastic syndromes. Hematol Oncol Clin North Am 1992;6:619–631.

Miller JS, Arthur DC, Litz CE: Myelodysplastic syndrome after autologous bone marrow transplantation: An additional late complication of curative cancer therapy. Blood 1994;83: 3780–3786.

Miller KB, Kim K, Morrison FS: Evaluation of low-dose ara-C versus supportive care in the treatment of myelodysplastic syndromes: An intergroup study by the Eastern Cooperative Oncology Group and the Southwest Oncology Group (abstract). Blood 1988;72:215a.

Molldrem J, Stetler-Stevenson M, Movroudis D, Young NS, Barret AJ: Antithymocyte globulin abrogates cytopenias in patients with myelodysplastic syndromes (abstract). Blood 1996;88:454a.

Pedersen-Bjergaard J, Philip P: Balanced translocations involving chromosome bands 11q23 and 21q22 are highly characteristic of myelodysplasia and leukemia following therapy with cytostatic agents targeting DNA-topoisomerase II. Blood 1991;78:1147–1148.

Rege KP, Janes SL, Saso R, Min T, Swansbury J, Powles RL, Treleaven JG: Secondary leukaemia characterised by monosomy 7 occurring post-autologous stem cell transplantation for AML. Bone Marrow Transplant 1998;21:853–855.

Runde V, De Witte F, Aul C, Gratwohl A, Niederwieser D, van Biezen A, Hermans J, Vernant J, Kolb H, Vossen J, Lönqvist B, Beelen D, Ferrant A, Arnold R, Cahn J, van Lint M, Verdonk L, Apperley J: Myelodysplastic syndromes (MDS) or leukemia following MDS (sAML) treated with allogenic bone marrow transplantation (BMT): A survey of the working party on chronic leukemia of the EBMT. Ann Hematol 1995;70(suppl II):A138.

Sandler ES, Friedman DJ, Mustafa MM, Winick NJ, Bowman PW, Buchanan GR: Treatment of Children with Epipodophyllotoxin-Induced Secondary Acute Myeloid Leukemia. American Cancer Society, 1997, pp 1049–1054.

Smith MA, Rubinstein L, Anderson JR, Arthur D, Catalano PJ, Freidlin B, Heyn R, Khayat A, Krailo M, Land BJ, Miser J, Shuster J, Vena D: Secondary leukemia or myelodysplastic syndrome after treatment with epipodophyllotoxins. J Clin Oncol 1999;17:569–577.

Traweek WT, Slovak ML, Nademanee AP: Clonal karyotypic hematopoietic cell abnormalities occurring after autologous bone marrow transplantation for Hodgkin's disease and non-Hodgkin's lymphoma. Blood 1994;84:957–963.

Yunis JJ, Rydell RE, Oken MM, Arnesen MA, Mayer MG, Lobell M: Refined chromosome analysis as an independent prognostic indicator in de novo myelodysplastic syndrome. Blood 1986;67:1721–1730.

Dr. Ursula Rüther, Paul-Lincke-Straße 4, D–70195 Stuttgart (Germany)

Rüther U, Nunnensiek C, Schmoll H-J (eds): Secondary Neoplasias following Chemotherapy, Radiotherapy, and Immunosuppression. Contrib Oncol. Basel, Karger, 2000, vol 55, pp 275–285

....

Immunological Aspects of the Pathogenesis of Tumors Associated with Epstein-Barr Virus: Vaccines for Prevention and Therapy

Gerlinde Benninger-Döring, Hans Wolf

Institut für Medizinische Mikrobiologie und Hygiene, Regensburg, Deutschland

Introduction

The Epstein-Barr virus (EBV), with its very efficient transference (usually by mouth) and its lifelong persistence in the host, is one of the most widespread viruses. It is present in more than 95% of adults all over the world. In the United States and Europe, one of the most common EBV-related illnesses among young people is infectious mononucleosis, which may present with marked clinical symptoms. Secondary EBV diseases include several human malignancies, such as the endemic form of African Burkitt's lymphoma, and, primarily in Asia and Africa, nasopharyngeal carcinoma. Also included are certain forms of Hodgkin's lymphoma [see chapter on 'Herpesviruses in Secondary Tumorigenesis', pp. 17–35]. Of special significance for the medical field is that lymphomas are increasingly appearing in organ recipients and are usually EBV-correlated [see chapter on 'Posttransplant Lymphoproliferative Disorder', pp. 305–346].

The role of humoral and cellular mechanisms in preventing disease has been investigated in several primate studies [reviewed in Wolf and Morgan, 1998]. Preliminary results for a preventive vaccine for humans show potential [Gu et al., 1995], so that further clinical trials are underway.

Correlates of the Protection Given by Vaccination

While studies and trials have not yet discovered the exact role of neutralizing antibodies, the cellular components of immune control are better understood. Cellular immune components, such as unspecific natural killer cells, and ADCC mechanisms that are mediated by the two glycoproteins gp110 and gp350/220 [Jilg et al.,

1994; Khyatti et al., 1991] have been described, as has cellular immune control via HLA class I-restricting cytotoxic T lymphocytes (CTL). These are targeted at proteins of latency [Rickinson and Moss, 1997] and at EBV antigens of the lytic replication phase [Bogedain et al., 1995; Steven et al.; 1997; Pepperl et al., 1998; Redchenko and Rickinson, 1999; Khanna et al., 1999a; Benninger-Döring et al., 1999]. Using tetrameric MHC molecules, it was demonstrated that during acute infection, up to 40% of the entire CD8+ cell population targets one single lytic antigen [Callan et al., 1998]. Even healthy virus carriers whose primary infection progressed asymptomatically had a high frequency of CD8+ CTL against lytic antigens [Tan et al., 1999; Benninger-Döring et al., 1999]. An overview of the immunologic control of EBV infection in the B-cell compartment is given in figure 1.

Circumventing Control by the Immune System

While co-evolving with its human host, EBV acquired certain characteristics that improve its potential for colonizing the B-cell compartment. How efficiently the virus infects a new host depends on its speed in reaching B cells and in increasing the number of EBV-infected cells before the host immune system can respond. The individual viral strategies are explained below.

Latency
After primary infection, EBV-infected B cells can persist latently in the B-cell compartment [Babcock et al., 1998]. Quiescent B cells are characterized by restricted gene expression, during which only EBNA1 and/or LMP2 are synthesized [Qu and Rowe, 1992; Thorley-Lawson et al., 1996]. Although LMP2 contains CTL epitopes [Lee et al., 1997], the immune system does not destroy these cells. This is because quiescent B cells lack the co-stimulatory surface molecule B7, which mediates ligation to CD28 and is essential for T-cell activation [Linsley and Ledbetter, 1993]. The number of EBV-infected peripheral B cells remains remarkably constant in the host for years, and is in the order of $10^1–10^3$ EBV-infected cells/10^7 B cells [Miyashita et al., 1997].

Immune Modulation by Cytokines
The BCRF1 reading frame expressed during lytic replication encodes for the viral interleukin (IL)-10 protein with an 80% homology with cellular IL-10. Like the cellular homolog, BCRF1 inhibits the production of interferon-γ by lymphocytes, and the production of IL-12 by macrophages. Viral IL-10 directly stimulates B-cell growth and inhibits dendritic cells from maturation. Via these mechanisms, BCRF1 affects T-cell response and B-cell growth, and may thereby enable EBV-infected

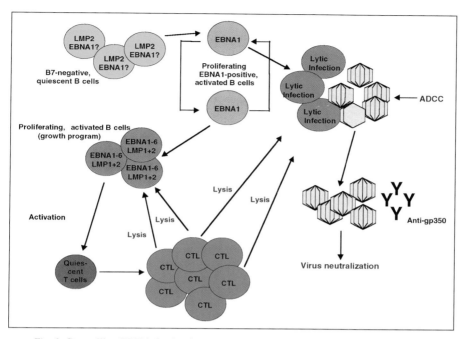

Fig. 1. Controlling EBV infection in the B-cell compartment [based on Khanna et al., 1995]. Virus-neutralizing anti-gp350/220 antibodies, as well as ADCC mechanisms, are involved in preventing viral spread. However, it is the HLA class I-restricted cytotoxic T cells that play the most important role in controlling EBV infection. Quiescent B cells, lacking the co-stimulatory activation marker B7, cannot be detected by CTL, and therefore form the reservoir for latent viruses [Babcock et al., 1998]. Exogenous signals can activate these cells and cause them to switch into the EBNA1-only phase [Thorley-Lawson et al., 1996]. Due to an internal glycine-alanine repeat, EBNA1 is not antigenic [Levitskaya et al., 1995]; hence, cells expressing EBNA1 only are not eliminated by the immune system. When in this mode, cells can switch directly into the lytic cycle or into the growth phase [Rowe et al., 1992]. The growth program is characterized by the expression of EBV nuclear antigens (EBNA1–6), as well as by that of latent membrane proteins LMP1 and LMP2. All of these proteins, except for EBNA1, are targeted and eliminated by cytotoxic T cells [Rickinson and Moss, 1997; Khanna et al., 1998]. The latest studies underscore the significance of the lytic antigens as targets of cytotoxic T cells. B cells that switch into the replicative phase are eliminated with great efficiency [Tan et al., 1999; Benninger-Döring et al., 1999]. All together, these immune control mechanisms maintain a biological balance between virus and host such that the virus persists in the healthy host for life, but without pathologic symptoms.

cells to survive longer. In addition, increased cellular IL-10 production by Hodgkin's lymphoma cells may be responsible for the reduced activity of cytotoxic T cells in Hodgkin's lymphoma [Ohshima et al., 1995].

Inhibition of HLA Class I Processing and Down-Regulation of T-Cell Molecules

Burkitt's lymphoma cells have a nonantigenic phenotype and cannot be eliminated by the immune system. Burkitt's lymphoma cells express EBNA1 as their only viral protein. EBNA1, in turn, contains a glycine-alanine repeat sequence that inhibits protein reduction via MHC class I processing [Levitskaya et al., 1995] . If EBNA1 is presented exogenously, then EBNA1-specific HLA class 1-restricted CTL can be detected in the blood of EBV-seropositive donors [Blake et al., 1997]. In vivo, the significance of this TAP-independent means of presenting and processing is unclear. Also characteristic of Burkitt's lymphoma cells is the down-regulation of TAP1 and TAP2 molecules [Rowe et al., 1995], as well as of MHC class I antigens on the cell surface [Jilg et al., 1991]. These changes do not affect the MHC class II presentation route. Via this route, EBV-specific CD4+ CTL can recognize processed and presented viral peptide epitopes and lyse Burkitt's lymphoma cells [Khanna et al., 1997a]. In addition, ICAM1 and LFA3 mediate T-cell adhesion, their absence or very low level of expression also inhibits immune elimination of cells with a Burkitt's lymphoma phenotype [Gregory et al., 1988].

Immunodominant Effects

For nasopharyngeal carcinomas and Hodgkin's lymphomas, antigen processing and presentation are intact. Even though these tumors cannot be eliminated efficiently, both types of tumors express only viral proteins EBNA1, LMP1 and LMP2. Both LMP1 and LMP2 contain CTL epitopes [Khanna et al., 1998; Lee et al., 1997]. The inability of the CTL system to access these tumors is explained from a weak LMP-specific immune response. In general, CTL response is restricted to a limited number of CTL epitopes, less than 10% of these are immunodominant [Wettstein and Bailey, 1982]. The hierarchy of antigenic CTL epitopes results from several limiting steps that lead to antigen presentation and T-cell recognition [Gallimore et al., 1998]. Accordingly, Levitsky et al. [1996] were able to demonstrate that the intensity of two HLA-A11-restricted, EBV-specific CTL responses correlated with the density of the epitopes on the antigen-presenting cell.

CTL-Epitope Variations

To escape detection by the immune system, many viruses mutate, altering the amino acid sequence and thus the quantity and quality of CTL epitopes. Such mutations impact either the bonding of the peptide epitope to the HLA complex, or the correlating T-cell receptor's recognition of the trinary complex. Immunodominant epitopes can be destroyed by point mutations in anchor positions, which prevents epitope-specific CTL from recognizing them. This kind of mutation has been observed in the anchor position of the HLA-A11-restricted EBNA3B$_{416-424}$ epitope in EBV isolates from China [de Campos-Lima et al., 1993, 1994]. HLA-A11 alleles are particularly frequent in the coastal populations of New Guinea and China. This correlation has led to the hypothesis that evolutionary pressure exerted by the immune system causes CTL epitopes to change and to provide a selective advantage for the virus. However, the same mutation appears in highland populations in New Guinea – but in conjunction with low HLA-A11 frequency – contradicting this hypothesis [Burrows et al., 1996]. Other studies of the B35.01 allele, which is common in West Africa and which presents the EBNA3A$_{458-466}$ epitope, also contradict this theory [Lee et al., 1995]. Amino-acid differences in CTL epitopes may be nothing more than geographic markers that did not develop due to selective pressure exerted by the host [Khanna et al., 1997c].

Therapy and Prevention: Work towards an EBV-Specific Vaccine

After primary contact, EBV remains in the host lifelong. The demonstration of viral DNA in peripheral blood cells or of EBV-specific antibodies does not necessarily indicate EBV-associated tumorigenesis. To demonstrate such an association, the tumor cells, such as in Hodgkin's or Burkitt's lymphoma, or in various lymphomas in immunocompromised patients, must first be cytologically or histologically identified. If viral genomes are detected in the tumor cells, tumor association with EBV can be assumed. For tissue specimens, viral genomes are detected by in-situ hybridization mostly using DNA probes. Viral gene activity such as EBER transcripts can be detected using in-situ hybridization with RNA probes. Finally, evidence may be gained immunohistochemically with monoclonal antibodies against viral antigens of the latency period (EBNA2, LMP1). In its early stages, it is difficult to detect nasopharyngeal carcinoma in situ. However, continued elevation of immunoglobulin class A antibodies against EBNA1, as well as against early proteins (EA) of the lytic cycle and structural proteins (VCA), are very early, reliable and prognostic markers [Foong et al., 1990; Zeng et al., 1982, 1983].

Chemotherapy cannot access the viruses latently persisting in quiescent B cells (which form the viral reservoir in the host), nor the latent viruses in the tumor cells. Thus, EBV infection can at present not be therapied systematically. Administration of nucleoside analogs such as acyclovir or ganciclovir – which inhibit lytic viral replication – is probably not beneficial in these cases. Thus, therapy of EBV-associated tumors involves surgical excision of the primary tumor, plus subsequent radiotherapy (for nasopharyngeal carcinoma) and/or chemotherapy (for nasopharyngeal carcinoma and Burkitt's lymphoma).

EBV-associated lymphomas occurring in immunosuppressed transplantees express the complete pattern of latent EBV antigens. The adoptive transfer of EBV-specific CTL of the donor can cause immunoblastic B-cell lymphomas occurring after bone marrow transplantation to regress [Rooney et al., 1995; Heslop et al., 1996]. CTL preparations can also be administered prophylactically to reduce the initial viral load and thus lessen the risk of lymphoma. Autologous or HLA-matched CTL preparations of the transplant recipient may be administered to aid in tumor regression after organ transplantation [Haque et al., 1998; Khanna et al., 1999b].

Prevention of EBV-Associated Diseases

Fifty percent of the patients with primary EBV infection manifest the symptoms of infectious mononucleosis, which increase markedly with patient age. This, in addition to the growing number of EBV-associated lymphoproliferative disorders and today's better comprehension of virally induced immune response, have strengthened the call for an EBV vaccine. In populations with high socioeconomic standards, such an EBV vaccine would be administered primarily as protection against infectious mononucleosis.

A vaccine that would lessen the initial viral load might suffice to greatly reduce or even suppress clinical symptoms in EBV-negative youth. Where a graft or a blood transfusion has led to a spontaneous lymphoproliferative disorder in posttransplant patients [Craig et al., 1993], reducing EB viral load should offer protection. For full-blown lymphoproliferative disorders, only expanded vaccination strategies seem promising, and therefore have to be tested separately. The most common EBV-associated tumors (Burkitt's lymphoma, nasopharyngeal carcinoma and Hodgkin's lymphoma) usually do not develop until years after primary infection. This primary infection is generally severe, or, as in the case of nasopharyngeal carcinoma [Zeng et al., 1982; 1983] and Burkitt's lymphoma [de Thé et al., 1978], is followed by lasting, markedly increased systemic EBV activity, as demonstrated by serologic parameters. Because the first therapeutic vaccines show promising results for hepatitis B [Coullin et al., 1999], similar protocols for EBV should be tested.

There have been two approaches to developing an EBV vaccine. The first involves developing a prophylactic vaccine based on the viral glycoprotein gp350 [Gu et al., 1995]. The second is based on the induction of an EBV-specific CTL immunity for therapy of lymphoproliferative disorders [Rooney et al., 1995].

EBV Vaccines Based on Viral Glycoprotein gp350

The first attempts to develop an EBV vaccine concentrated on the viral glycoprotein gp350, because this protein mediates the binding to the cellular EBV receptor CD21. Also, this dominant antigen of the viral envelope is the target of virus-neutralizing antibodies. In the Tamarin model, EBV vaccine substances consisting of gp350 glycoprotein or recombinant vectors expressing this antigen offer protection against EBV-induced B-cell lymphomas [Morgan, 1992]. Studies involving a recombinant gp350 live vaccine administered to EBV-negative infants in China showed that in the course of 3 years, only 44% of the vaccinated group seroconverted, while all of the control group were EBV-positive after 1 year [Gu et al., 1995; reviewed in Wolf and Morgan, 1998]. More recent studies describe CTL epitopes in glycoprotein gp350 and the use of these peptide epitopes to successfully immunize mice [Khanna et al., 1999a].

Induction of an EBV-Specific CLT Immunity
Latent Antigens. HLA class-I-restricted CTL play the key role in mediating T-cell immunity during latency and the replicative phase of EBV. From the biological point of view, a vaccination strategy based on CTL epitopes seems promising. Corresponding preliminary clinical studies have been conducted with the HLA-B8-restricted peptide sequence FLRGRAYGL (EBNA3A$_{325-333}$). Here, the murine model demonstrated the efficacy of a vaccination based on immunodominant CTL epitopes [Scalzo et al., 1995]. Because epitope selection is HLA-specific, HLA's polymorphism is the main barrier to developing a vaccine based only on CTL epitopes. Introducing multiple peptide epitopes of various HLA restrictions into a vaccine vector enables CTL to recognize multiple epitopes, and may circumvent some of these problems [Thomson et al., 1995].

Early Lytic Proteins. EBV persists in quiescent B cells, and from this stage can switch directly to the lytic cycle – without expression of further latent antigens. For this reason, CTL epitopes of latent EBV antigens, as well as those of lytic antigens, must be taken into consideration when developing vaccines. Strong evidence for this approach comes from careful studies on the analysis of viral mRNA and protein species in clinical samples [Prang et al., 1997] and are confirmed by quantitative CTL analysis in clinical specimens [Benninger-Döring et al., 1999; Callan et al., 1998].

The cells of EBV-associated tumors, such as Burkitt's lymphoma, nasopharyngeal carcinoma and Hodgkin's disease, have a very limited pattern of expression. There are four possible approaches to controlling them: (1) Prophylactic EBV vaccination that does not necessarily prevent primary infection completely for the entire life of the host, but instead modulates infection such that the immune system can hold clinical symptoms down to a minimum. (2) A modulatory vaccination administered after infection to persons at a high risk of developing EBV-associated neoplasms. As is the case for nasopharyngeal carcinoma or Burkitt's lymphoma, this increased risk could be calculated on the basis of regional or individual factors or perhaps indications derived by specific serodiagnosis. (3) Where nasopharyngeal carcinoma is already manifest, it must be determined why those tumor cells which present antigens sufficiently have not been detected or eliminated by CTL against expressed genes (LMP1, LMP2, BZLF1, BARF0 and possibly slight amounts of structural proteins such as gp350). (4) Vaccination for Burkitt's lymphoma would have to override the Burkitt's lymphoma phenotype and to force antigen presentation. A possible mediator is the CD40 surface molecule, which can increase TAP expression in Burkitt's lymphoma cells [Khanna et al., 1997b].

References

Babcock GJ, Decker LL, Volk M, Thorley-Lawson DA: EBV persistence in memory B cells in vivo. Immunity 1998;9:395–404.

Benninger-Döring G, Pepperl S, Deml L, Modrow S, Wolf H, Jilg W: Frequency of CD8-positive T lymphocytes specific for lytic and latent antigens of Epstein-Barr virus in healthy virus carriers. Virology 1999;264:289–297.

Blake N, Lee S, Redchenko I, Thomas W, Steven N, Leese A, Steigerwald-Mullen P, Kurilla M, Frappier L, Rickinson A: Human CD8+ T cell responses to EBV EBNA1: HLA class I presentation of the (Gly-Ala)-containing protein requires exogenous processing. Immunity 1997;7:791–802.

Bogedain C, Wolf H, Modrow S, Stuber G, Jilg W: Specific cytotoxic T lymphocytes recognize the immediate-early transactivator Zta of Epstein-Barr virus. J Virol 1996;69:4872–4879.

Burrows JM, Burrows SR, Poulsen LM, Sculley TB, Moss DJ, Khanna R: Unusually high frequency of Epstein-Barr virus genetic variants in Papua New Guinea that can escape cytotoxic T-cell recognition: Implications for virus evolution. J Virol 1996;70: 2490–2496.

Callan MF, Tan L, Annels N, Ogg GS, Wilson JD, O'Callaghan CA, Steven N, McMichael AJ, Rickinson AB: Direct visualization of antigen-specific CD8+ T cells during the primary immune response to Epstein-Barr virus in vivo. J Exp Med 1998;187:1395–1402.

Couillin I, Pol S, Mancini M, Driss F, Brèchot C, Tiollais P, Michel ML: Specific vaccine therapy in chronic hepatitis B: Induction of T cell proliferative responses specific for envelope antigens. J Infect Dis 1999;180:15–26.

Craig FE, Gulley ML, Banks PM: Posttransplantation lymphoproliferative disorders. Am J Clin Pathol 1993;99:265–276.

de Campos-Lima PO, Gavioli R, Zhang QJ, Wallace LE, Dolcetti R, Rowe M, Rickinson AB, Masucci MG: HLA-A11 epitope loss isolates of Epstein-Barr virus from a highly A11+ population. Science 1993;260:98–100.

de Campos-Lima PO, Levitsky V, Brooks J, Lee SP, Hu LF, Rickinson AB, Masucci MG: T cell responses and virus evolution: Loss of HLA A11-restricted CTL epitopes in Epstein-Barr virus isolates from highly A11-positive populations by selective mutation of anchor residues. J Exp Med 1994;179:1297–1305.

De The G, Geser A, Day NE, Tukei PM, Williams EH, Beri DP, Smith PG, Dean AG, Bronkamm GW, Feorino P, Henle W: Epidemiological evidence for causal relationship between Epstein-Barr virus and Burkitt's lymphoma from Ugandan prospective study. Nature 1979;274: 756–761.

Foong YT, Cheng HM, Sam CK, Dillner J, Hinderer W, Prasad U: Serum and salivary IgA antibodies against a defined epitope of the Epstein-Barr virus nuclear antigen are elevated in nasopharyngeal carcinoma. Int J Cancer 1990;45:1061–1064.

Gallimore A, Hengartner H, Zinkernagel R: Hierarchies of antigen-specific cytotoxic T-cell responses. Immunol Rev 1998;164:29–36.

Gregory CD, Murray RJ, Edwards CF, Rickinson AB: Downregulation of cell adhesion molecules LFA-3 and ICAM-1 in Epstein-Barr virus-positive Burkitt's lymphoma underlies tumor cell escape from virus-specific T cell surveillance. J Exp Med 1988;167:1811–1824.

Gu SY, Huang TM, Ruan L, Miao YH, Lu H, Chu CM, Motz M, Wolf H: First EBV vaccine trial in humans using recombinant vaccinia virus expressing the major membrane antigen. Dev Biol Stand 1995;84:171-177.

Haque T, Amlot PL, Helling N, Thomas JA, Sweny P, Rolles K, Burroughs AK, Prentice HG, Crawford DH: Reconstitution of EBV-specific T cell immunity in solid organ transplant recipients. J Immunol 1998;160:6204–6209.

Heslop HE, Ng CY, Li C, Smith CA, Loftin SK, Krance RA, Brenner MK, Rooney CM: Long-term restoration of immunity against Epstein-Barr virus infection by adoptive transfer of gene-modified virus-specific T lymphocytes. Nat Med 1996;2:551–555.

Jilg W, Bogedain C, Mairhofer H, Gu SY, Wolf H: The Epstein-Barr virus-encoded glycoprotein gp 110 (BALF 4) can serve as a target for antibody-dependent cell-mediated cytotoxicity. Virology 1994;202:974–977.

Jilg W, Voltz R, Markert-Hahn C, Mairhofer H, Münz I, Wolf H: Expression of class I major histocompatibility complex antigens in Epstein-Barr virus-carrying lymphoblastoid cell lines and Burkitt-lymphoma cell lines. Cancer Res 1991;51:27–32.

Khanna R, Burrows S, Moss DJ: Immune regulation in Epstein-Barr virus-associated diseases. Microbiol Rev 1995;59:387–405.

Khanna R, Burrows SR, Thomson SA, Moss DJ, Cresswell P, Poulsen LM, Cooper, L: Class I processing-defective Burkitt's lymphoma cells are recognized efficiently by CD4+ EBV-specific CTLs. J Immunol 1997a;158:3619–3625.

Khanna R, Cooper L, Kienzle N, Moss DJ, Burrows SR, Khanna KK: Engagement of CD40 antigen with soluble CD40 ligand up-regulates peptide transporter expression and restores endogenous processing function in Burkitt's lymphoma cells. J Immunol 1997b;159:5782–5785.

Khanna R, Slade RW, Poulsen L, Moss DJ, Burrows SR, Nicholls J, Burrows JM: Evolutionary dynamics of genetic variation in Epstein-Barr virus isolates of diverse geographical origins: Evidence for immune pressure-independent genetic drift. J Virol 1997c;71:8340–8346.

Khanna R, Burrows SR, Nicholls J, Poulsen LM: Identification of cytotoxic T cell epitopes within Epstein-Barr virus (EBV) oncogene latent membrane protein 1 (LMP1): Evidence for HLA A2 supertype-restricted immune recognition of EBV-infected cells by LMP1-specific cytotoxic T lymphocytes. Eur J Immunol 1998;28:451–458.

Khanna R, Sherritt M, Burrows SR: EBV structural antigens, gp350 and gp85, as targets for ex vivo virus-specific CTL during acute infectious mononucleosis: Potential use of gp350/gp85 CTL epitopes for vaccine design. J Immunol 1999a;162:3063–3069.

Khanna R, Bell S, Sherritt M, Galbraith A, Burrows SR, Rafter L, Clarke B, Slaughter R, Falk MC, Douglass J, Williams T, Elliott SL, Moss DJ: Activation and adoptive transfer of Epstein-Barr virus-specific cytotoxic T cells in solid organ transplant patients with posttransplant lymphoproliferative disease. Proc Natl Acad Sci USA 1999b;96:10391–10396.

Khyatti M, Patel PC, Stefanescu I, Menezes J: Epstein-Barr virus (EBV) glycoprotein gp350 expressed on transfected cells resistant to natural killer cell activity serves as target for EBV-specific antibody-dependent cellular cytotoxicity. J Virol 1991;72:1622–1626.

Lee SP, Morgan S, Skinner J, Thomas WA, Jones SR, Sutton J, Khanna R, Whittle HC, Rickinson AB: Epstein-Barr virus isolates with the major HLA B35.01-restricted cytotoxic T lymphocyte epitope are prevalent in a highly B35.01-positive African population. Eur J Immunol 1995;25:102–110.

Lee SP, Tierney RJ, Thomas WA, Brooks JM, Rickinson AB: Conserved CTL epitopes within EBV latent membrane protein 2: A potential target for CTL-based tumor therapy. J Immunol 1997;158:3325–3334.

Levitskaya J, Coram M, Levitsky V, Imreh S, Steigerwald-Mullen PM, Klein G, Kurilla MG, Masucci MG: Inhibition of antigen processing by the internal repeat region of the Epstein-Barr virus nuclear antigen-1. Nature 1995;375:685–688.

Levitsky V, Zhang QJ, Levitskaya J, Masucci MG: The life span of major histocompatibility complex-peptide complexes influences the efficiency of presentation and immunogenicity of two class I-restricted cytotoxic T lymphocyte epitopes in the Epstein-Barr virus nuclear antigen 4. J Exp Med 1996;183:915–926.

Linsley PS, Ledbetter JA: The role of the CD28 receptor during T cell responses to antigen. Annu Rev Immunol 1993;11:191–212.

Masucci MG, Ernberg I: Epstein-Barr virus: Adaptation to a life within the immune system. Trends Microbiol 1994;2:125–130.

Miyashita EM, Yang B, Babcock GJ, Thorley-Lawson DA: Identification of the site of Epstein-Barr virus persistence in vivo as a resting B cell [published erratum appears in J Virol 1998;72: 9419]. J Virol 1997;71:4882–4891.

Morgan AJ: Epstein-Barr virus vaccines. Vaccine 1992;10:563–571.

Ohshima K, Suzumiya J, Akamatu M, Takeshita M, Kikuchi M: Human and viral interleukin-10 in Hodgkin's disease, and its influence on CD4+ and CD8+ T lymphocytes. Int J Cancer 1995;62:5–10.

Pepperl S, Benninger-Doring G, Modrow S, Wolf H, Jilg W: Immediate-early transactivator Rta of Epstein-Barr virus (EBV) shows multiple epitopes recognized by EBV-specific cytotoxic T lymphocytes. J Virol 1998;72:8644–8649.

Prang NS, Hornef MW, Jäger M, Wagner WJ, Wolf H, Schwarzmann F: Lytic replication of Epstein-Barr virus in the peripheral blood: Analysis of viral gene expression in B-lymphocytes during infectious mononucleosis and in the normal carrier state. Blood 1997;89:1665–1677.

Qu L, Rowe DT: Epstein-Barr virus latent gene expression in uncultured peripheral blood lymphocytes. J Virol 1992;66:3715–3724.

Redchenko IV, Rickinson AB: Accessing Epstein-Barr virus-specific T-cell memory with peptide-loaded dendritic cells. J Virol 1999;73:334–342.

Rickinson AB, Moss DJ: Human cytotoxic T lymphocyte responses to Epstein-Barr virus infection. Annu Rev Immunol 1997;15:405–431.

Rooney CM, Smith CA, Ng CY, Loftin S, Li C, Krance RA, Brenner MK, Heslop HE: Use of gene-modified virus-specific T lymphocytes to control Epstein-Barr-virus-related lymphoprolife-ration. Lancet 1995;345:9–13.

Rowe M, Lear AL, Croom-Carter D, Davies AH, Rickinson AB: Three pathways of Epstein-Barr virus gene activation from EBNA1-positive latency in B lymphocytes. J Virol 1992;66: 122–131.

Rowe M, Khanna R, Jacob CA, Argaet V, Kelly A, Powis S, Belich M, Croom-Carter D, Lee S, Burrows SR, Trowsdale J, Moss DJ, Rickinson AB: Restoration of endogenous antigen processing in Burkitt's lymphoma cells by Epstein-Barr virus latent membrane protein-1: Co-ordinate up-regulation of peptide transporters and HLA class I antigen expression. Eur J Immunol 1995;25:1374–1384.

Scalzo AA, Elliott SL, Cox J, Gardner J, Moss DJ, Suhrbier A: Induction of protective cytotoxic T cells to murine cytomegalovirus by using a nonapeptide and a human-compatible adjuvant (Montanide ISA 720). J Virol 1995;69:1306–1309.

Steven NM, Annels NE, Kumar A, Leese AM, Kurilla MG, Rickinson AB: Immediate early and early lytic cycle proteins are frequent targets of the Epstein-Barr virus-induced cytotoxic T cell response. J Exp Med 1995;185:1605–1617.

Tan LC, Gudgeon N, Annels NE, Hansasuta P, O'Callaghan CA, Rowland-Jones S, McMichael A, Rickinson A, Callan MFC: A re-evaluation of the frequency of CD8+ T cells specific for EBV in healthy virus carriers. J Immunol 1999;162:1827–1835.

Thomson SA, Elliott SL, Sherritt MA, Sproat KW, Coupar BE, Scalzo AA, Forbes CA, Ladhams, AM, Mo XY, Tripp RA, Doherty PC, Moss DJ, Suhrbier A: Recombinant polyepitope vaccines for the delivery of multiple CD8 cytotoxic T cell epitopes. J Immunol 1996;157:822–826.

Thorley-Lawson DA, Miyashita EM, Khan G: Epstein-Barr virus and the B cell: That's all it takes. Trends Microbiol 1996;4:204–208.

Wettstein PJ, Bailey DW: Immunodominance in the immune response to 'multiple' histocompatibility antigens. Immunogenetics 1982;16:47–58.

Wolf HJ, Morgan AJ: Epstein-Barr virus vaccines; in Medveczky et al (eds): Herpesviruses and Immunity. New York, Plenum Press, 1998.

Zeng Y, Zhang LG, Li HY, Jan MG, Zhang Q, Wu YC, Wang YS, Su GR: Serological mass survey for early detection of nasopharyngeal carcinoma in Wuzhou City, China. Int J Cancer 1982;29:139–141.

Zeng Y, Zhong JM, Li LY, Wang PZ, Tang H, Ma YR, Zhu JS, Pan WJ, Liu YX, Wei ZN: Follow-up studies on Epstein-Barr virus IgA/VCA antibody-positive persons in Zangwu County, China. Intervirology 1983;20:190–194.

Prof. Dr. Hans Wolf, Institut für Medizinische Mikrobiologie und Hygiene,
Franz-Josef-Strauß-Allee 11. D–93053 Regensburg (Germany)
Tel. +49 941 944-6400, Fax -6402, E-mail Hans.Wolf@klinik.uni-regensburg.de

Rüther U, Nunnensiek C, Schmoll H-J (eds): Secondary Neoplasias following Chemotherapy,
Radiotherapy, and Immunosuppression. Contrib Oncol. Basel, Karger, 2000, vol 55, pp 286–304

....

Live Attenuated Varicella Vaccine

Anne A. Gershon

Department of Pediatrics, Columbia University College of Physicians & Surgeons,
New York, NY, USA

Background: Varicella-Zoster Virus

Varicella-zoster virus (VZV) is one of the eight herpesviruses that cause infection in humans. VZV was first isolated in tissue culture in the 1950s by Weller and co-workers [99–102], and subsequently recognized to be a herpesvirus capable of causing latent infection. *Varicella* results from primary infection with VZV. The typical varicella patient manifests with fever, malaise and a generalized rash lasting about 5 days. Generally, the infection is mild, self-limited, and without complications, especially in normal hosts. It usually consists of maculopapular lesions that progress rapidly to vesicles, pustules and crusts; the rash is characteristically pruritic. The preponderance of skin lesions is present on the face, head and trunk. At the time of the rash of varicella, it is thought that VZV infects nerve endings in the skin, from which latent infection is established. For most individuals, virus latency persists for decades without symptoms. Overall, about 15% of individuals who live into old age may develop zoster.

Zoster results when latent VZV reactivates; it is therefore a secondary infection with VZV. A previous history of varicella is a prerequisite for development of zoster, although in rare cases, zoster patients give no history of the illness. Presumably, such patients had an asymptomatic case of varicella, which is thought to occur in about 5% of individuals. Zoster occurs in individuals with a low cell-mediated immune (CMI) response to VZV; typically, their antibody titers are high at onset of illness [3, 47]. Patients with zoster experience a unilateral vesicular rash localized to 1–3 dermatomes; the rash may be accompanied by fever and pain, particularly in the elderly. Zoster is typically a disease of adults, in contrast to varicella, which is mainly seen in children.

That varicella and zoster are caused by the same infectious agent was established over 100 years ago, when vesicular fluid from zoster patients was injected into children with the result that the children developed varicella that was usually mild [29]. Additional details concerning zoster have recently come to light. From autopsy specimens it was determined that VZV DNA and RNA can be present in dorsal root ganglia, both in neurons and satellite cells in individuals with a history of varicella but no history of zoster [71]. Reactivation of VZV in neurons has actually been visualized using in situ hybridization [71]. During latent infection, at least 5 of the 68 genes of VZV are expressed. In addition, at least 5 regulatory and other early proteins are also expressed, but in an aberrant location in the neuron. Normally, these 5 proteins are expressed in the nucleus of a VZV-infected cell, where they regulate the expression of other VZV genes. However, during latent infection, they are expressed in the cytoplasm of the cell. The expression of these proteins in the cytoplasm of latently infected cells, rather than in the nucleus, is hypothesized to play a role in controlling latent VZV infection [72].

Epidemiology and Pathogenesis

The incubation period of *varicella* is 10–21 days, during which time it is thought that at least two viremic phases occur. The first viremia delivers virus to the viscera, where multiplication takes place. This additional viral burden is thought to result in a second viremic phase, during which the virus reaches the skin and results in the rash [42]. Most otherwise healthy children with varicella develop about 300 skin lesions, although the range may be from just a few vesicles to more than 1,000 [77]. Adolescents and adults are more likely to develop more extensive varicella rashes and have more complications than children.

Laboratory abnormalities associated with varicella in healthy hosts include elevations of liver function tests (common), and effects on the bone marrow, such as lymphopenia, thrombocytopenia and granulocytopenia (rare) [29]. In households, primary cases are likely to be less severe than secondary cases [77]. In countries with temperate climates, most cases of varicella occur in childhood, usually in the first decade of life, and varicella is more common in winter and early spring than at other times of the year. In countries with tropical climates, varicella is less common in childhood, so that adults are more likely to develop the infection than children [29]. Second attacks of varicella are unusual but have been described, even in healthy hosts [37, 55].

The most common complication of varicella is bacterial superinfection, which is most likely caused by *Staphylococcus aureus* or *Streptococcus pyogenes*. Bacterial superinfections often involve the skin, and there may be an invasive component with resulting pneumonia, sepsis with shock, arthritis, fascitis and osteomyelitis. Central nervous system (CNS) complications of varicella include cerebellar ataxia (1 in 5,000 cases) and encephalitis (1 in 100,000 cases).

According to the Centers for Disease Control (CDC) in Atlanta, GA, there are an estimated 4 million cases of varicella and 10,000 hospitalizations due to this illness in the US annually. On average, at least 100 individuals die yearly in the US from varicella; about half of them persons who were healthy before developing varicella. Despite the licensure of varicella vaccine in 1995 in the US, there has been little impact on varicella incidence and epidemiology in the US. With the increased emphasis on vaccination, however, the CDC is hopeful that by the year 2010, 90% of children between the ages of 19 and 36 months will be immunized against varicella. It is predicted that then, the incidence of varicella would decrease significantly and the epidemiology of varicella and zoster would change considerably.

Varicella is a highly contagious disease, with most cases being clinically apparent. Following household exposure to varicella, the clinical attack rate in susceptibles approaches 90% [77]. Zoster is also contagious to others (as varicella), although the degree of contagion is probably about one quarter that of varicella. The possibility of spread of VZV from individuals with varicella and zoster among patients and staff in hospitals has made varicella a major problem for infection control. Prevention of nosocomial varicella is extremely time-consuming and costly [59, 95, 96].

The following individuals are at high risk of developing severe varicella: adults, immunocompromised patients, newborn infants and pregnant women. All of these individuals have lower primary CMI responses to VZV than otherwise healthy children, which may account for their tendency to develop severe varicella. These individuals are at risk of developing extensive skin rashes accompanied by hemorrhage, pneumonia and disseminated intravascular coagulation [28, 75]. Immunocompromised patients such as those with leukemia, lymphoma and other malignancies, as well as organ transplantees or patients receiving high doses of steroids, are at particular risk of developing severe or disseminated varicella. In fact, in the pre-antiviral drug era, the incidence of severe disseminated varicella in children with leukemia was 30% [25]. Although rare fatalities from varicella in HIV-infected children have been recorded, varicella in HIV-infected children does not seem to be as severe as in those with leukemia [23].

Zoster is most likely to develop on the thorax (50%); other common sites of rash are the face and lumbosacral areas. In contrast to varicella, which occurs mainly in winter and spring, zoster occurs with equal frequency all year. Zoster is most common in persons over 50 years of age; its incidence increases steadily with each additional decade of life. Immunocompromised patients are at a much higher risk of developing zoster; often as high as 35% over an interval of a few years. The highest recorded incidence of zoster, a rate of 70%, was observed in HIV-infected children who developed varicella when their CD4 levels were < 15% [31].

In addition to clinical zoster, subclinical reactivation of VZV may occur, as well as unilateral pain in a dermatomal distribution in the absence of any skin rash, termed zoster sine herpete [2]. Using a polymerase chain reaction (PCR) assay, sub-clinical zoster manifested by viremia was demonstrated in 19% of patients after bone marrow transplantation [110]. Viremia has also been observed in the absence of a generalized rash in immunocompromised patients with zoster, and as many as 10–40% of immunocompromised patients are at risk of developing viremia with dissemination of VZV. Clinically, these patients appear to have coexisting zoster and varicella [2].

Headache, pleocytosis in the cerebrospinal fluid (CSF) – and, in older patients especially, cerebral angiitis – are important complications of zoster involving the CNS. Other nervous system complications include neurogenic bladder, motor deficits and transverse myelitis. Additional complications include keratitis, uveitis and facial nerve palsy, especially when the initial rash involves the face. Postherpetic pain – a syndrome in the area of the healed skin rash developing about 1 month after the onset of the rash of zoster – is a frequent complication in individuals over 60 years of age. This pain may be especially difficult to treat and may last up to 1 year; its pathogenesis is poorly understood [2]. HIV-infected patients may have unusual features of zoster including retinitis, encephalitis without rash, and chronic zosteriform rashes [2].

Passive Immunization against Varicella

Passive immunization may be successfully carried out by administering varicella-zoster immune globulin (VZIG) [14, 32]. An injection of VZIG given within 5 days of exposure to susceptibles provides preformed specific antibodies that usually modify or prevent varicella. VZIG is superior to regular immune globulin for this purpose because the antibody titer of VZIG is about 10 times higher [77]. VZIG is recommended for individuals at high risk of developing severe varicella if they have had intimate exposure to an individual with an active VZV infection [17]. VZIG is expensive, painful for the patient, and affords protection for only about 2–3 weeks after its administration. VZIG has no role in preventing or controlling zoster because zoster develops despite high antibody titers to VZV.

Antiviral Therapy for VZV Infections

Three antiviral drugs are now available for treatment of VZV infections: acyclovir (ACV), valacyclovir (VCV), and famciclovir (FCV) [2]. These drugs inhibit VZV DNA replication by acting as a chain terminator and inhibiting DNA polymerase, mainly in virus-infected cells. These drugs therefore have little associated toxicity. Because of poor gastrointestinal absorption, oral ACV has not proven very useful for treatment of varicella. It usually shortens the course of illness by about 1 day, but it has no effect on viral shedding [24]. Intravenous ACV is used for treatment of (potentially) severe varicella in immunocompromised patients [106, 107]. When administered orally, both VCV and FCV result in therapeutic drug levels, making them useful for treating adult zoster [79, 88, 90]. Neither VCV nor FCV has been used to treat varicella, or administered to children. There are no data published on the efficacy of orally administered ACV in immunocompromised children with varicella.

Although there are reports of using ACV prophylactically to prevent varicella, there is little information about the drug for this indication, especially with regard to long-term immunity [9]. Resistance to ACV has been reported in HIV-infected patients, in which instance foscarnet, which is more toxic than ACV, is recommended for high-risk patients [26, 78, 83]. Thus, antiviral drugs have not proven useful for control of VZV since they are recommended for established infection only, and do not prevent spread of virus to others.

History of Varicella Vaccine

Varicella vaccine was developed in the early 1970s [87]. The parent virus came from an otherwise healthy 3-year-old boy with varicella whose family name was Oka, hence the designation of the strain. The virus was attenuated by approximately 30 passages in various cell cultures (including WI-38 cells) at various temperatures. The vaccine is now marketed by four pharmaceutical companies (Merck & Co., Inc., Varivax®; SmithKline Beecham Biologicals, Varilrix/Priorix®; Pasteur Mérieux Connaught, and Biken). All are derived from the original Oka strain, but they vary in exact passage number in WI-38 cells, dose of virus (1,000–10,000 plaque-forming units, pfu), and stabilizers. The Merck varicella vaccine is licensed for use in the US and the SmithKline Beecham vaccine is licensed widely in Europe and Asia. The vaccines have not been directly compared, but their behavior is presumed to be quite similar because they all originated from the Oka strain.

The Oka strain can be distinguished from wild-type VZV by several characteristics. These include increased sensitivity to 39 °C in the vaccine strain; lower infectivity of the wild-type strain in guinea pig fibroblast cell culture, and differences in DNA cleavage patterns [28]. Restriction fragment length polymorphisms (RFLP), which can be demonstrated by PCR, have proven useful to distinguish between vaccine and wild-type VZV in the US [51, 63, 80]. In Japan, these differences are not consistent since there is circulation of apparent Oka strain virus. However, the PCR technique should be useful in most other countries where Oka strains are not circulating [62]. The molecular basis of attenuation of the Oka strain is unknown, but may involve alterations of one of the glycoproteins of VZV, gC in the Oka strain [57, 58, 74].

Safety and Tolerability of Varicella Vaccine

Initial clinical trials on varicella vaccine were carried out in Japan. The first vaccinees were 70 healthy children who received a dose of 100–2,000 pfu of the Oka strain. No significant vaccine reactions were noted in these children. Subsequently, children hospitalized with a wide variety of illnesses including hepatitis, nephrotic syndrome, nephritis and meningitis were immunized because they were exposed to varicella while hospitalized [87]. Other than the occasional observation of mild rash and fever, there were no adverse effects of vaccination or nosocomial spread of varicella [87]. Additional Japanese studies indicated that vaccinees developed and maintained antibodies to VZV for as long as 2 years, even if they were receiving steroid therapy [5, 6, 8, 84].

Subsequent to the studies in Japan, numerous clinical trials in healthy children in the US indicated that varicella vaccine is extremely safe. The most common adverse event following vaccination is transient pain and redness at the injection site, which occurs in about 20% of vaccinees. About 10% may also experience transient fever [35, 104]. A generalized rash and/or some papules and vesicles at the injection site follows immunization in about 5% of vaccine recipients 1–6 weeks later (average 1 month) [35, 104]. Rashes occurring less than 14 days after vaccination are highly likely to be caused by wild-type VZV, which presumably the vaccinee was incubating at the time of vaccination [105].

The development of a rash following vaccination is a potential risk factor for transmission of the vaccine strain to susceptible contacts. Contact cases have been mild and no clinical reversion to virulence has been observed. Transmission to others following vaccination of healthy persons has been reported only very rarely [63, 80]. In one of the two such reports cited herein, vaccine virus was transmitted from a 12-month-old child with 30 skin lesions to his pregnant mother [80]. The mother developed mild clinical varicella with approximately 100 skin lesions in which vaccine-type virus was identified. At that time, several million doses of Merck varicella vaccine had been distributed to healthy persons in the US, indicating that the risk of transmission of vaccine virus from healthy vaccinees to others must be exceedingly rare. The other report of transmission of vaccine virus from one healthy person to another involved SmithKline Beecham vaccine in a clinical trial [63]. Transmission of vaccine-type VZV to others in leukemic children can occur, but is about one quarter as transmissible as is natural varicella [51, 89]. Transmission of vaccine-type virus is much less likely to occur from healthy vaccinated persons than from immunocompromised vaccinees.

Further studies of adverse events in the post-licensure vaccine era in the US are ongoing. In studies conducted by Merck and the FDA, there have been extremely rare reports of pneumonia, ataxia, anaphylaxis and thrombocytopenia temporally related to vaccination [82]. In many instances, it is difficult to judge whether these events were truly caused by the vaccine.

Adverse events in healthy vaccinated adults are very similar to those reported in healthy children [35, 40, 45].

Initial Safety Studies in Immunocompromised Patients

Immunization of Japanese children with an underlying malignancy soon followed. This approach was important because at that time, antiviral drugs were not available, and it was recognized that immunocompromised children could die of varicella while being treated for their primary disease. Maintenance chemotherapy was withheld for 1 week before and 1 week after immunization. Approximately 350 children were vaccinated, and the only significant adverse effect was development of maculopapular or mild vesicular rash in about 20%. Most developed detectable antibodies, and if exposed to VZV, did not develop varicella [48, 53, 84].

American Safety Studies in Immunocompromised Patients

After the obvious success in Japan in immunocompromised children, investigators in the US began to consider clinical trials in immunocompromised patients [56]. Clinical trials in children with underlying leukemia were begun in the US in the late 1970s [1, 15, 38]. The largest of these trials, which was carried out between 1979 and 1990, was sponsored by the National Institute of Allergy and Infectious Diseases and conducted by the Collaborative Varicella Vaccine Study Group. In this study, 575 US and Canadian children with underlying leukemia were immunized. 511 of the children were still receiving maintenance chemotherapy, which was stopped for 1 week before and 1 week after immunization [30, 35]. At immunization, children had to: have been in continuous remission from leukemia for at least 1 year; have no detectable antibodies to VZV; have a positive response to mitogens in vitro, and have more than 700/mm^3 circulating lymphocytes. Although 1 dose of vaccine had been planned, due to a failure to seroconvert after 1 dose in almost 20% and the loss of detectable VZV antibody after 1 year in about 5%, 2 doses of vaccine 3 months apart were ultimately given to most children. A seroconversion to VZV occurred in 82% of leukemic children after 1 dose, and in 95% after 2 doses [28, 36, 38, 41]. Approximately 50% of the children still receiving maintenance chemotherapy (usually 6-mercaptopurine, methotrexate, vincristine, and prednisone) developed a mild to moderate rash about 1 month following immunization, with most rashes occurring after the first dose. Approximately 40% of the children who developed the rash were treated with high oral doses (900 mg/m^2 4 times/day) of ACV until the rash was healed. Approximately 40% of these children had to be hospitalized (usually for less than 1 week) to receive the ACV intravenously. In children no longer receiving chemotherapy, rash occurred in only about 5%, and none required treatment with ACV. Other transient adverse effects attributed to the vaccine included upper respiratory tract symptoms, neutropenia and thrombocytopenia, appearing in about 5%. There was no observed increase in the rate of relapse of leukemia in those vaccinees who had their chemotherapy withheld for 2 weeks. A retrospective analysis of rash in children on maintenance chemotherapy led to the recommendation that they not be given steroids for at least 2 weeks after immunization, nor other anticancer therapy for 1 week after immunization [73].

Smaller studies in children with leukemia and other forms of childhood malignancy have also indicated that while the rate of vaccine-associated rash is higher than that seen in healthy children and adults after vaccination, even moderately severe rashes are unusual in these vaccinees [1, 15]. One exception was a study of vaccination of children with lymphoma and lymphosarcoma in Japan, in which the rate and severity of vaccine-associated rash was unacceptable and the vaccine study was therefore discontinued in these children [85]. In studies carried out in Europe on children with uremia prior to renal transplantation, the vaccine was very well tolerated, with responses similar to those seen in healthy children [12, 111].

A small safety study of varicella vaccine in about 40 HIV-infected children with relatively normal CD4 counts was recently conducted by the Pediatric AIDS Clinical Trials Group in the US [67]. These children tolerated a 2-dose schedule of immunization extremely well with no serious adverse events. The major side effect of vaccination was development of a minor vaccine-associated rash in 5%. 83% of these children developed a positive immune response (antibodies and/or CMI), but no protective efficacy data are available from this small study. It had already been determined that even natural varicella in these children does not lead to more rapid development of AIDS [31]. The rationale behind immunization of HIV-infected children when their CD4 lymphocytes remain intact is to immunize them when their primary immune response is likely at its best. HIV-infected children who contract varicella when they have low CD4 counts have an extremely high risk of developing zoster. One HIV-infected child who was inadvertently immunized with almost undetectable levels of CD4 lymphocytes developed a severe disseminated infection from the Oka strain of VZV [11].

Zoster in Vaccinees

From the beginning, there was concern that the incidence of zoster might increase through immunization, although it was hoped that the incidence might be low or even absent after vaccination. While zoster is normally rare or unusual in healthy populations, it is common in immunocompromised patients with a history of varicella. It was therefore possible to determine, in immunocompromised patients, whether the incidence of zoster changed as a result of immunization. A number of studies showed that the incidence of zoster was decreased, not increased, in vaccinees [16, 47, 49, 50, 65, 86]. In the Collaborative Vaccine Study, which included a control group of children with leukemia who had natural varicella, the incidence of zoster was significantly lower in 96 leukemic children after vaccination (2%) than in 96 vaccinated leukemic children after natural varicella (15%) (p = 0.01) [47].

A similar decrease in the incidence of zoster following immunization was observed more recently in children who underwent renal transplantation in France. Over a 10-year interval, the incidence of zoster was lower in vaccinated children (7% of 212 vaccinees) than in those with past natural varicella prior to transplantation (13% of 415 children); zoster was even more common, 38%, in 49 children who developed varicella following renal transplantation [13]. Development of zoster in vaccinees has been related to the presence of VZV skin lesions, either as a vaccine-associated rash or breakthrough varicella [35, 46, 47]. Perhaps there is less opportunity for VZV to establish latent infection following vaccination compared to natural infection. Or, perhaps the fewer skin lesions provide less opportunity for latent infection to occur. Other possibilities are that the attenuated vaccine strain is less able to establish latency in neurons than wild-type virus, or that it is less able to reactivate than wild-type VZV. That the vaccine virus can cause zoster in both healthy and immunocompromised patients has been established [69, 108].

Immunogenicity and Efficacy of Varicella Vaccine

Both humoral and CMI responses to VZV have been examined in vaccinees. Antibodies to VZV are measured by a variety of methods with various degrees of sensitivity. These include the fluorescent antibody to membrane antigen (FAMA) assay, which, while highly sensitive and specific [34, 109], is used only as a research tool. Nor is the exquisitely sensitive glycoprotein (gp) ELISA assay, developed by Merck & Co., commercially marketed [76]. Commercially available ELISAs are not sensitive enough to detect all individuals who have responded to varicella vaccine [22]. Yet despite their limitations, these assays have proven useful in evaluating the immunogenicity of varicella vaccine. Seroconversion rates approaching 100% were observed for immunized children and adults with the gp ELISA assay [60, 105]. In healthy children, 98% seroconverted after 1 dose of vaccine [54], and in studies of healthy adults, 94% seroconverted after 2 doses [40]. In healthy persons, the presence of detectable FAMA antibodies during the year before close exposure to VZV is associated with protection from clinical illness. In a study of 58 healthy individuals with antibodies detectable by FAMA at the time of household exposure to chickenpox, none became ill. However, of 28 individuals with no detectable FAMA antibodies at household exposure, all developed varicella [34]. In over 25 years of experience with FAMA performed in one laboratory by the same person, only 1 VZV FAMA-positive healthy vaccinee has been observed to develop clinical VZV infection after a household exposure, and this woman developed only 1 vesicle [39].

Follow-up studies of healthy children who were immunized have indicated that persistence of antibodies is the rule. 90% of 36 American children vaccinated between 1984 and 1987 had detectable VZV FAMA antibody titers between 6 and 10 years later [54]. 100% of 25 Japanese young adults who were vaccinated 17–20 years previously had antibodies detectable by FAMA [7]. Measured by gp ELISA, persistence of VZV antibodies for up to 5 years was demonstrated in over 500 American children [2, 18, 54, 61, 92, 93]. VZV antibody titers increase over time in healthy immunized children, presumably due to exposure to wild-type VZV and boosting of immunity [7, 54].

CMI to VZV can be measured by several methods, including skin testing and lymphocyte stimulation against VZV antigen. Results of these assays usually parallel FAMA titers. Follow-up studies in vaccinated healthy children have demonstrated persistence of CMI for as long as 5 years after vaccination [92, 93, 112].

The protective efficacy of varicella vaccine in healthy children was evaluated in two double-blind studies and in open-label studies by observing the outcome when vaccinees had had household exposure to varicella. The latter approach is feasible because after exposure to VZV in a family, about 90% of varicella susceptibles develop clinical chickenpox [77]. In a double-blind randomized placebo-controlled trial conducted on Merck varicella vaccine in 1984, 956 seronegative children aged 1–14 years were enrolled and monitored for 2 years [61, 97, 98]. There were 468 children who were vaccinated with 17,000 pfu [35], and 446 seronegative children who received a placebo [97, 98]. In the vaccinated, 94% seroconverted. During the first year afterwards, the vaccine was 100% effective in preventing chickenpox [98]. During the second year, a few vaccinees contracted mild varicella, and vaccine efficacy was 96% [61, 97]. During the following 7 years, over 95% of vaccinees remained free of varicella [61].

A second double-blind placebo-controlled trial involving 513 healthy young children was performed in Finland using vaccine produced by SmithKline Beecham [91]. The children were divided into three groups. One third were given a high-dose vaccine (10,000 or 15,850 pfu/dose), one third were given a low-dose vaccine (630 or 1,260 pfu/dose), and one third were given a placebo. 94–100% of vaccinated children seroconverted. After about 30 months, there were 5 cases of varicella in the high-dose group, an attack rate of 3%. There were 19 cases in the low-dose group, an attack rate of 11.4%. There were 41 cases in the placebo group, an attack rate of 26% (p ≤ 0.005 for each group). In the vaccinated groups, therefore, the higher dose conferred better protection than the lower dose.

Several open-label investigations of vaccine efficacy comparing the occurrence of varicella to natural rates of chickenpox for various ages of children and protection after household exposure have indicated approximately 90% efficacy against varicella [60, 105]. A 5-year case-control study of the effectiveness of varicella vaccine in clinical practice in the US is in progress; in the first study year, the licensed Merck vaccine was 85% effective in four pediatric practice groups [81].

The efficacy of varicella vaccine is lower in adults than in children, probably because the CMI response to VZV is less vigorous in adults than it is in children [28, 75]. Open-label efficacy studies in adults, based on household exposure to varicella, indicate that the vaccine is about 75% protective against varicella [33, 39, 40, 45]. Moreover, adults need 2 doses of vaccine to reach a seroconversion rate of > 90% [33, 39, 40, 45]. Side effects of vaccination are similar to those observed in children, and the vaccine is extremely safe, even if multiple doses are administered [33, 39, 40, 45].

Although children often have an increase in VZV antibody titer with time, vaccinated adults may lose detectable VZV antibodies after some months to years. Of 40 healthy adults, 18% had become seronegative 7–13 years after immunization; in contrast, only about 5% of vaccinated children lost antibodies after a similar interval [28, 54]. Also, in adult vaccinees, geometric mean titers (GMTs) may not increase over time [4, 28, 54].

Approximately 10% of vaccinated children and 25% of vaccinated adults have been observed to develop varicella months to years after immunization. This is normally a mild form of infection; only about one tenth of the number of skin lesions expected usually develop, and there are few associated symptoms such as fever [33, 39, 40, 45, 94]. In addition, about 5% of vaccinees may experience a 'no take' and may develop a full-blown illness [40]. Vaccinees who have lost detectable antibodies are at risk of developing breakthrough varicella, but silent re-seroconversions after exposure have also been observed [40, 54].

Waning immunity in individuals who originally seroconverted to VZV after immunization, termed secondary vaccine failure, has thus far been difficult to document. Significant is that in 343 adults and 143 children, neither the incidence nor the severity of varicella was observed to increase up to 120 months after immunization [28, 54].

Efficacy in Immunosuppressed Vaccinees

The efficacy of varicella vaccine was high in immunocompromised leukemic children participating in the Collaborative NIAID Study. During a 10-year period, there were 123 family exposures to varicella, with 17 cases of breakthrough chickenpox – a protection rate of 86% [28, 36, 41]. Varicella occurred in 39 vaccinated children, most of whom did not have household exposure to chickenpox. Children with varicella experienced a modified illness, with an average of 96 skin lesions (range 1–640). Normally, more than 300 lesions would be expected on average in an otherwise healthy child with varicella. None of the leukemic children who developed varicella despite immunization required treatment with antiviral drugs.

Vaccine efficacy was also examined in the 212 French children who were immunized prior to renal transplantation. Over several years, the incidence of varicella, 26/212 (12%), was lower in vaccinees than in a similar group that was not vaccinated: 22/49 (45%). The disease was also milder in vaccinees, with no deaths, while there were 3 deaths from varicella in the unvaccinated. Four of 415 (10%) uremic children with past varicella developed a second attack, which was similar to the attack rate in vaccinees [13].

Thus, varicella vaccine appears to be almost as effective in immunocompromised children as in healthy children, although immunocompromised children usually need to be given 2 doses of vaccine. It is probably unsafe to immunize some highly immunocompromised children, such as those with leukemia, while they are receiving induction chemotherapy. Other populations, such as those with lymphoma and lymphosarcoma, may not tolerate immunization. In the US, these problems can perhaps be avoided by immunizing all healthy children after their first birthday. With this strategy, most children who eventually become immunocompromised due to disease will have pre-existing immunity to varicella.

Benefits of Active Immunization

The many advantages of active immunization would accrue to both individuals and society. In the US, universal vaccination of healthy susceptibles over 1 year of age has been recommended by the American Academy of Pediatrics, the Public Health Service Advisory Committee on Immunization Practices (ACIP), and the American Association of Family Physicians [17, 20, 21]. Although varicella vaccine was licensed for general use in 1995, more than 4 years ago, only about 25% of healthy young American children have been immunized, albeit with considerable variability of immunization rates in different locales. However, it is predicted that by the year 2000, 90% of young American children will have been vaccinated.

Vaccinated persons are expected to achieve long-term protection against varicella and possibly against zoster as well. Theoretically, this should protect them against complications of varicella and zoster, such as nosocomial varicella, invasive streptococcal infections, congenital varicella syndrome, and varicella in adults. Children vaccinated today may possibly have less zoster when they become elderly. Those children immunized when healthy are predicted to have residual immunity to VZV should they subsequently become immunocompromised for a variety of medical reasons. These are all benefits that passive immunization and antiviral therapy, while useful in certain situations, cannot provide.

Society may also benefit from the widespread use of varicella vaccine. Medical costs of treating varicella and zoster, particularly complications, should be significantly reduced. Varicella vaccine has been shown to be cost-effective. Huse et al. [52] calculated an annual net savings in the US of USD 6.6 million with universal use of varicella vaccine. Lieu et al. [70] reported that for every dollar spent on immunization, USD 2 in medical costs alone would be saved, and USD 5 of work-time otherwise lost. A study in Germany revealed savings of almost DEM 1.5 annually by vaccinating 12-year-olds [10].

Since active immunization lessens viral shedding and spread, incidence of varicella should decrease markedly, even in children who have not been vaccinated. This phenomenon was observed in a day-care setting in the US involving approximately 3,000 children, where the decrease in incidence of disease was proportionally greater than the increase in use of the vaccine [19].

Potential disadvantages of routine use of varicella vaccine are theoretical. Immunity could wane over time after immunization, but, as noted above, there is little evidence that this occurs. There is also concern that decreased opportunity for exposure to the virus would result in less immune boosting, which could contribute to waning immunity and even lead to a possible increase in the incidence of zoster [27]. Realistically, it has been pointed out that failure to immunize over 85% of the population may allow significant circulation of wild-type VZV, and might result in an increase of adult varicella in individuals *not immunized* as children [43]. Therefore, once public health policy recommends immunization of all children, as in the US, it is imperative that vaccine coverage for children approaches 100% [44, 103].

Vaccine Recommendations in the US

Children aged 12 months to 12 years receive 1 dose of vaccine, and for those who have reached their 13th birthday, 2 doses 4–8 weeks apart are recommended. Antibody titers need not be determined when immunizing children and adolescents. However, adults who are vaccinated should be tested for VZV antibodies before and after immunization. This is important because most adults who believe themselves to be susceptible to varicella, at least in countries with a temperate climate, are actually seropositive [64]. Contraindications to vaccination include immunocompromisation, allergy to vaccine components and pregnancy.

At present, except for selected children with acute leukemia in remission, immunocompromised children should only be immunized under research protocols [21]. Varicella vaccine can be obtained for children with leukemia in remission on a compassionate-use basis in the US [21]. Varicella vaccine is being researched to determine if it can prevent zoster by boosting immunity to VZV [66, 68].

Conclusions

Varicella vaccine has proven highly effective in preventing chickenpox in healthy and immunocompromised children and in healthy adults. It can also prevent zoster as well. The vaccine is extremely safe and well tolerated, with only mild reactions reported, although – very rarely – more severe complications of vaccination have been observed. It is predicted that complications of varicella will be lower following immunization. Although waning immunity in healthy vaccinated children has not been well documented and is probably not significant, studies on this possibility are ongoing. As the first vaccine against herpesviruses to be licensed and widely used, it is clearly a success story and should serve as a model for the investigation and analysis of future vaccines against these human pathogens.

References

1 Arbeter A, Granowetter L, Starr S, Lange B, Wimmer R, Plotkin S: Immunization of children with acute lymphoblastic leukemia with live attenuated varicella vaccine without complete suspension of chemotherapy. Pediatrics 1990;85:338–344.
2 Arvin A, Gershon A: Live attenuated varicella vaccine. Annu Rev Microbiol 1996;50:59–100.
3 Arvin AM, Pollard RB, Rasmussen L, Merigan T: Selective impairment in lymphocyte reactivity to varicella-zoster antigen among untreated lymphoma patients. J Infect Dis 1978;137:531–540.
4 Asano Y, Nagai T, Miyata T, et al. Long-term protective immunity of recipients of the Oka strain of live varicella vaccine. Pediatrics 1985;75:667–671.
5 Asano Y, Nakayama H, Yazaki T, Ito S, et al: Protective efficacy of vaccination in children in four episodes of natural varicella and zoster in the ward. Pediatrics 1977;59:8–12.
6 Asano Y, Nakayama H, Yazaki T, et al: Protection against varicella in family contacts by immediate inoculation with live varicella vaccine. Pediatrics 1977;59:3–7.
7 Asano Y, Suga S, Yoshikawa T, et al: Experience and reason: Twenty-year follow-up of protective immunity of the Oka live varicella vaccine. Pediatrics 1994;94:524–526.
8 Asano Y, Takahashi M: Clinical and serologic testing of a live varicella vaccine and two-year follow-up for immunity of the vaccinated children. Pediatrics 1977;60:810-814.
9 Asano Y, Yoshikawa T, Suga S, et al: Postexposure prophylaxis of varicella in family contact by oral acyclovir. Pediatrics 1993;92:219–222.
10 Beutels P, Clara R, Tormans G, Vandoorslaer E, Van Damme P: Costs and benefits of routine varicella vaccination in German children. J Infect Dis 1996;174:S335–S341.
11 Blackwood A: Pneumonia from varicella vaccine in HIV (in preparation).
12 Broyer M, Boudailliez B: Varicella vaccine in children with chronic renal insufficiency. Postgrad Med J 1985;61(suppl 4):103–106.
13 Broyer M, Tete MT, Guest G, Gagnadoux MF, Rouzioux C: Varicella and zoster in children after kidney transplantation: Long-term results of vaccination. Pediatrics 1997;99:35–39.
14 Brunell P, Ross A, Miller L, Kuo B: Prevention of varicella by zoster immune globulin. New Engl J Med 1969;280:1191–1194.

15   Brunell PA, Shehab Z, Geiser C, Waugh JE: Administration of live varicella vaccine to children with leukemia. Lancet 1982;ii:1069–1073.

16   Brunell PA, Taylor-Wiedeman J, Geiser CF, Frierson L, Lydick E: Risk of herpes zoster in children with leukemia: Varicella vaccine compared with history of chickenpox. Pediatrics 1986;77:53–56.

17   Centers for Disease Control: Prevention of varicella: Recommendations of the Advisory Committee on Immunization Practices (ACIP). MMWR Morb Mortal Wkly Rep 1996;45: 1–36.

18   Clements DA, Armstrong CB, Ursano AM, Moggio M, Walter EB, Wilfert CM: Over five-year follow-up of Oka/Merck varicella vaccine recipients in 465 infants and adolescents. Pediatr Infect Dis J 1995;14:874–879.

19   Clements D, Moreira SP, Coplan P, Bland C, Walter E: Postlicensure study of varicella vaccine effectiveness in a day-care setting. Pediatr Infect Dis J 1999;18:1047–1050.

20   Committee on Infectious Diseases: Live attenuated varicella vaccine. Pediatrics 1995;95: 791–796.

21   Committee on Infectious Diseases: Report of the Committee on Infectious Diseases. Elk Grove Village/IL, American Academy of Pediatrics, 1997.

22   Demmler G, Steinberg S, Blum G, Gershon A: Rapid enzyme-linked immunosorbent assay for detecting antibody to varicella-zoster virus. J Infect Dis 1988;157:211–212.

23   Derryck A, LaRussa P, Steinberg S, Capasso M, Pitt J, Gershon A: Varicella and zoster in children with human immunodeficiency virus infection. Pediatr Infect Dis J 1998;17:931–933.

24   Dunkel L, Arvin A, Whitley R, et al: A controlled trial of oral acyclovir for chickenpox in normal children. N Engl J Med 1991;325:1539–1544.

25   Feldman S, Hughes W, Daniel C: Varicella in children with cancer: 77 cases. Pediatrics 1975; 80:388–397.

26   Fillet AM, Dumont B, Caumes E, Visse B, Agut H, Bricaire F, Huraux JM: Acyclovir-resistant varicella-zoster virus: Phenotypic and genetic characterization. J Med Virol 1998;55:250– 254.

27   Garnett GP, Grenfell BT: The epidemiology of varicella-zoster infections: A mathematical model. Epidemiol Infect 1992;108:495–511.

28   Gershon A: Varicella-zoster virus: Prospects for control. Adv Pediatr Infect Dis 1995; 10:93–124.

29   Gershon A, LaRussa P: Varicella-zoster virus; in Katz S, Gershon A, Hotez P (eds): Krugman's Textbook of Pediatric Infectious Disease. St Louis, Mosby, 1998.

30   Gershon A, LaRussa P, Steinberg S: Varicella vaccine: Use in immunocompromised patients; in White RE (ed): Infectious Disease Clinics of North America. Philadelphia, Saunders, 1996.

31   Gershon A, Mervish N, LaRussa P, et al: Varicella-zoster virus infection in children with underlying HIV infection. J Infect Dis 1997;175:1496–1500.

32   Gershon A, Steinberg S, Brunell P: Zoster immune globulin: A further assessment. N Engl J Med 1974;290:243–245.

33   Gershon A, Steinberg S, Gelb L, NIAID Collaborative Varicella Vaccine Study Group: Live attenuated varicella vaccine: Use in immunocompromised children and adults. Pediatrics 1986;78(suppl):757–762.

34   Gershon A, Steinberg S, LaRussa P: Detection of antibodies to varicella-zoster virus by latex agglutination. Clin Diag Virol 1994;2:271–277.

35   Gershon A, Takahashi M, White CJ: Live attenuated varicella vaccine; in Plotkin S, Orenstein W (eds): Vaccines, ed 3. Philadelphia, Saunders, 1999, pp 475–507.

36   Gershon AA, LaRussa P, Steinberg S: Live attenuated varicella vaccine: Current status and future uses. Semin Pediatr Infect Dis 1991;2:171–178.

37 Gershon AA, Steinberg S, Gelb L, NIAID Collaborative Varicella Vaccine Study Group: Clinical reinfection with varicella-zoster virus. J Infect Dis 1984;149:137–142.

38 Gershon AA, Steinberg S, Gelb L, NIAID Collaborative Varicella Vaccine Study Group: Live attenuated varicella vaccine: Efficacy for children with leukemia in remission. JAMA 1984;252:355–362.

39 Gershon AA, Steinberg S, LaRussa P, Hammerschlag M, Ferrara A, NIAID Collaborative Varicella Vaccine Study Group: Immunization of healthy adults with live attenuated varicella vaccine. J Infect Dis 1988;158:132–137.

40 Gershon AA, Steinberg S, NIAID Collaborative Varicella Vaccine Study Group: Live attenuated varicella vaccine: Protection in healthy adults in comparison to leukemic children. J Infect Dis 1990;161:661–666.

41 Gershon AA, Steinberg S, NIAID Collaborative Varicella Vaccine Study Group: Persistence of immunity to varicella in children with leukemia immunized with live attenuated varicella vaccine. N Engl J Med 1989;320:892–897.

42 Grose CH: Variation on a theme by Fenner. Pediatrics 1981;68:735–737.

43 Halloran E, Cochi S, Lieu T, Wharton M, Fehrs L: Theoretical epidemiological and morbidity effects of routine immunization of preschool children with varicella vaccine in the United States. Am J Epidemiol 1994;140:81–104.

44 Halloran ME: Epidemiologic effects of varicella vaccination. Infect Clin North Am 1996;10:631–656.

45 Hardy I, Gershon A: Prospects for use of a varicella vaccine in adults. Infect Dis Clin North Am 1990;4:160–173.

46 Hardy IB, Gershon A, Steinberg S, LaRussa P, et al: Incidence of zoster after live attenuated varicella vaccine, International Conference on Antimicrobial Agents and Chemotherapy, Chicago, 1991.

47 Hardy IB, Gershon A, Steinberg S, LaRussa P: The incidence of zoster after immunization with live attenuated varicella vaccine. A study in children with leukemia. N Engl J Med 1991;325:1545–1550.

48 Hattori A, Ihara T, Iwasa T, et al: Use of live varicella vaccine in children with acute leukemia or other malignancies (letter). Lancet 1976;ii:210.

49 Hayakawa Y, Torigoe S, Shiraki K, Yamanishi K, Takahashi M: Biologic and biophysical markers of a live varicella vaccine strain (Oka): Identification of clinical isolates from vaccine recipients. J Infect Dis 1984;149:956–963.

50 Hayakawa Y, Yamamoto T, Yamanishi K, Takahashi M: Analysis of varicella zoster virus DNAs of clinical isolates by endonuclease HpaI. J Gen Virol 1986;67:1817–1829.

51 Hughes P, LaRussa PS, Pearce JM, Lepow ML, Steinberg SP, Gershon A: Transmission of varicella-zoster virus from a vaccinee with underlying leukemia, demonstrated by polymerase chain reaction. J Pediatr 1994;124:932–935.

52 Huse DM, Meissner C, Lacey MJ, Oster G: Childhood vaccination against chickenpox: An analysis of benefits and costs. J Pediatr 1994;124:869–874.

53 Izawa T, Ihara T, Hattori A, Iwasa T, Kamiya H, Sakurai M, Takahashi M: Application of a live varicella vaccine in children with acute leukemia or other malignant diseases. Pediatrics 1977;60:805–809.

54 Johnson C, Stancin T, Fattlar D, Rome LP, Kumar ML: A long-term prospective study of varicella vaccine in healthy children. Pediatrics 1997;100:761–766.

55 Junker AK, Angus E, Thomas E: Recurrent varicella-zoster virus infections in apparently immunocompetent children. Pediatr Infect Dis J 1991;10:569–575.

56   Kempe CH, Gershon AA: Varicella vaccine at the crossroads. Pediatrics 1977;60:930–931.

57   Kinchington PR, Ling P, Pensiero M, Gershon A, Hay J, Ruyechan WT: A possible role for gpV in the pathogenesis of varicella-zoster virus. Adv Exp Med Biol. New York, Plenum Press, 1990, vol 278, pp 83–92.

58   Kinchington PR, Ling P, Pensiero M, Ruyechan WT, Hay J: The glycoprotein products of varicella-zoster virus gene 14 and their defective accumulation in a vaccine strain (Oka). J Virol 1990;64:540–548.

59   Krasinski K, Holzman R, LaCoutre R, Florman A: Hospital experience with varicella-zoster virus. Infect Control Hosp Epidemiol 1986;7:312–316.

60   Krause P, Klinman DM: Efficacy, immunogenicity, safety, and use of live attenuated chickenpox vaccine. J Pediatr 1995;127:518–525.

61   Kuter BJ, Weibel RE, Guess HA, Matthews H, Morton DH, Neff BJ, Provost PJ, Watson BA, Starr SE, Plotkin SA: Oka/Merck varicella vaccine in healthy children: Final report of a 2-year efficacy study and 7-year follow-up studies. Vaccine 1991;9:643–647.

62   LaRussa P, Steinberg S, Arvin A, Dwyer D, Burgess M, Menegus M, Rekrut K, Yamanishi K, Gershon A: PCR and RFLP analysis of VZV isolates from the USA and other parts of the world. J Infect Dis 1998;178(suppl 1):64–66.

63   LaRussa P, Steinberg S, Meurice F, Gershon A: Transmission of vaccine strain varicella-zoster virus from a healthy adult with vaccine-associated rash to susceptible household contacts. J Infect Dis 1997;176:1072–1075.

64   LaRussa P, Steinberg S, Seeman MD, Gershon AA: Determination of immunity to varicella by means of an intradermal skin test. J Infect Dis 1985;152:869–875.

65   Lawrence R, Gershon A, Holzman R, Steinberg S, NIAID Varicella Vaccine Collaborative Study Group: The risk of zoster after varicella vaccination in children with leukemia. N Engl J Med 1988;318:543–548.

66   Levin M: Can herpes zoster be prevented? Eur J Clin Microbiol Infect Dis 1996;15:1–3.

67   Levin M, Gershon A, Weinberg A, et al: Administration of Varicella Vaccine to HIV-Infected Children. Retroviral Conference, Chicago, 1999.

68   Levin M, Murray M, Zerbe G, White CJ, Hayward AR: Immune responses of elderly persons 4 years after receiving a live attenuated varicella vaccine. J Infect Dis 1994;170:522–526.

69   Liang MG, Heidelberg KA, Jacobson RM, McEvoy MT: Herpes zoster after varicella immunization. J Am Acad Dermatol 1998;38:761–763.

70   Lieu T, Cochi S, Black S, Halloran ME, Shinefield HR, Holmes SJ, Wharton M, Washington AE: Cost-effectiveness of a routine varicella vaccination program for US children. JAMA 1994;271:375–381.

71   Lungu O, Annunziato P, Gershon A, Staugaitis SM, Josefson D, La Russa P, Silverstein SJ: Reactivated and latent varicella-zoster virus in human dorsal root ganglia. Proc Natl Acad Sci USA 1995;92:10980–10984.

72   Lungu O, Panagiotidis C, Annunziato P, Gershon A, Silverstein S: Aberrant intracellular localization of varicella-zoster virus regulatory proteins during latency. Proc Natl Acad Sci USA 1998;95:780–785.

73   Lydick E, Kuter BJ, Zajac B, Guess H, NIAID Collaborative Varicella Vaccine Study Group: Association of steroid therapy with vaccine-associated rashes in children with acute lymphocytic leukaemia who received Oka/Merck varicella vaccine. Vaccine 1989;7:549–553.

74   Moffat JF, Zerboni L, Kinchington P, Grose C, Kaneshima H, Arvin A: Attenuation of the vaccine Oka strain of varicella-zoster virus and role of glycoprotein C in alpha-herpesvirus virulence demonstrated in the SCID-hu mouse. J Virol 1998;72:965–974.

75 Nader S, Bergen R, Sharp M, Arvin A: Comparison of cell-mediated immunity to varicella-zoster virus in children and adults immunized with live attenuated varicella vaccine. J Infect Dis 1995;171:13–17.

76 Provost PJ, Krah DL, Kuter BJ, Morton DH, Schofield TL, Wasmuth EH, White CJ, Miller WJ, Ellis RW: Antibody assays suitable for assessing immune responses to live varicella vaccine. Vaccine 1991;9:111–116.

77 Ross AH, Lencher E, Reitman G: Modification of chickenpox in family contacts by administration of gamma-globulin. N Engl J Med 1962;267:369–376.

78 Safrin S, Berger T, Gilson I, Wolfe PR, Wofsy CB, Mills J, Biron KK: Foscarnet therapy in five patients with AIDS and acyclovir-resistant varicella-zoster infection. Ann Intern Med 1991;115:19–21.

79 Saltzman R, Boon R: The safety of famciclovir in patients with herpes zoster. Curr Ther Res 1995;56:219–225.

80 Salzman MB, Sharrar R, Steinberg S, LaRussa P: Transmission of varicella-vaccine virus from a healthy 12-month-old child to his pregnant mother. J Pediatr 1997;131:151–154.

81 Shapiro ED, LaRussa PS, Steinberg S, Gershon A: Protective efficacy of varicella vaccine. 36th Annual Meeting Infectious Diseases Society of America, Denver, 1998, Abstr 78.

82 Sharrar R, LaRussa P, Galea S, et al: An analysis of the first eighteen months of reported adverse experiences associated with the administration of varicella vaccine. (Submitted.)

83 Smith K, Kahlter DC, Davis C, James WD, Skelton HG, Angritt P: Acyclovir-resistant varicella zoster responsive to foscarnet. Arch Dermatol 1991;127:1069–1071.

84 Takahashi M: Vaccine development. Infect Dis Clin North Am 1996;10:469–488.

85 Takahashi M, Gershon A: Varicella vaccine; in Mortimer E, Plotkin S (eds): Vaccines, ed 2. Philadelphia, Saunders, 1994, pp 387–417.

86 Takahashi M, Gershon A: Varicella vaccine; in Levine M, Woodrow GC, Kaper JB, Cobon GS (eds): New Generation Vaccines, ed 2. New York, Dekker, 1997, pp 647–658.

87 Takahashi M, Otsuka T, Okuno Y, Asano Y, Yazaki T, Isomura S: Live vaccine used to prevent the spread of varicella in children in hospital. Lancet 1974;ii:1288–1290.

88 Thackeray AM, Field HJ: Differential effects of famciclovir and valacyclovir on the pathogenesis of herpes simplex virus in a murine infection model including from latency. J Infect Dis 1995;173:291–299.

89 Tsolia M, Gershon A, Steinberg S, Gelb L: Live attenuated varicella vaccine: Evidence that the virus is attenuated and the importance of skin lesions in transmission of varicella-zoster virus. J Pediatr 1990;116:184–189.

90 Tyring S, Barbarash RA, Nahlik JE, Cunningham A, Marley J, Heng M, Jones T, Rea T, Boon R, Saltzman R: Famciclovir for the treatment of acute herpes zoster: Effects on acute disease and post-herpetic neuralgia. Ann Intern Med 1995;123:89–96.

91 Varis T, Vesikari T: Efficacy of high titer live attenuated varicella vaccine in healthy young children. J Infect Dis 1996;174:S330–S334.

92 Watson B, Boardman C, Laufer D, Piercy S, Tustin N, Olaleye D, Cnaan A, Starr SE: Humoral and cell-mediated immune responses in healthy children after one or two doses of varicella vaccine. Clin Infect Dis 1995;20:316–319.

93 Watson B, Gupta R, Randall T, Starr S: Persistence of cell-mediated and humoral immune responses in healthy children immunized with live attenuated varicella vaccine. J Infect Dis 1994;169:197–199.

94 Watson BM, Piercy SA, Plotkin SA, Starr SE: Modified chickenpox in children immunized with the Oka/Merck varicella vaccine. Pediatrics 1993;91:17–22.

95 Weber DJ, Rotala WA, Parham C: Impact and costs of varicella prevention in a university hospital. Am J Publ Health 1988;78:19–23.

96 Weber DJ, Rutala WA, Hamilton H: Prevention and control of varicella-zoster infections in health care facilities. Infect Control Hosp Epidemiol 1996;17:694–705.

97 Weibel R, Kuter B, Neff B, Rothenberger CA, Fitzgerald AJ, Connor KA, Morton D, McLean AA, Scolnick EM: Live Oka/Merck varicella vaccine in healthy children: Further clinical and laboratory assessment. JAMA 1985;254:2435–2439.

98 Weibel R, Neff BJ, Kuter BJ, et al: Live attenuated varicella virus vaccine: Efficacy trial in healthy children. N Engl J Med 1984;310:1409–1415.

99 Weller TH: Serial propagation in vitro of agents producing inclusion bodies derived from varicella and herpes zoster. Proc Soc Exp Biol Med 1953;83:340–346.

100 Weller TH: Varicella and herpes zoster: Changing concepts of the natural history, control, and importance of a not-so-benign virus. N Engl J Med 1983;309:1362–1368,1434–1440.

101 Weller TH, Coons AH: Fluorescent antibody studies with agents of varicella and herpes zoster propagated in vitro. Proc Soc Exp Biol Med 1954;86:789.

102 Weller TH, Witton HM: The etiologic agents of varicella and herpes zoster. Serological studies with the viruses as propagated in vitro. J Exp Med 1958;108:869–890.

103 Wharton M: The epidemiology of varicella-zoster virus infections. Infect Dis Clin North Am 1996;10:571–581.

104 White CJ: Clinical trials of varicella vaccine in healthy children. Infect Dis Clin North Am 1996;10:595–608.

105 White CJ: Varicella-zoster virus vaccine. Clin Infect Dis 1997;24:753–763.

106 Whitley RJ, Gnann JW: Acyclovir: A decade later. N Engl J Med 1992;327:782–789.

107 Whitley RJ, Straus S: Therapy for varicella-zoster virus infections: Where do we stand? Infect Dis Clin Pract 1993;2:100–108.

108 Williams DL, Gershon A, Gelb LD, Spraker MK, Steinberg S, Ragab AH: Herpes zoster following varicella vaccine in a child with acute lymphocytic leukemia. J Pediatr 1985;106:259–261.

109 Williams V, Gershon A, Brunell P: Serologic response to varicella-zoster membrane antigens measured by indirect immunofluorescence. J Infect Dis 1974;130:669–672.

110 Wilson A, Sharp M, Koropchak C, Ting S, Arvin A: Subclinical varicella-zoster virus viremia, herpes zoster, and T lymphocyte immunity to varicella-zoster viral antigens after bone marrow transplantation. J Infect Dis 1992;165:119–126.

111 Zamora I, Simon JM, Da Silva ME, Piqueras AI: Attenuated varicella vaccine in children with renal transplants. Pediatr Nephrol 1994;8:190–192.

112 Zerboni L, Nader S, Aoki K, Arvin AM: Analysis of the persistence of humoral and cellular immunity in children and adults immunized with varicella vaccine. J Infect Dis 1998;177: 1701–1704.

Anne A. Gershon, MD, 650 W. 168th Street, New York, NY 10032 (USA)
Tel. +1 212-305 9445, Fax -342 5218, E-mail aag1@columbia.edu

Rüther U, Nunnensiek C, Schmoll H-J (eds): Secondary Neoplasias following Chemotherapy, Radiotherapy, and Immunosuppression. Contrib Oncol. Basel, Karger, 2000, vol 55, pp 305–346

······························

Posttransplant Lymphoproliferative Disorder – New Approaches to Monitoring and Management

H. A. Leitch[a], M. Cantarovich[b], J. E. Mangel[a], P. Laneuville[a]

Divisions of [a]Hematology and [b]Transplantation, Department of Medicine, McGill University Health Center, Montreal, Que., Canada

Introduction

It has been recognized since the 1960s that lymphoid neoplasms following organ transplantation are occurring with increased frequency [1, 2]. Approximately 2% of organ transplant recipients develop posttransplant lymphoproliferative disorder (PTLD), compared to an incidence of non-Hodgkin's lymphoma (NHL) of 0.1–9 per 100,000 in the general population. This corresponds to a 20- to 120-fold increase of NHL following transplantation. In one analysis, PTLD occurred 49 times more frequently in patients following transplantation than in age-matched controls [3]. The incidence of PTLD varies according to type of organ transplanted and type and intensity of immunosuppression. It has been estimated as follows: kidney, 1.0%; liver, 2.2%; heart, 3.4%; lung, 7.9%; bone marrow transplantation (BMT), overall < 1%; T-cell-depleted bone marrow graft, 12%; use of anti-CD3 antibody, 14%, and HLA-mismatched and T-cell-depleted graft, 24% [4]. In renal transplant recipients, the absolute risk of lymphoma is increased 350-fold [5]. Mortality is high, ranging from 40 to 50% [6–8]. PTLD and its treatment are associated with a significant risk of allograft loss, which may be as high as 60% [9].

The risk of PTLD is highest in the first year following transplantation, and falls subsequently [10]. Among 45,141 kidney transplant recipients, the risk was 0.2% in the first year, and 0.04% in subsequent years. Of 7,634 heart transplants, 1.2% developed PTLD in the first year and 0.4% per year thereafter. Of 69 patients with PTLD following solid-organ transplantation, 67% presented within 12 months, and only 14% presented more than 4 years following transplantation [11]. A wide regional variation in rates of PTLD has been noted. Rates appear to be higher in North America than in Europe, which may be related to different immunosuppressive regimens [12].

Ninety-three percent of PTLDs are non-Hodgkin's in type. Malignant cells are of B lineage in 86% and T-cell in 14% [3]. Over half are at an advanced stage, and two thirds involve extranodal sites. In NHL in the general population, one quarter to one half are extranodal. Whereas 1% of NHL involves the central nervous system (CNS), its involvement is seen in 28% of PTLD. PTLD involving the CNS is almost uniformly fatal. The incidence of CNS PTLD has declined with the use of immunosuppressive regimens containing cyclosporine, as has the incidence of extranodal disease [3]. Up to 18% of PTLD involves the allograft, and this incidence may vary according to the organ transplanted. Involvement of transplanted liver, kidney or lung has been described in 8.6, 17, and 60% of cases, respectively [reviewed in 13].

While some aspects of the biology and management of PTLD have become increasingly clear in recent years, in many ways it remains an elusive entity. Much of the literature is in the form of case reports, small to medium-sized case series, and retrospective reviews; there are few prospective studies. Collection of data is hampered by the lack of a central registry; reporting to registries such as the Cincinnati Transplant Tumor Registry (CCTR) and the European Collaborative Transplant Study is voluntary [13].

While the relative significance of these factors is unclear, the transplant population likely differs between centers. What is more, immunosuppression has evolved: prior to 1980, corticosteroids, azathioprine and antilymphocyte globulins were the main drugs used in clinical practice. In the 1980s, cyclosporine and anti-CD3 monoclonal antibodies became available, followed by tacrolimus (FK-506). In the 1990s, the introduction of mycophenolate and new monoclonal antibodies completed the armamentarium. These agents are used in various combinations and are variably quantified, making the relative contribution of each to the development of PTLD difficult to evaluate. Several systems for the classification of PTLD are in use, and treatment of PTLD is rarely standardized. Thus, many aspects of PTLD, such as predisposing factors, incidence, prognosis and optimal treatment, remain to be clarified.

Several excellent recent reviews discuss in detail the incidence of PTLD, classification systems and the influence of immunosuppressive regimens [4, 14–16]. This chapter reviews the present literature, with a focus on prognostic factors, new therapies, the effect of standardized treatment strategies, the role of Epstein-Barr virus (EBV) in pathogenesis, and the possible contribution of molecular changes to the evolution of PTLD.

Etiology

EBV-Associated Malignancies

EBV is a herpes virus that has been associated with several malignancies, including endemic or African Burkitt's lymphoma (BL), nasopharyngeal carcinoma, Hodgkin's disease and X-linked lymphoproliferative disease [17]. More recently, EBV has been associated with lymphoproliferations arising in the setting of immune deficiency, including human immunodeficiency virus-associated NHL (HIV-NHL). The majority of PTLD, as in HIV, are B-cell, and 70–90% are EBV-positive, depending on the series and probably on the detection technique in addition. EBV has been implicated in several additional T-cell lymphoproliferations, including T-cell PTLD, hemophagocytic syndrome-associated T-cell lymphocytosis, nasal T-cell lymphoma, and peripheral T-cell lymphoma of angioimmunoblastic lymphadenopathy (AILD) [17].

EBV and PTLD

The association between EBV and PTLD was recognized in the 1980s [18], and has been supported by several lines of evidence, including epidemiologic data, serologic and molecular genetic measurements of neutralizing antibodies, cytotoxic T-lymphocyte activity, and viral load [4, 19–21]. It was noted early that a higher incidence of PTLD occurred following transplantation in organ recipients who were EBV-seronegative prior to transplant and who received an organ from a seropositive donor [22, 23]. In North America, 90% of adults exhibit humoral immunity to EBV, as compared to 20% of children; the incidence of PTLD is particularly high in children [24]. Most data suggest that EBV is present in the latent form in PTLD, but there may be a role for the replicative form of infection in tumorigenesis. This has led to the addition of acyclovir to therapeutic maneuvers for PTLD [4, 13].

EBV Infectious Cycle and the Establishment of Latency

EBV is a double-stranded, enveloped DNA virus [13]. Upon primary exposure, the virus establishes replicative and cytolytic infection in the oropharyngeal mucosa. This phase may be associated with symptoms of infectious mononucleosis, including exudative pharyngitis, or may be subclinical. As humoral and cellular immunity are established in the immunocompetent host, viral infection becomes latent. A well-documented reservoir for latent infection is the B lymphocyte [4].

The cellular receptor for EBV is glycoprotein CD21, which binds the viral outer envelope glycoprotein gp350/220 and results in cellular internalization of the viral particle. Expression of virally encoded proteins is induced, resulting in replicative or lytic infection. Many of the details of lytic infection are uncertain, due to the lack of an appropriate tissue culture model [13]. After the emergence of cytotoxic T lymphocytes (CTL) specific for EBV-infected cells, lytically infected cells are rapidly cleared, a phenomenon termed regression [25]. Latently infected cells, however, persist for life, owing in part to the lack of CTL response to the viral product EBNA-1, which is important in maintaining latent infection [26]. Because of the lack of expression of most viral proteins, latently infected cells are not driven to proliferate. However, an autocrine loop is established, whereby B-cell growth factors such as interleukin-6 (IL-6) are produced, promoting cell survival [reviewed in 13]. EBV infection upregulates the expression of the nuclear proto-oncogene *bcl-2,* an inhibitor of apoptosis, or programmed cell death, an additional signal in favor of cell survival. Expression of viral proteins ensures continued stimulation of the immune system, resulting in a balance between EBV latency and immune surveillance. A compromise to such immunity disrupts this balance and may permit reactivation of viral replication, which may result in expansion of the pool of virally infected lymphocytes. Consistent with this model, T-cell-mediated regression is not seen in some patients receiving immunosuppressive therapy [27, 28].

Latent infection involves maintenance of a viral episome, a circular viral genome that is not integrated into cellular DNA and is maintained separately in the cell nucleus. The viral DNA circularizes to form an episome during primary infection, via random homologous recombination of terminal repeat sequences. This leads to a unique number of repeat sequences within each episome, which can be identified by molecular techniques such as Southern blot analysis. In this way, clonality can be identified [29]. During latent infection, one in 10^6–10^8 B cells harbors EBV under normal conditions [13].

A limited set of viral gene products is expressed during latent infection: 9 out of a total of the 80–100 gene products encoded by the viral genome. These are termed latent membrane proteins (LMP, LMP1, LMP2A and LMP2B), and EBV nuclear antigens (EBNA, EBNA-1, EBNA-2, EBNA-3A, EBNA-3B, EBNA-3C and EBNA-LP). EBNA-1 is essential for maintenance of the viral episome [30]. Under some conditions, a switch from latent infection to active replication may be triggered, and may result in the expression of several B-cell stimulatory cytokines. Early antigens (EA), a set of nonstructural proteins involved in the synthesis of viral DNA, are expressed, as are viral structural proteins termed viral capsid antigen (VCA), required for the packaging and egress of viral particles. EBER-1 and -2 are ribonucleic acids which in situ hybridization can target for identification in affected tissues [31].

Latent membrane proteins (LMP) are expressed during latent infection, and have transforming properties in vitro. LMP1 is a viral analog of the tumor necrosis factor (TNF) family of receptors, and is involved in the transmission of growth signals from the cell membrane to the nucleus via cytoplasmic TNF-associated factors (TRAFs). This results in expression of transcription factor NFκB-controlled cellular genes, and upregulation of cell proliferation [reviewed in 32, 33].

There are several patterns of LMP expression which are associated with distinctive EBV-associated tumors. The most restricted pattern, termed latency type I, involves the expression of EBNA-1 only, and is associated with endemic Burkitt's lymphoma. Latency type II refers to the expression of EBNA-1, LMP1, LMP2A and LMP2B, and is associated with Hodgkin's disease and nasopharyngeal carcinoma. Latency type III refers to the expression of all nine EBNAs and LMPs, and is associated with PTLD and HIV-NHL [17].

The expression of LMP is essential for the maintenance of long-term immunity to EBV, which is largely cell-mediated. Under certain conditions, LMP expression may be downregulated, decreasing the antigenic targets which stimulate ongoing immunity, and possibly the molecular signaling pathway that promotes cell division. Recent evidence suggests that expression of EBNA-1 itself alters the ability of the immune system to effectively process and present antigen [34], possibly by influencing protein degradation. In these ways, EBV adapts cellular machinery to evade the immune response and promote its own survival.

Primary EBV infection results in the stimulation of anti-VCA IgM. Anti-VCA IgG appears later and, under normal circumstances, persists for life. Anti-EA antibodies appear during primary infection and recovery, then wane, but may persist in chronic infection. Anti-EBNA antibodies appear during recovery and persist [13].

EBV plays an important role in oncogenesis and malignant cell transformation. Several latency-associated proteins have been linked with transformation of lymphoblastic cell lines in vitro; most notably EBNA-1, a protein which binds specifically to sequences at the episome origin of replication, and is thus involved in the control of viral replication. Expression of EBNA-1 has been shown in vitro to (1) cause loss of contact inhibition and anchorage dependence; (2) promote growth in low-serum medium, and (3) result in B-cell activation and expression of adhesion molecules [35, 36]. Downregulation of EBNA-1 occurs in BL, suggesting that upregulation of c-myc gene expression from the t(8;22) translocation characteristic of BL might make cell survival independent of EBNA-1-mediated cell stimulatory functions [reviewed in 33]. This model correlates with the observation, in a series of PTLDs, that those which were polyclonal or oligoclonal exhibited no clonal cytogenetic abnormalities, whereas those that were monoclonal exhibited several. These included the Burkitt's translocations involving c-myc, trisomies of chromosomes 9 or 11, abnormalities involving the cellular proto-oncogene bcl-6, and rearrangement of the immunoglobulin heavy chain locus [32]. Cytogenetics correlated with histology, with oligoclonal or normal cytogenetics found in polymorphic or centroblastic morphology, Burkitt's translocation associated with Burkitt's morphology, and other molecular abnormalities with immunoblastic morphology [37]. Several other cytogenetic abnormalities have been reported in patients with monoclonal disease [25]. Thus, EBV may drive polyclonal B-cell proliferation, creating an environment in which further genetic changes are possible and thereby result in outgrowth of a malignant clone.

EBV infection of B lymphocytes involves the expression of B-cell growth factors and growth factor receptors. One factor negatively regulating B-cell growth is interferon-α (IFN-α), which has been used in several series to treat PTLD [38–42]. Deletions of the IFN-α gene were demonstrated in 4 of 9 cases of PTLD associated with EBV infection [43]. This suggests deletion of downregulatory cytokines as a mechanism for malignant outgrowth in PTLD, and provides a rationale for the observed success of therapy with IFN-α.

The EBV open reading frame BCRF1 is highly homologous to the sequence of human interleukin-10 (IL-10), and expression of the BCRF protein has shown similar biologic activity to IL-10. IL-10 suppresses NK-cell function, as well as tumor cytotoxicity by monocytes and macrophages [44]. In a series of renal transplants, it was demonstrated by enzyme-linked immunosorbent assay that serum IL-10 was elevated, and clearly preceded the clinical onset of PTLD.

Relationship of EBV Viral Load to the Development of PTLD

It was recently demonstrated that an increase in EBV viral load in conjunction with a decrease in antibodies directed against EBV proteins correlates to the development of PTLD [19]. The semiquantitative polymerase chain reaction (PCR) assay to amplify EBV sequences showed that a series of patients who did not develop PTLD exhibited a less than 10-fold increase in viral load in peripheral blood leukocytes when compared to normal healthy EBV carriers. Transplant recipients who underwent primary EBV infection exhibited an up to 400-fold increase in viral load over immunocompetent individuals with primary EBV infection, and a 4,000-fold increase in viral load over normal healthy carriers. Of patients who developed PTLD, a viral load increase of up to a million-fold over normal healthy carriers was seen, corresponding to a 25-fold or higher level of viremia compared to transplant recipients who did not develop PTLD. This was associated with a concomitant decrease in anti-EBNA antibodies.

These results were confirmed in a second study. Using 5′ nucleotidase TaqMan assay to detect EBV DNA in serial peripheral blood mononuclear cells of solid-organ transplant recipients, it was shown that an increase in viral load correlated to development of PTLD. Zero of 18 control patients had detectable levels of EBV DNA, as compared to 15 of 16 patients with PTLD [45]. EBV DNA levels decreased following therapy, and copy numbers were 5–10 times higher in patients with extensive disease than in those with limited disease.

In another series, by PCR amplification of EBV sequences, 7 of 10 patients with high EBV copy number following BMT developed PTLD, as compared to zero of 16 patients with low copy number [46]. Conversely, 10 of 11 patients with low levels spontaneously reverted to PCR negativity, while only 1 of 10 patients with high copy number had a spontaneous decline in viral load and remained clinically well. A second patient with high copy number and clinical PTLD was treated with donor leukocyte infusion (DLI) from the original bone marrow donor, with a decline in viral load and clinical improvement.

In a series of pediatric liver transplant patients, 7 patients who developed PTLD were identified, and viral load sequentially followed [47]. Mean viral load at the time of diagnosis of PTLD was high, and fell with treatment. Low viral load corresponded to an increased risk of graft rejection, presumably related to an increasingly intact immune response. Finally, in a series of 60 patients followed for up to 11 years after kidney transplantation, 100- to 1,000-fold expansion of circulating EBV-positive B lymphocytes was common at 3–6 months. In this series, however, no patient developed PTLD [48].

Thus, in several centers, monitoring of EBV viral load was useful for predicting patients likely to develop PTLD, and for identifying patients who might benefit from early clinical intervention. EBV viral load might be a marker of the relative efficiency of immunity directed against EBV. For example, in BMT, the majority of PTLDs arise in the first 6 months after transplant [20]. In a study designed to evaluate cell-mediated immunity to EBV following BMT, cytotoxic T-lymphocyte precursor (CTLp) frequencies were quantified by limiting dilution analysis in 26 recipients of marrow grafts [21]. At 3 months following transplantation, only 5 of 13 patients had CTLp frequencies in the range of normal controls, but by 6 months, the number had risen to 9. One patient with low CTLp frequency at 4 months following transplantation developed PTLD which responded to DLI. Thus, although the frequency of PTLD in this series was low, the period at which a deficiency of EBV-specific cell-mediated immunity was demonstrated corresponds to the period of highest risk for PTLD following BMT.

Attempts have been made to identify the cell of origin of EBV-related PTLD during B-cell ontogeny. By analysis of immunoglobulin (Ig) genes for somatic hypermutation, the post-germinal center B lymphocyte was implicated as the cell of origin of monomorphic PTLD [37], suggesting that germinal center selection might be important in its development. Ig genes of cells derived from polymorphic PTLD are currently under analysis.

While the majority of cases of PTLD associated with EBV may be secondary to a reactivation of EBV infection, a minority are associated with primary infection, particularly in children. Primary EBV infection following transplantation increases the risk of PTLD 24-fold [22]. Recently, an EBV-negative patient received an organ from an EBV-negative donor, and subsequently developed EBV-associated PTLD. It was demonstrated through restriction fragment length polymorphism analysis that the EBV strain had originated with a unit of packed red blood cells [49]. The blood donor had experienced an episode of clinical mononucleosis 15 months prior to donation. These data suggest a role for leukodepletion of blood products destined for EBV-negative recipients, and for identification of donors with a history of infectious mononucleosis.

Finally, the development of PTLD might be dependent on the strain of EBV involved in infection of the immunocompromised host. There have been isolated reports of detection of type B EBV in the tissues of patients with PTLD [50], but a role for coinfection with two viral types has been suggested. In a recent series, all of the patients in which EBV was associated with PTLD expressed type A EBV [51]. This is a viral type associated with more efficient in vitro immortalization of B lymphocytes, better survival of cultured cells, and more frequent infection of peripheral blood leukocytes in vivo [52]. These results point towards a pathogenic role for the type A viral strain, and suggest that patients infected with this strain might require close monitoring for early detection of PTLD and more concerted attempts at prevention and treatment.

EBV-Negative PTLD

Eleven PTLDs not associated with EBV were recently compared to EBV-related PTLDs [53]. By molecular and immunohistochemical techniques, 8 of 11 EBV-negative PTLDs were B-cell and 3 were T-cell. Of 21 PTLDs associated with EBV in this series, all but 1 were B-cell. The EBV-negative PTLDs were characterized by late onset (180–10,220 vs. 60–2,100 days), disseminated disease, poor outcome, and little or no response to reduction of immunosuppression, suggesting more intensive therapeutic interventions might be required in this group.

In one study, most EBV-negative PTLDs were monomorphic [54], suggesting that monomorphic PTLDs may not require EBV stimulation for support of cell survival. It has been suggested that late-occurring EBV-negative PTLD may represent a separate disease entity. Others maintain that these are PTLDs at an end of the spectrum in which cell survival is independent of requirement for EBV [14].

Other Etiologic Agents and Genetic Changes

In a retrospective analysis, 13 of 40 patients seronegative for EBV at the time of liver transplantation developed PTLD. Cytomegalovirus (CMV) disease was found to be the risk factor, with a relative risk of 7.3 [23]. Eleven patients developed CMV disease; 7 of these had PTLD. The development of PTLD was associated with more severe CMV disease, with 5 of 7 manifesting CMV pneumonitis, as compared to zero of 4 without PTLD. This may be related to the direct immunosuppressive effects of CMV, particularly on cell-mediated immunity [55]. Factors which were not significant included sex, age, ABO blood group, HLA antigen type, HLA antigen match, surgical factors, use of acyclovir prophylaxis, cumulative level of immunosuppression, and number of transfusions.

In a series of 381 adult nonrenal solid-organ recipients, the risk of development of PTLD was increased 24-fold in EBV-seronegative recipients. This risk was magnified 4- to 6-fold by CMV sero-mismatch [22].

A study investigating transactivation of viruses within the herpes family provides a rationale for an increased risk of PTLD observed in patients coinfected with EBV and CMV. Using Ig avidity testing, 13 of 56 (23%) of EBV-seropositive

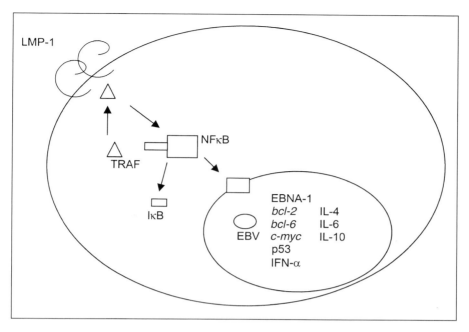

Fig. 1. Cellular pathway of EBV-supported growth stimulation. The EBV product LMP is an analog of the TNF family of receptors. A transmembrane protein, aggregation of LMP-1 results in binding of the cytoplasmic TRAF. This results in TRAF-induced degradation of IκB and liberation of the transcription factor NFκB, which is translocated to the nucleus. The transcription of NFκB-controlled genes results, favoring cell survival and division. Cellular and viral proto-oncogenes and tumor suppressor genes implicated in PTLD include EBNA-1, *bcl-2, bcl-6, c-myc,* p53, IFN-α, and possibly others [adapted from 32].

patients undergoing CMV primary infection showed serologic evidence of EBV activation, with a rise in titer of EBV-specific antibodies [23]. Conversely, of CMV-seropositive patients undergoing EBV primary infection, zero of 22 patients showed reactivation of CMV. Thus, CMV appears to stimulate EBV activity. In the immuno-suppressed host, this stimulation could support dysregulated proliferation of EBV-infected cells and clonal outgrowth. It may thus be important to match organs and blood transfusions to donor EBV and CMV status whenever possible.

Proto-oncogenes and cytokines associated with PTLD include *bcl-2,* a known inhibitor of programmed cell death, which strongly correlated with immunohisto-chemical staining for LMP1 in a series of 17 cases [56]. IL-6 is a B-cell growth factor known to be elevated in PTLD [57]; IL-6 plasma bioactivity was transiently elevated in 17 of 18 cases [58]. *bcl-6* is a nuclear proto-oncogene involved in the control of germinal center formation and T-helper type 2 inflammatory responses [59], and frequently mutated in several de novo and HIV-associated NHLs. In a series of 57 PTLDs, mutations in the *bcl-6* gene were identified in 33 (58%). The presence of mutation correlated with shorter survival and refractoriness to therapeutic maneuvers [60].

Finally, serum levels of interleukin-4 (IL-4), a B-cell stimulatory cytokine, are elevated at diagnosis of PTLD, whereas levels of IFN-α are decreased [61]. Immunosuppression with cyclosporine is associated with increased levels of IL-4; in this way, IL-4 might play a role in the association between treatment with cyclosporine and the development of PTLD [61]. Thus, several cellular growth factors, proto-oncogenes and cytokines have been implicated in the development of PTLD.

The cell signaling pathway that results in transcription of NFκB-controlled genes in PTLD is summarized in figure 1. Aggregation of LMP1 on the cell membrane results in activation of TRAF via the LMP1 cytoplasmic tail. TRAF, in turn, degrades IκB, releasing NFκB, which translocates to the cell nucleus, where it is active as a transcription factor. Alteration in expression of cellular and possibly viral genes supports cell survival, and creates an environment in which malignant transformation may occur [32].

Classification and Pathophysiology

Classification Systems

Several systems for the classification of PTLD have been proposed and modified [reviewed in 62]. Common to these is the use of morphologic, immunophenotypic and molecular genetic techniques to separate lesions into low-grade (polymorphic and/or polyclonal) versus high-grade (monotypic and/or monoclonal). However, this separation has failed to predict clinical behavior and prognosis, and thus its utility in defining appropriate therapy is unclear. Polyclonal lymphoproliferations have been documented to behave in a malignant and rapidly progressive manner, and conversely, monoclonal proliferations have responded to conservative measures [15]. Thus, while the current practice is to document morphology and cellular and viral clonality, treatment schemes are designed to correspond to clinical behavior.

Classification is further complicated by the following: (1) Occult clonality can be detected in patients with polymorphic lesions; (2) separate PTLD lesions from one individual patient may be polyclonal and others monoclonal, and (3) patients with clonal disease may harbor more than one separate clone [63–65].

A recently revised system incorporates features of previous classification systems and identifies both cellular and viral clonality, as well as genetic lesions in known cellular proto-oncogenes and tumor suppressor genes. This system is attractive in that it incorporates a rational biologic basis for tumor progression in which infection of B cells results in polyclonal expansion to a point at which one or several clones are able to grow out under reduced immune surveillance, and viral clonality is demonstrated. Further evolution involves cellular genetic alterations, resulting in truly malignant behavior [16]. Specific categories include: (1) Plasmacytic hyperplasia, which is usually confined to the oropharynx or lymph nodes, is polyclonal, and manifests multiple cellular and viral clones. In this category, no alterations in cellular genes are seen. (2) Polymorphic hyperplastic or lymphomatous lesions arise in nodal or extranodal sites, are clonal, are infected by a single EBV clone, and do not have alterations in cellular genes. (3) Immunoblastic lymphoma or myeloma present with widely disseminated disease, are monoclonal, have a single clone of EBV, and exhibit alterations in one or more cellular genes [16]. In this series, classification corresponded to clinical aggressiveness. However, a large clinical series is warranted to further delineate morphologic and molecular factors that predict clinical aggression.

The morphologic variability of PTLD is illustrated in a recent report. In this case, initial histopathology was consistent with an EBV-associated T-cell PTLD involving the spleen and bone marrow. Upon reduction of immunosuppression, the emergence of B-cell PTLD rich in plasma cells was observed in bone marrow and liver. Genotypic studies confirmed the presence of two cellular clones; one with a T-cell receptor-β chain rearrangement, and one with an Ig heavy chain joining region rearrangement [66]. Multiple EBV clones were demonstrated. This case illustrates the difficulties inherent in morphologic classification of PTLD on the basis of isolated tissue biopsy and histology, and the importance of performing repeat biopsy on recurrence or progresssion, or on multiple sites of involvement.

In a summary of a recent workshop, classification was simplified and unified by including the following categories: early lesions, polymorphic, monomorphic, plasmacytoma-like, and T-cell-rich large B-cell/Hodgkin-like lesions. Monomorphic lesions are further subclassified according to recognized classification of NHL, with PTLD status specified [14].

Early lesions correspond to polyclonality and are generally polymorphic; however, polymorphic lesions are not necessarily polyclonal. EBV is typically present, usually without clonality. These PTLDs display a range of clinical behavior from spontaneous regression to fatality. Polymorphic lesions exhibit the full range of B-cell maturation, with clonality demonstrated by examination of Ig gene rearrangements and EBV terminal repeats. These PTLDs may regress with reduction in immunosuppression, or may progress [14].

Monomorphic PTLDs are often monoclonal, and have the morphology of high-grade lymphoma. Most are of diffuse large-cell or immunoblastic type, while some have the morphology of BL. Ig genes and EBV are clonal. Some have mutations in cellular proto-oncogenes and tumor suppressor genes such as *ras* and p53. Some may respond to reduced immunosuppression, a minority with lasting response. This category may identify a subgroup in which truly malignant behavior is more frequent and aggressive therapeutic interventions are warranted.

EBV-negative PTLDs occur a median of 7 years following transplantation, compared to 1 year for EBV-positive cases [14]. It has been suggested that these may not represent true PTLDs. Others maintain that EBV-negative tumors are probably transplant-related, and that analysis of these lymphoproliferations is important in elucidating mechanisms of lymphomagenesis that bypass the association with EBV [14].

Consensus recommendations for pathologic workup include morphology, immunophenotyping for lineage and clonality, and, where feasible, molecular genetic studies for the presence of EBV, and cellular and viral clonality [14]. Further classification may additionally require information on transplant organ type, immunosuppressive regimen, sites and stage of disease, and, possibly, donor vs. host origin. Diagnostic and staging evaluations, as well as studies for delineating clinical-pathological correlation and monitoring the efficacy of therapeutic interventions, are summarized in table 1.

Guidelines on cytologic features in body fluids or fine-needle aspirates which support the diagnosis of PTLD have been provided by one group [67]. These share many cellular features with conventional lymphoma. Here, a key to recognition of PTLD was knowledge of the clinical history. Fine-needle aspirate specimens appeared polymorphic, whereas histologic specimens from the same site were monomorphic, emphasizing the importance of excisional biopsy in the evaluation of PTLD. The presence of PTLD in body fluids implied a worse prognosis: 4 patients with PTLD in ascites, effusions or cerebrospinal fluid all died within 3 months of diagnosis.

Several recent reports illustrate the difficulties in distinguishing between PTLD, benign lymphoid proliferation and graft rejection; both can cause nonspecific symptoms and graft dysfunction [68, 69]. This distinction is important, since initial treatment of PTLD – reduction of immunosuppression – is diametrically opposed to the management of rejection by increasing immunosuppression. Thus, timely tissue diagnosis is critical.

Donor/Recipient Origin

Donor or host origin of lymphoproliferation can be determined using molecular techniques, including analysis of genetic polymorphism, EBV clonality, microsatellite instability, HLA typing, fluorescence in situ hybridization, cytogenetics and DNA fingerprinting. For the most part, PTLDs in recipients of solid organs are of host origin, whereas in recipients of bone marrow grafts, PTLD usually arises from grafted donor hematopoietic cells. There are exceptions, which are discussed below.

Table 1. Workup of PTLD

Diagnosis	Strong clinical suspicion	
	Tissue biopsy	Histology
		Cellular clonality, e.g., microsatellite instability
		EBV presence and clonality, e.g., terminal repeats
Staging	As for NHL	Image chest, abdomen, pelvis
		Image head, cerebrospinal fluid analysis, if indicated
		Gallium scan
		Bone marrow biopsy
		Chemistry
Additional studies	EBV viral load	
	Analysis for monoclonal peak	
	Donor/recipient origin	
	Cytogenetic changes	
	Specific oncogenes	

Most studies of donor/host PTLD type refer to the cell of origin. There are, however, documented cases in which donor EBV has been transmitted via the organ graft, resulting in infection of host cells and ultimately PTLD [70]. This occurred in a patient who was EBV-seronegative prior to transplant, and is in contrast to the more usual finding of recipient EBV PTLD arising in patients who were seropositive prior to transplant.

Recent reports include the following: a B-lymphoblastic EBV-associated PTLD in the allograft 4 months following lung transplantation was shown to be of donor origin by HLA analysis [71]. Two intrahepatic PTLDs were of donor origin by microsatellite analysis. Both were clonal B-cell and EBV-associated, and occurred 5 and 3 months following liver transplantation [72]. A monoclonal B-cell PTLD, EBV-associated and localized to the liver graft, arose 8 months following liver transplantation. Donor origin was demonstrated by fluorescence in situ hybridization for sex chromosome identification [73]. One patient developed monoclonal B-cell PTLD confined to the porta hepatis 4.5 months following transplantation. Donor origin was demonstrated by PCR for DNA sequence polymorphism [74].

Following a sex-mismatched transplant, an EBV-positive polymorphic B-cell PTLD occurred 7 months after transplantation of a single lung, and was localized to the allograft [75]. This PTLD was found to be of donor origin by fluorescence in situ hybridization for the Y chromosome. A B-cell EBV-positive PTLD localized to the allograft was detected 5 months after renal transplantation with an HLA-mismatched kidney, and was determined to be of donor origin by cytogenetic analysis and DNA fingerprinting [76].

Finally, in one remarkable report, kidneys grafted from the same donor into 2 recipients resulted in B-cell EBV-positive PTLD in both. Both recipients had been EBV-seronegative prior to grafting, while the donor had evidence of primary EBV infection at the time of donation. PTLD was diagnosed 38 and 65 days following transplantation; both followed a fulminant and fatal course despite therapeutic interventions including graft nephrectomy [77].

In a series of 7 patients analyzed by microsatellite instability, 2 were of donor origin [78], and both were B-cell in type. In one series, 10 of 11 patients who had received solid organs had PTLD of recipient origin by detection of genetic polymorphism [79]. The one PTLD of donor origin occurred in the recipient of a liver allograft and was localized to the liver. In contrast, only 3 of the 10 PTLDs of recipient origin were localized. In one analysis, 4 out of 4 patients with donor origin PTLD were alive and disease-free, in contrast to only 6 of 18 patients with PTLD of recipient origin. These observations suggest that PTLD expressing alloantigens might present a better target for cell-mediated immunity and be more easily controlled by the host immune system. Neither series provides information on whether tumors of donor origin arose at a different interval following transplantation compared to tumors of recipient origin.

The finding of PTLD of donor origin is not surprising, considering that donor lymphocytes in the graft are capable of reconstituting long-term hematopoiesis at distant sites [80, 81]. The probability of development of PTLD of donor origin might be related to the degree of HLA mismatch between the host and grafted organ [72]. However, few reports provide information adequate for analysis of this feature. Of 6 cases in which donor origin was definitively documented following solid-organ transplantation, all occurred early, within 8 months, all were B-cell in type, EBV-related, and localized to the allograft. This is in contrast to the finding that 13% [15] to 40% of PTLDs as a whole are localized to the allograft, and suggests that factors specific to the graft itself might play a role in limiting PTLD. In a series of 25 PTLDs following renal transplantation, 9 involved the allograft, and 3 were confined to the grafted organ [82]. A better outcome for PTLD of donor origin in solid-organ transplantation is an established fact, and it has been suggested that workup of PTLD is not complete without evaluation of donor vs. host origin [83].

The disseminated disease seen in the 2 cases of PTLD arising after transplantation of kidneys from a single donor might be related to the transmission of active lytic primary EBV infection into an immunocompromised host. Thus, EBV matching is desirable in organ transplantation, and when not possible, careful follow-up of EBV-negative patients receiving EBV-positive organs is warranted. Further evaluation of antiviral prophylactic regimens in this group would also be of considerable value.

In contrast to the localized disease and better outcome seen in solid-organ transplant recipients, PTLD arising after BMT, while generally of donor origin, has an almost uniformly poor outcome [20]. In a recent summary, 23 patients were evaluated for PTLD origin following BMT. All 23 were of donor origin, and EBV-positive. PTLD arose 54–1,000 days following transplantation, with all but 1 case arising within 6 months [84]. In 1 case, autopsy performed on the immunocompetent donor – who had died of other causes – revealed no evidence of lymphoma. This supports the role of immune suppression in the development of PTLD. The poor outcome of PTLD following BMT is a situation which might improve with the therapeutic use of DLI or anti-EBV-specific T-cell lines (see 'Treatment').

PTLD following BMT

In a recent series of allogeneic BMT, 25 of 2,395 patients developed PTLD, for an overall incidence of 1.2% (including both allogeneic and autologous BMT); 2.0% for allogeneic BMT; 3.3% for BMT from unrelated donors, and 1.6% for related donors [41]. Risk factors for PTLD included T-cell depletion and HLA mismatch. All tumors were associated with EBV, and mortality was 92%. Two patients survived, and were among a group of 7 who received treatment with IFN-α.

In a smaller series of allogeneic BMT, 8 of 428 patients developed PTLD, for an incidence of 1.9% [85]. Six patients with PTLD had received grafts from unrelated donors, 5 of which were T-cell-depleted. Median time to presentation was 90 days following transplantation, and all cases presented within 10 months. Localized disease presented greater than 200 days following transplantation, whereas advanced disease presented earlier, at a mean of 80 days, and within the 6-month window in which cellular immunity to EBV generally is low [21]. One patient recovered; this patient had localized disease. All PTLD were EBV-positive, and of 7 tested, all were monoclonal.

Most cases of PTLD following BMT occur in recipients of allogeneic grafts. However, there are 7 reported cases of PTLD following autologous stem cell transplantation. Five cases were monomorphic B-cell PTLD and 2 were polymorphous. All 7 cases were EBV-positive [86–88]. Most cases were fatal. The case with a favorable outcome was one of 2 with polymorphous morphology, and one of 3 with limited disease [85]. Many cases presented within 90 days following BMT, or during the time of lowest immunity to EBV.

Unusual Histology

While the majority of monotypic PTLDs are diffuse large-cell or immunoblastic, several other morphologic variants have been described. These comprise BL, T-cell lymphoma including Ki-1 lymphoma and $\gamma\delta$ lymphoproliferation, myeloma and Hodgkin's disease. Although BL occurs with increased frequency in other forms of immune deficiency such as HIV infection [89], it is less common following transplantation. Recently, a case was reported in which a patient developed polyclonal B-cell PTLD 3 years after cardiac transplantation [90]. Although there was an initial response to decreased immunosuppression and acyclovir, the PTLD subsequently progressed rapidly. Investigations demonstrated a monoclonal EBV-positive PTLD harboring the translocation t(8;14)(q24;q32) characteristic of BL. In keeping with the diagnosis of BL, LMP1 was expressed by the malignant cells, and no expression of other latency-associated proteins was found. The patient responded well to combination chemotherapy, and was in remission for 4 years following diagnosis. Unlike African BL, North American BL, aside from in the HIV population, is infrequently associated with EBV. The association with EBV in this case, in addition to the evolution from polyclonality to monoclonality, suggests that this was truly a case of lymphoproliferation related to transplantation.

T-cell PTLD is less frequent than B-cell; about 10–20% of cases are T-cell in origin. Of T-cell PTLD, however, clonal EBV has been demonstrated in the malignant cells in some cases. Several recent reports illustrate the variety of T-cell lymphoma that can be seen following transplantation.

Following renal transplantation, 2 patients presented with T-cell lymphoma at 10 and 15 years. In both cases, clonality was demonstrated for the T-cell receptor β. One case was EBV-negative, and both cases were negative for HTLV-1. The third case presented 1 year after cardiac transplantation with an anaplastic large-cell (Ki-1, CD30+) EBV-negative lymphoma. All 3 patients died – 2 during combination chemotherapy, and 1 patient 2 days after presentation – before diagnostic workup was complete [91]. In the same report, features of 22 cases of T-cell PTLD are summarized. Several features in common were noted, including a propensity for extranodal presentation and poor survival, usually in days to weeks. EBV might be less frequently associated with T-cell PTLD; of 15 cases tested, 5 were positive. The majority of cases presented several years following transplantation, with only a few in the early weeks. No apparent relationship between time of presentation and EBV positivity was seen.

A second case of Ki-1-positive PTLD was reported. In this case, the lymphoproliferation was clonal for B cells, but was T-cell-rich, the T cells demonstrating positivity for CD30 [92]. Although Ki-1-positive, since clonality in this case was of B-cell origin, it might be more accurate to classify this PTLD as B cell in type.

One of 61 (1.6%) PTLDs at a single center was T-cell in phenotype in another series [93]. Analysis of this case demonstrated cellular clonality and EBV positivity. It is suggested that criteria for diagnosis of EBV-related T-cell PTLD should include consistent morphology, evidence of T-cell clonality, lack of evidence of B-cell clonality, presence of EBV, and lack of predisposing causes other than transplantation.

There are 2 reported cases of γδ T-cell PTLD after renal transplantation, and 1 following BMT [94]. By immunohistochemistry, the first case was positive for the

T-cell receptor γ; the patient died despite combination chemotherapy. The second case was positive for both γ and δ, and the patient responded well to decreased immunosuppression.

In summary, several generalizations can be made about T-cell PTLD. It appears to be less common than B-cell PTLD, may be less frequently associated with EBV, appears to have a worse prognosis; and occurs later after transplantation.

Extramedullary plasmacytoma and myeloma are reported only rarely following transplantation [95, 96]. CD21, the cellular EBV receptor, is rarely expressed by mature plasma cells, which may account for the low incidence of myeloma in this setting [95]. Of 10 reported cases, all but 1 myeloma occurred at an interval greater than 1.5 years, and up to 12 years. Median survival in this group was poor, only 4–6 months. The long-term risk of myeloma in transplant patients is increased 2.3-fold over that of the general population [97]. Thus, although myeloma occurs less frequently than do other types of PTLD, it appears to be more frequent than in the general population, and indicates poor survival. The association with EBV is less certain than for other types of PTLD, and remains to be defined.

Hodgkin's disease is rare following transplantation; only 6 cases have been reported in recent years. Five followed renal or combined renal and pancreas transplantation [98, 99], and one followed allogeneic BMT [100]. Two patients with renal grafts presented with stage IA Hodgkin's disease at 19 months and 5 years. The patient who received combined renal and pancreatic grafts presented with stage IVB disease at 20 months [99]. This patient had had a previous PTLD at 4 months after transplant, which was successfully treated with anti-B-cell monoclonal antibody therapy. In all 3 cases, EBV was present in Reed-Sternberg cells by EBER analysis. The histologic subtypes of Hodgkin's disease were not reported.

Two cases of Hodgkin's disease were associated with cadaveric renal transplantation [98]. One report discusses a stage IIB nodular sclerosing Hodgkin's disease presenting 5 years prior to renal transplantation; the transplant was performed 4 years following complete remission. There was no recurrence of Hodgkin's disease at 15 months following transplantation, in keeping with previous reports of 8 patients who underwent renal transplantation after complete remission of Hodgkin's disease [101]. The second patient presented with stage IA mixed cellularity Hodgkin's disease 6 years after renal transplantation, and was in complete remission 2 years following diagnosis and treatment [98].

The report of a case of stage IIB nodular sclerosing Hodgkin's disease following allogeneic BMT for chronic myelogenous leukemia brings the total number to 3 [100]. In this instance, the patient presented with Hodgkin's disease 8 years following BMT; Reed-Sternberg cells were positive for EBV. The diagnosis of Hodgkin's disease coincided with reappearance of the *bcr-abl* transcript by PCR analysis. It is unclear whether this reappearance plays a significant role in the emergence of Hodgkin's disease, but it may be related to Hodgkin's disease-associated immunosuppression. The patient was undergoing combination chemotherapy at the time of reporting, with disappearance of the *bcr-abl* transcript. The intervals between BMT and presentation of Hodgkin's disease were 2 and 4 years in the previously reported cases, compared to 8 years in this instance. The patient had previously been treated with IFN-α and DLI for reappearance of the *bcr-abl* transcript. While numbers are small and no conclusions can be drawn, these therapeutic measures may have played a role in prolonging the interval between transplantation and presentation of Hodgkin's disease.

These cases bring the total number of reported cases of Hodgkin's disease following renal transplantation to 14, and to 3 following BMT. This makes it difficult to draw conclusions regarding relative incidence, stage and subtype. Hodgkin's disease should be diagnosed with caution in this setting, as many PTLDs are reported to contain Reed-Sternberg-like cells [14].

Risk Factors and Predictors of Prognosis

The increased risk for PTLD in EBV-seronegative transplant recipients is well recognized, and has been reviewed elsewhere [9]. The magnitude of risk is estimated at 23–50%, versus 1–2% in the transplant population as a whole. Many patients who develop PTLD after seroconversion exhibit signs of active EBV infection. As many as 37% of pediatric transplant patients undergo primary EBV infection in the posttransplant period [6]. Thus, as many as 8.5–18.5% of pediatric transplant recipients may be at high risk of developing PTLD.

Other factors which have been reviewed include the intensity and type of immunosuppressive regimen. An increased incidence of PTLD became apparent following the introduction of cyclosporine. This may be related to its anti-T-cell effect, or to a direct mutagenic effect [3]. In children, the incidence of PTLD is 2–4% in patients receiving cyclosporine alone. This risk increases to 10–14% in those receiving the anti-CD3 monoclonal antibody OKT3 as prophylaxis and/or treatment for rejection [6]. The cyclosporine-treated group developed PTLD significantly sooner after transplantation (15 months) than did the group receiving conventional immunosuppression (48 months). This risk has been partially abrogated by routine monitoring of cyclosporine blood levels. Reduction or withdrawal of cyclosporine results in regression of PTLD in up to one third of cases [reviewed in 3]. It remains to be determined whether the risk will increase with newer immunosuppressive medications such as FK-506, mycophenolate mofetil, and new monoclonal antibodies.

Two additional factors that are markers for the degree of immunosuppression have been linked to the development of PTLD in pediatric BMT recipients. Recipients of non-HLA-identical bone marrow transplants were at greater risk for

PTLD than were recipients of HLA-identical grafts (14 vs. 0%, respectively). In addition, T-cell numbers lower than 50/µl at 1 month and 100/µl at 2 months were associated with increased risk (6 of 18 or 33%, p < 0.04; 6 of 21 or 29%, p < 0.1) [102].

The former practice of T-cell depletion of bone marrow grafts in order to reduce the incidence of graft-versus-host disease resulted in an increased incidence of PTLD. Of note, there was no increase in PTLD in patients receiving bone marrow from which B cells were depleted concomitantly. Here, it is presumed that the removal of B cells resulted in decreased EBV viral load. The use of anti-T-cell antibodies in immunosuppression induction poses an additional risk. These antibodies are still commonly used to manage rejection episodes. The presence and magnitude of risk of PTLD under these circumstances may be increased with a cumulative dose of OKT3 > 75 mg, whereas a similar effect with antilymphocyte globulin is not well defined. Also unclear is the relative contribution of various components of maintenance immunosuppression [reviewed in 4].

Risk factors for aggression and outcome appear to include site of involvement of PTLD. PTLD confined to the allograft may correlate to improved survival: in one series of 9 PTLDs involving transplanted kidneys, 3 were confined to the allograft. Two of these resolved with reduced immunosuppression. Of the 6 cases which were more widespread, 4 were fatal and 3 required allograft nephrectomy [82].

Appearance of PTLD in a body fluid portends a poor outcome, because it signals the presence of extensive disease [67]. Of 4 patients in whom PTLD was detected in peritoneal fluid (1 patient), pleural fluid (2) or CSF (1), all died within 3 months of detection.

Time to onset of PTLD may be important in predicting outcome. In a series of 607 heart, lung and combined heart-lung transplantations, mortality of early-onset PTLD was 36% (less than 1 year in 13 patients), whereas that of late onset was 70% (greater than 1 year in 7 patients) [8]. Eighty-nine percent of a group of patients who presented with PTLD within 1 year of transplantation responded to reduced immunosuppression, and mortality was 36%. Conversely, fewer than 10% of those who presented later than 1 year responded to reduced immunosuppression, and their mortality was 70% [4, 8].

Finally, clonality does not correlate to outcome or response to therapy, which underscores the importance of evaluation of clinical behavior in estimating prognosis and making therapeutic decisions [103].

In summary, factors that increase the risk of developing PTLD include EBV seronegativity prior to transplant, immunosuppressive regimen, and in BMT recipients, HLA mismatch and T-cell depletion. In these patients, increased vigilance for PTLD is warranted. Risks for adverse outcome include site and extent of involvement, involvement of the CNS or of body fluids, and time to onset of PTLD. In these patients, increased aggression of therapeutic maneuvers may improve outcome.

Paraproteins in the Identification of Patients at Risk for PTLD

Several groups have attempted to delineate laboratory factors to predict the development of PTLD. These include the detection of serum paraproteins and viral load.

In a retrospective analysis of 86 liver transplant patients, the prevalence of abnormal serum protein detection by immunofixation electrophoresis was 44% [104]. All paraproteins were newly detected following transplantation; the majority within the first year. Thirty percent of patients had a monoclonal Ig peak; half of these were permanent. The appearance of a permanent monoclonal peak was correlated with the occurrence of viral infections including CMV and EBV, suggesting a role for repeated antigenic stimulation in the occurrence of gammopathy. Three of 13 patients with permanent monoclonal Ig developed PTLD and died. This group of patients with permanent monoclonal paraproteins might thus be appropriate for intensive monitoring in an attempt to detect PTLD early. A survival benefit to early detection, however, has yet to be demonstrated.

A second group of liver transplant recipients underwent routine serum protein electrophoresis following transplantation. Twelve of 149 developed monoclonal or oligoclonal peaks at a mean of 5.8 months following transplantation; 6 of these were transient, while 6 were permanent (1.8%). Two of the 6 patients with permanent peaks developed PTLD [105]. By isoelectric focusing, 21 of 327 (6%) recipients of kidney or combined kidney-pancreas transplants developed monoclonal or oligoclonal peaks at 27–125 months following transplantation. Eight of these patients (38%) developed PTLD [106].

Using high-resolution electrophoresis, a high incidence of monoclonal Ig was detected in a group of 84 renal transplant recipients, both prior to (66.6%) and following transplantation (85.5%) [107]. By immunofixation, monoclonal Ig were found in 21.4% of cases. Although patients who developed PTLD were excluded from this study, it appears that the high baseline incidence of paraproteins may reduce the discriminative value of screening for patients at high PTLD risk by this method.

Finally, in a group of 99 patients undergoing kidney or combined kidney-pancreas grafts, monoclonal peaks were detected by immunofixation in 82% of patients, 52% by 6 months following transplantation [108]. Monoclonal Ig were more frequently detected in patients who had experienced episodes of allograft rejection, and in patients with CMV infection. In most cases, 1–3 monoclonal peaks were detected; more than 4 peaks were detected in 2 patients. Both of these patients had B-cell PTLD diagnosed within days of paraprotein detection, a short interval that makes the predictive value of detecting multiple peaks uncertain.

Thus, the utility of screening for paraproteins to identify patients at risk for PTLD differs between studies and remains unproven. The occurrence of monoclonal Ig appears to be higher in patients who subsequently develop PTLD, particularly in the presence of multiple peaks. However, in some studies, a minority (1.8–6%) of patients develop monoclonal paraproteins, necessitating screening of a large population in order to detect the few at increased risk. By more sensitive techniques, paraproteins were detected in the majority, reducing the discriminative value of this approach. Any beneficial effect of screening this population would require testing at regular intervals to allow time for appropriate clinical intervention. The literature does not contain guidelines on the appropriate workup, monitoring or management of patients who evince a monoclonal peak.

Identification of EBV Sequences in Biopsy Specimens

In a series of 4 PTLDs following liver transplantation, 3 were EBV-related. While biopsies at the time of PTLD diagnosis showed numerous cells positive for PTLD, few were positive in biopsies taken up to several months prior to diagnosis. However, EBV-positive cells were identified both in biopsy specimens from patients who did not develop PTLD and from healthy donors with chronic EBV infection [109]. Thus, the utility of this method to predict patients at risk for PTLD was limited.

An earlier series of pediatric liver transplant recipients was analyzed by in situ hybridization of liver biopsy specimens for EBER-1 sequences. EBER-1 positivity was detected in 17 of 24 patients (71%) 2 days to 22 months prior to the onset of PTLD [31]. This was in contrast to the positivity rate of 2 out of 20 (10%) controls. Thus, in this study, this method appeared to have some predictive value for the development of PTLD. However, it is likely to be superseded by analysis of EBV viral load in peripheral blood (see below).

Direct and Indirect Quantification of EBV Viral Load

Several groups have demonstrated that the development of PTLD correlates to an increase in EBV viral load, as detected by PCR amplification of EBV sequences from peripheral blood lymphocytes. Risk of contracting PTLD and extent of disease correlated to EBV copy number, and treatment of PTLD resulted in decreased viral load [19, 45–48]. Thus, determination of EBV viral load appears useful for monitoring patients likely to develop PTLD, and for identifying patients who might benefit from clinical intervention. The hypothesis that early detection leads to improved outcome, however, remains to be confirmed (see 'EBV').

Following BMT, the majority of PTLDs arise in the first 6 months [20]. In a study designed to evaluate cell-mediated immunity to EBV after transplant, CTLp frequencies were quantified by limiting dilution analysis in 26 recipients of marrow grafts from EBV-positive donors [21]. At 3 months, only 5 of 13 patients had CTLp frequencies in the range of normal controls; by 6 months, the number had risen to 9. One patient with low CTLp frequency at 4 months following transplantation developed PTLD, which responded to DLI. Although the frequency of PTLD in this series was low, the period of deficient EBV-specific cell-mediated immunity corresponded to the period of highest frequency of PTLD, which presumably develops via an unchecked proliferation of EBV-infected B-cell clones.

Treatment

Although treatment protocols are under evaluation, no consensus on approach has been reached. In the absence of clear guidelines, therapy is individualized to the clinical situation and type of organ transplant. More cautious reduction in immunosuppression is advisable in transplants of organs vital to maintain life. For example, in renal transplantation, the patient may resume dialysis in the event of allograft loss. For the same reason, there has been hesitation to employ some therapies for certain transplant types. Precipitation of acute vascular graft rejection of renal allografts has been reported in patients who were treated with IFN-α, possibly due to upregulation of cellular expression of HLA antigens [13]. This observation has led to reluctance to use IFN-α for PTLD occurring in the setting of nonrenal organ transplantation.

Evaluation of treatment protocols is hampered when clinical series include inhomogeneous groups of patients: there may be patients presenting with PTLD at variable time intervals following the transplantation, and/or with different types of grafts. Moreover, these grafts may be maintained on variable immunosuppressive regimens. Often, there are variable types and extents of PTLD involvement. Because multiple treatments are often used concomitantly, the impact of a particular treatment type is difficult to discern [13]. A prospective clinical trial with correlative biologic studies, coordinated by the Southwest Oncology Group and the Eastern Cooperative Oncology Group, is currently underway [4].

Treatment options include conventional approaches such as reduction of immunosuppression, surgical resection or radiation therapy for limited disease, antiviral agents and cytotoxic chemotherapy. More recent additions to the therapeutic arsenal include IFN-α with or without intravenous immunoglobulins (ivIg), monoclonal antibodies directed against B-cell determinants, EBV-specific cellular immunotherapy and hematopoietic cell transplantation. Mortality using conventional approaches is usually 40–50% [110]. Long-term outcome with newer approaches remains to be defined.

In this section, treatment of the largest group of PTLDs – namely, those that are NHL in type – is discussed, with the exception of BL and T-cell lymphoma. Treatment of rare forms of PTLD, including BL [90], T-cell lymphoma [91–94], plasmacytoma/myeloma [95–97] and Hodgkin's disease [98–101], is based on a small number of cases and is beyond the scope of this review.

Reduction of Immunosuppression

While a variable proportion of PTLD responds to reduced immunosuppression, there is valid concern about this approach precipitating graft rejection. In a series of pediatric liver transplants, 36 patients developed PTLD. All patients were treated with reduced immunosuppression, with a minority receiving other treatments in addition. Of the 32 survivors, 23 experienced acute graft rejection, whereas 2 developed chronic rejection, an incidence of 70% [111].

The appropriate extent and duration of reduced immunosuppression is not well defined [4]. It has ranged from the discontinuation of all immunosuppression to the discontinuation of azathioprine, while steroids are continued, and cyclosporine or FK-506 is continued in reduced dosage. This variability in approach leads to uncertainty as to the efficacy of reducing immunosuppression in patients with PTLD.

Antiviral Agents

There is no strong evidence that treatment with antiviral agents such as acyclovir alters the course of PTLD. In a trial of BMT recipients, prophylactic acyclovir had no effect on the incidence of subsequent PTLD [12]. As acyclovir targets herpesvirus thymidine kinase, it is specific for replicative infection. Although some investigators suspect a role for reactivation of latent infection in the development of PTLD, this is unproven [112]. However, as acyclovir generally has little toxicity, it is included in many therapeutic protocols on the basis that it may be beneficial, and with little risk of harm to the patient.

Other antivirals have been used on both a prophylactic and therapeutic basis. In 1 case of EBV-positive B-polymorphous hyperplasia following heart and lung transplant, immunosuppression was maintained during PTLD treatment, since there had been a recent rejection episode. The patient was treated with foscarnet for 28 days, with complete regression of PTLD and no recurrence at 8 months [113]. While an interesting result, the classification of this case as hyperplasia implies lack of clonality, and possibly reduced clinical aggression. Thus, the PTLD might have been one that was prone to regression with minimal intervention, and the value of treatment with foscarnet is uncertain.

Pediatric liver transplant patients at high risk for PTLD received preemptive therapy with intravenous ganciclovir for 100 days or more [114]. Eighteen EBV-seronegative patients received a transplant from an EBV-seropositive donor. Viral load was serially monitored by PCR analysis of peripheral blood leukocytes, with reduction in immunosuppression for a rise in viral load. PTLD was treated by discontinuing immunosuppression and reinstituting ganciclovir. Using this approach, 2 patients developed PTLD; both patients had been included in the group of 22 patients considered as low-risk. While promising, the numbers in this series are small. Further studies will be required to determine whether CMV prophylaxis with ganciclovir results in a consistently reduced incidence of PTLD.

It should be noted that there is evidence of transactivation of EBV by CMV infection (see 'EBV'). Thus, of patients who respond to antiviral therapy, it is possible that the effect on EBV-driven lymphoproliferation is indirectly mediated via downregulation of CMV.

Biologic Response Modifiers

IFN-α exhibits growth inhibitory effects on PTLD both in vitro and in a severe combined immunodeficiency mouse model [115]. Its effects on EBV occur via downregulation of EBNA-1, which is involved in controlling replication of the viral episome [116]. Other possible mechanisms of growth inhibition by IFN-α include induction of terminal plasmacytic differentiation, which has been observed in vitro. Cell-mediated cytotoxicity may be induced, and the tumor blood supply may be compromised via induction of vasculitis. IFN-α downregulates cell cycling by influencing several cellular proto-oncogenes and tumor suppressor genes, it promotes apoptosis via an effect on *bcl-2,* upregulates natural killer cell-mediated cytotoxic activity, and upregulates expression of MHC, which may have an effect on cellular antitumor immunity [117, 118].

An early report of the utilization of IFN-α describes a pediatric patient following double lung transplantation who developed PTLD in the graft [39]. The PTLD did not respond to reduction of immunosuppression and antiviral medications, and the patient was treated with daily subcutaneous injections of IFN-α. At 4 weeks, graft function had improved, and IFN-α was tapered over a period of 8 months. The patient remained in remission at 18 months.

The response to therapy in this case was correlated to levels of IL-4 and IL-10. IL-4 is a product of TH2 cells, and stimulates B lymphocytes, including EBV-infected cells. Levels of IL-4 and IL-10 were high in bronchiolar lavage specimens, and declined with therapy. Levels of IL-2 and IFN-γ, both TH1 products, were low. These results suggest that treatment with IFN-α may have resulted in regression of PTLD via an inhibition of TH2 cells, or alteration in the balance between TH2 and TH1 cells, in addition to direct antiviral effects.

A case of monoclonal B-cell PTLD following renal transplantation failed to respond to treatment with reduction of immunosuppression, antiviral therapy, and ivIg. It did regress with IFN-α given 3 times weekly for a period of 3 months, and the patient remained in remission at 1 year [40]. In this report, characteristics of 13 patients treated with IFN-α are summarized, including the 2 patients described above. Ten patients had monoclonal PTLD, and 8 of the PTLDs were positive for EBV. Eight patients achieved complete remission, with partial remission in an additional 2. There were 3 deaths due to progression of PTLD [40].

One report describes 2 patients who developed diffuse large-cell PTLD of B-cell type following heart and liver transplantation [42]. Neither responded to reduced immunosuppression, but both achieved complete remission with a combination of

IFN-α and ivIg. Three and 7 months were required to achieve complete remission, which was durable at 47 and 33 months. Both patients were maintained on low-dose prednisone and cyclosporine, and neither experienced allograft rejection.

In one series, IFN-α was discontinued early in 2 of 16 patients because of rapidly progressive disease and multisystem organ failure. Of 14 patients who received IFN-α for 6–9 months, 8 achieved complete remission; 5 of these 8 died of unrelated causes without evidence of PTLD. Two relapsed with a different PTLD clone [110]. Four patients developed neutropenia responsive to granulocyte colony-stimulating factor, and 4 patients developed rejection, resulting in loss of the kidney-pancreas graft in 1. Seven patients in a series of 25 who developed PTLD following BMT were treated with IFN-α [41]. Mortality in this series was 92% overall, with 2 survivors. Both survivors had been treated with IFN-α.

Thus, treatment with IFN-α results in lasting remission in some patients, including many who did not respond to conservative measures. Toxicity was generally low, although the risk of allograft rejection must be noted. Infusion of ivIg has been used in conjunction with IFN-α for the treatment of PTLD [38, 42]. To our knowledge, there are no data delineating the contribution of ivIg to this regimen. Mechanism of action and the beneficial effect of ivIg in PTLD remain to be defined.

Chemotherapy

Various combination chemotherapeutic regimens have been employed in the treatment of PTLD. Therapy in this setting often has high morbidity due to infectious complications and other considerations. For example, cardiac allografts appear to be particularly sensitive to anthracycline cardiotoxicity, a phenomenon that necessitated the discontinuation of doxorubicin in 57% of patients in one series [119].

In a series of 10 high-grade B-cell PTLDs following liver transplantation, 4 patients received combination chemotherapy with CHOP (cyclophosphamide, adriamycin, vincristine, prednisone) or VAPEC-B (adriamycin, cyclophosphamide, intrathecal methotrexate, vincristine, bleomycin, etoposide, prednisone). Of the 6 patients who did not receive chemotherapy, survival ranged from 9 days to 30 months. The 4 patients who received chemotherapy survived for 4–48 months; 2 out of 4 survived to the time of writing. Side effects of chemotherapy included neutropenic sepsis and reactivation of hepatitis B infection in 1 patient, resulting in acute liver failure and death [120]. In other series, 4 out of 4 patients treated with CHOP achieved complete remission, with survival of 30 months [121]. Five out of 7 patients treated with Pro-MACE-Cyta-BOM (cyclophosphamide, adriamycin, etoposide, prednisone, cytarabine, bleomycin, vincristine, methotrexate, leucovorin) achieved remission, with survival of 42 months [119].

One report describes a patient who developed high-grade B-cell PTLD localized to the larynx 5 years following sibling HLA-identical, T-cell-depleted BMT for chronic myelogenous leukemia. This patient was treated with three cycles of CHOP, resulting in complete regression of the lesion. He remained in complete remission 11 months following chemotherapy [122].

There is a single report of autologous BMT for the treatment of PTLD. An EBV-associated diffuse large-cell lymphoma, localized to the abdomen, developed 88 months following HLA-mismatched renal transplantation. Therapy with CEEP (cyclophosphamide, vindesine, epiadriamycin, prednisolone) and MIME (methotrexate, ifosfamide, mitoxantrone, etoposide) in alternating cycles for four courses was given with complete remission resulting after two courses. The patient received BEAM (BCNU, cytarabine, etoposide, melphalan) conditioning, followed by autologous BMT. Immunosuppression with cyclosporine was resumed at 2 months following BMT [123].

Complete remission rate of PTLD treated with chemotherapy (about two thirds to three quarters) is in approximately the same range as can be expected for NHL. However, there are no large-series reports on long-term outcome. Thus, treatment with combination chemotherapy may not result in improved survival [124]. Because of the ongoing requirement for immunosuppression after organ transplantation, the relapse rate following chemotherapy for PTLD may well be higher than for NHL. This is illustrated by the case of PTLD treated with autologous BMT, in which reintroduction of immunosuppression may have been implicated in subsequent relapse [123].

Adoptive Cellular Immunotherapy

A promising therapeutic approach involves the transfer of cellular immunity from the donor to the transplant recipient. Adoptive immunity has been used for the prevention and treatment of EBV-related PTLD, and is based on the premise that cellular immune responses can be targeted at EBV-infected cells. Cellular immune responses to EBV are diverse, and include the generation of both HLA-restricted and more broadly reactive immunity. Lysis of EBV-infected cells of identical HLA type occurs, but in some cases, lysis of EBV-infected cells of allogeneic type occurs in addition [125]. Adoptive transfer of EBV CTL has been demonstrated to prevent the development of lymphoma and prolong survival in a severe combined immunodeficiency mouse model [126, 127]. More recently, this therapeutic strategy has been extended to human transplant recipients [125].

One consideration in the design of EBV-reactive cell populations is the limited number of antigens processed and presented by particular HLA types. Because of this, many trials incorporate into a therapeutic mix a number of EBV-specific CTL lines. Most studies of adoptively transferred CTL have been conducted in bone marrow transplant recipients. In this setting, PTLD are almost invariably of donor origin, and of malignant monomorphic diffuse large B-cell in type.

In initial studies, unfractionated donor peripheral blood leukocytes were used as a source of cellular immunity directed toward EBV. Although regression of PTLD was observed, DLI was associated with inflammatory responses that resulted in respiratory failure and, in 2 patients, in death [125]. Regression of PTLD has been noted as early as 2–4 weeks following infusion of 0.5–1×10^6 T cells/kg [128].

More recent studies have investigated the use of EBV-specific T-cell lines prepared in vitro. Because lines containing CD8 lymphocytes, although specific for EBV, have shown limited ability to expand in vivo and generate effective immune responses, more recent strategies involve the use of a mixture of CD4 and CD8 lines in order to provide T-cell help for CD8 killing of EBV-infected cells. Donor-derived EBV-transformed lymphoblastoid cell lines are prepared in vitro and cultured in the presence of donor T cells. Thirty-six recipients of T-cell-depleted marrow grafts were treated by this method in an attempt to prevent the development of PTLD. No PTLD was observed in this series, in contrast to the expected incidence of 14%. EBV-specific CTL lines marked with the *neo* gene were detected at up to 2 years following infusion. In patients in whom a rise in viral load was detected by PCR, an increase in the level of *neo*-marked cells followed. Subsequently, a decline in EBV viral load was seen. This implies an expansion of *neo*-marked EBV-specific clones in response to EBV-infected cells, resulting in control of EBV viral load [129, 130]. These results are confirmed in more recent series [131]. Thus, infusion of EBV-specific CTL lines appears to effectively prevent an exuberant expansion of EBV-infected clones, and possibly the development of PTLD.

Two patients with PTLD were treated by this method; both achieved complete remission. One patient experienced an inflammatory response accompanied by tissue edema. On histologic examination, *neo*-marked cells were detected, suggesting selective homing of EBV-specific CTL to the site of PTLD [129].

A drawback to this technique is the time required for preparation of cell lines. Three to 4 weeks are required to prepare lymphoblastoid lines used for antigen presentation, and an additional 3–4 weeks for expansion of CTL. Thus, this method is impractical for patients in whom PTLD is rapidly progressive [129]. The labor involved in preparing lines for all patients in anticipation of PTLD could well be prohibitive, although the cost is on the order of that involved for prophylaxis of other viral infections in this population. Preparation time may be shortened by utilizing cultures of dendritic cells for antigen presentation, which can be prepared in 3–4 days.

Although only a low incidence of graft-versus-host disease (GVHD) was seen in this trial, it remains a concern. Several groups have attempted to overcome this complication by transduction into CTL lines of a suicide gene. In the event of severe GVHD, the CTL could be selectively destroyed by exposure to an agent which activates the suicide gene. An alternative method to minimize the risk of GVHD involves cell culture techniques which result in loss of alloreactive T cells over time [125]. The production of specific T-cell lines opens the possibility of treating host-derived PTLD in recipients of solid-organ transplants by the expansion of host-derived CTL ex vivo.

By culturing cells in IL-2-rich medium, autologous lymphocyte-activated killer (LAK) cells reactive against a high-grade monoclonal PTLD in a renal transplant recipient were produced ex vivo. Reinfusion of LAK induced resolution of PTLD within 5 months, with no recurrence at 13 months. There was no GVHD, and no effect on allograft function. As is the case for DLI, it has been suggested that LAKs are effective only in EBV-positive tumors [132].

Anti-B-Cell Antibodies

A promising development in the therapy of B-cell PTLD is the use of mono-clonal antibodies directed against B-cell surface markers. These are used in an attempt to restore immune balance by decreasing tumor burden. Antibodies direct-ed to the cell surface markers CD21, CD24 and CD37 have resulted in clinical improvement in several reported cases, although these tended to be oligoclonal PTLD, and no effect was seen in PTLD involving the CNS [13]. Complete remis-sions were rare; however, survival may be improved, at least in the short term. In a series of 28 patients with PTLD, there were 10 survivors. Eight of these 10 patients had received anti-B-cell antibody therapy with monoclonals directed toward CD21 or CD24 [54], which are no longer available. Other antibodies directed against B cells are currently being tested for this and other applications, such as those with specificity for the cell surface marker CD20 (see below).

A series of 58 patients with B-cell PTLD following bone marrow or solid-organ transplantation were treated with anti-CD21 or anti-CD24 antibodies daily for 10 days. Complete remission was achieved in 36 of 59 (61%) cases of PTLD [133]. Median time to complete remission was 15 days. Relapse was seen in 3 patients, and overall survival rate was 46% at a median of 61 months of follow-up. Survival was not as good in BMT recipients; 35% as compared to 55% for recipients of solid organs, and no bone marrow transplantee survived beyond 1 year. Risk factors for poor response, in addition to BMT, included multiorgan involvement, late onset and CNS disease. Side effects of therapy included fever, chills and neutropenia.

One group describes chimeric antibodies incorporating two human Fc regions, which interact with effector cells of the immune system, into a complex with one murine Fab, or antigen-directed region, for reasons of stability. Two such constructs were linked, incorporating Fab regions of separate specificity, and resulting in improved antibody-dependent cellular cytotoxicity and cell-mediated toxicity in vitro. Four patients were treated with weekly or biweekly infusions of such an anti-body construct for a period of 1–4 weeks. This resulted in complete remission of monotypic diffuse large-cell PTLD in 3 patients, durable for 14–15 months [134].

An immunoblastic monoclonal PTLD localized to a renal graft was treated with decreased immunosuppression, surgical debulking, and monoclonal antibody thera-py. Infusions of anti-CD37 and steroids were given monthly for 3 months, and resulted in disappearance of PTLD by day 100 [135].

Results of antibody therapy in PTLD involving the CNS are poor. One patient presented with CNS symptoms 6 months following renal transplantation. Two large lesions within the CNS proved to be immunoblastic PTLD. The patient was treated with three weekly intrathecal injections of anti-CD21 monoclonal antibody, with initial dramatic clinical improvement and 75% reduction in tumor mass. However, relapse occurred 3 months later. A second course of intrathecal anti-CD21 was ineffective, and despite chemotherapy and radiation therapy, the patient died [136]. CNS disease occurs in 14–20% of B-cell PTLDs; the use of anti-B-cell monoclonal antibodies in this setting may be limited.

A recent report describes the use of Rituximab [137], a humanized murine monoclonal antibody with specificity for CD20, in the treatment of PTLD. In this series, 32 patients were treated with 2–8 infusions of 375 mg/m^2 with or without reduction in immunosuppression. Complete remission was attained in 54%, including 5 of 6 bone marrow graft recipients. Partial remission was attained in an additional 5%, and 81% of patients were alive at a median of 5 months of follow-up. Therapy was tolerated well [138]. There have been no reported episodes of graft failure with monoclonal antibody therapy.

Thus, while follow-up is short in the study of patients treated with anti-CD20, remission appeared to be induced in a significant proportion of patients. Even if late relapses should occur, this therapy may well buy time needed to implement further workup and treatment options that would not otherwise be feasible.

Standardized Approach to Therapy

Two groups have described a standardized approach to the treatment of PTLD. In one series, using therapy targeted to the individual, complete remission was achieved in 16 of 26 patients with no relapses at 3–21 months of follow-up [139]. A standardized stepwise therapeutic approach designed by the same group is to be evaluated in a multicenter open phase II trial [139]. A second report describes a 'quintuple approach' used in a series of 6 patients. This consisted of reduced immunosuppression, antivirals, IFN-α, ivIg, and anti-CD19 monoclonal antibodies. Five PTLDs were monoclonal, and 4 out of 6 patients received all treatments. All attained complete remission, which was maintained at 9–62 months. Two patients did not receive IFN-α out of concern for possible graft loss; however, one lost the graft regardless. The 6th patient relapsed after 4 months of complete remission, was treated with CHOP chemotherapy, and was alive at 17 months [140].

In one series, a sequential approach to therapy was employed. It consisted of reduced immunosuppression in conjunction with surgical resection or radiation therapy, followed by a trial of IFN-α, followed by combination chemotherapy as needed. Seven patients received chemotherapy, of whom 5 achieved complete remission. One patient died of uncontrolled PTLD; however, there were a number of deaths from sepsis and other causes [110]. Overall, 9 patients were alive and disease-free at the time of writing, and 10 had died. Thus, while providing rational guidelines to therapy, this approach resulted in survival rates (47%) similar to those seen using previous individualized approaches.

Summary and Recommendations

Current knowledge regarding the biology of, and therapeutic approach to, PTLD is based largely on case reports and small case series, with few clinical trials. The incidence of PTLD varies according to type of organ transplanted and immunosuppressive regimen. Several systems classify PTLD on the basis of histology and cellular and viral clonality. For the most part, however, this classification has failed to predict clinical aggression and outcome, and further clinical-pathological correlations in large series are warranted.

Clinical risk factors for PTLD include EBV seronegativity prior to transplant, and coinfection with CMV, which possibly acts through transactivation of EBV. Laboratory predictors of the emergence of PTLD include detection of serum paraproteins, and more recently and convincingly, evaluation of viral load in the peripheral blood.

Therapy of PTLD using conventional approaches has resulted in suboptimal response rates, high rates of graft rejection, and dismal long-term survival. New and promising approaches to therapy include biologic response modifiers, adoptive transfer of cytotoxic T lymphocytes and cell lines, and antibodies directed against B-cell determinants. The optimal use and long-term outcome of these therapies remain to be defined. Indications for each therapy will likely become increasingly refined over the next several years, and will probably be determined in conjunction with improved methods of clinical and molecular surveillance for PTLD.

Large prospective trials which correlate histology, clonality, cellular genetic changes, viral load and clinical aggression to remission rate, relapse rate and long-term outcome are warranted in order to elucidate predictors of outcome and optimal therapeutic strategies. This type of trial is currently being coordinated by the Southwest Oncology Group and the Eastern Cooperative Oncology Group, and by a European group [4, 139].

As much clinical and molecular information as possible should be collected for each case of PTLD. This includes histologic evaluation of tissue from excisional biopsy material, determination of cellular and viral clonality, preferably by molecular techniques, and evaluation of further cytogenetic and molecular changes. Demographic information should be gathered, EBV and CMV serologic status documented, and EBV viral load should be followed if possible. Clinical EBV and CMV infection should be monitored and documented. Staging and site of disease should be documented, as should degree of HLA match, and immunosuppressive

Table 2. Therapeutic options in PTLD

Therapy	Time to response	Response rate	Early mortality	Long-term outcome	References
Decreased immunosuppression	3–6 weeks	0–80%	30–60%	10–30% OS	Reviewed in 4, 13
Antiviral agents[1]	ND	ND	None	ND	Reviewed in 4, 13
Surgical resection[2]	Immediate	100%		ND	
Radiation therapy[2]	Days to weeks	100%		ND	
Interferon-α +/- ivIg[3]	3–20 weeks	52%	7%	33% CR>1 year	39–41, 109
Anti-B-cell monoclonal antibodies[4]	1–2 weeks	59%	None	46% OS at 5 years	132, 133
Adoptive cellular therapy[5]	2–4 weeks	Close to 100%	None	ND	128, 131
Chemotherapy[6]	1 week	85%	15%	30–42 months MS	119–122

OS = Overall survival; MS = median survival; CR = complete remission; ND = not determined.

[1] Antiviral agents are used in conjunction with decreased immunosuppression, and independent effect is impossible to delineate.

[2] Reported for use in limited disease; may also be used for local control.

[3] Based on a total of 27 patients.

[4] Based on a total of 96 patients.

[5] Based on a total of 38 patients.

[6] Based on a total of 13 patients.

regimen. Complete remission rate, relapse rate and long-term outcome should be reported. Patients should be entered on cooperative prospective protocols wherever feasible.

Table 2 summarizes the therapeutic approaches available, expected time to response, and expected long-term outcome. In the absence of firm clinical-pathological correlation, a therapeutic approach such as that summarized in figure 2 is recommended. This approach considers transplant type and the potential conse-

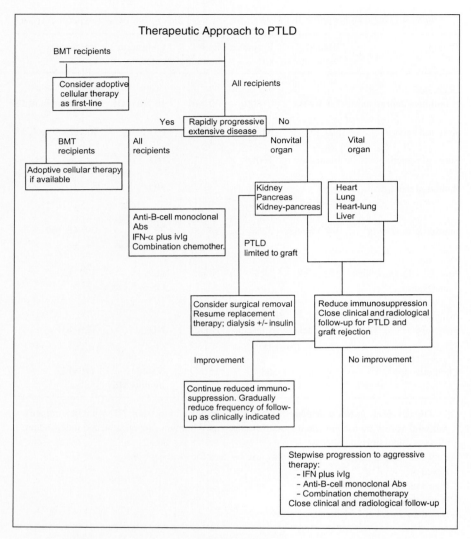

Therapeutic Approach to PTLD

BMT recipients

All recipients

Consider adoptive cellular therapy as first-line

Yes — Rapidly progressive extensive disease — No

BMT recipients

All recipients

Nonvital organ

Vital organ

Adoptive cellular therapy if available

Anti-B-cell monoclonal Abs
IFN-α plus ivIg
Combination chemother.

Kidney
Pancreas
Kidney-pancreas

Heart
Lung
Heart-lung
Liver

PTLD limited to graft

Consider surgical removal
Resume replacement therapy; dialysis +/- insulin

Reduce immunosuppression
Close clinical and radiological follow-up for PTLD and graft rejection

Improvement

No improvement

Continue reduced immunosuppression. Gradually reduce frequency of follow-up as clinically indicated

Stepwise progression to aggressive therapy:
– IFN plus ivIg
– Anti-B-cell monoclonal Abs
– Combination chemotherapy
Close clinical and radiological follow-up

Fig. 2. Therapeutic approach to PTLD. Some BMT recipients may respond to conservative measures, but cellular therapy should be considered as first-line therapy where feasible. This is particularly important in the case of rapidly progressive or extensive disease, which has high mortality. In more slowly progressive disease, a trial of conservative measures may be warranted, such as reduction of immunosuppression and treatment with antiviral agents. If conservative measures do not succeed, a stepwise trial of more aggressive measures is warranted. The consequences of rejection of the transplanted organ must be considered. Measures which might precipitate rejection of a graft essential for survival should be reserved for failure of other measures. It should be noted that the clinical rapidity of PTLD progression is highly variable; the extent and frequency of restaging and repeat biopsy must be tailored to the clinical situation.

quences of allograft loss. Treatment is determined largely on the basis of clinical aggression: more aggressive strategies with higher potential morbidity are used early for patients with PTLD at a high risk of imminent mortality.

Future attempts at ameliorating the effect of PTLD may focus on prevention. Preventive strategies include the use of more specific and reduced immunosuppression, use of monoclonal antibody therapy or DLI to decrease viral load, or may involve immunization of seronegative patients against EBV. An attempt at avoiding introduction of organs or blood products from EBV-seropositive donors into EBV-seronegative recipients should be considered. When this is not possible, special attention should be paid to CMV sero-status. While no good vaccine for EBV is currently available, several approaches are under development. These are largely aimed at preventing or limiting the extent of primary infection by induction of neutralizing antibodies, which would be of possible benefit to seronegative transplant recipients if immunization at an appropriate time interval prior to transplantation was feasible. Malignancy associated with viral latency, including PTLD, might be more likely to benefit from the delivery of epitopes such as the viral structural proteins gp350 and gp85 [141] in order to stimulate cell-mediated immunity. As many viral epitopes are HLA-restricted, the delivery of either epitopes tailored to the individual's HLA type, or of a mixture of multiple epitopes, may be necessary [142]. Finally, therapy directed at blocking the action of latency-associated genes is under study in vitro [13]. These strategies, while promising, are unlikely to be available for clinical use in the near future [143].

Summary

Posttransplant lymphoproliferative disorder (PTLD), or lymphoid malignancy following organ transplantation, has occurred with increasing frequency in recent years. The majority of PTLD are non-Hodgkin's lymphomas, and many are associated with Epstein-Barr virus (EBV) infection. PTLD comprises a spectrum of cellular and viral clonality, and a spectrum of clinical aggression. Treatment has ranged from reduction of immunosuppression to combination chemotherapy. More recently, cellular, cytokine-mediated, and antibody-mediated immunomodulatory approaches have been undertaken. This review summarizes current data regarding classification of PTLD, the role of EBV in pathogenesis and delineation of clonality, prognostic factors, classical and innovative treatment approaches, and the implementation of standardized treatment strategies.

References

1 McKhann CF: Primary malignancy in patients undergoing immunosuppression for renal transplantation. Transplantation 1969;8:209–212.

2 Penn I, Hammond W, Brettschneider L, Starzl TE: Malignant lymphomas in transplantation patients. Transplant Proc 1969;1:106–112.

3 Penn I: The changing pattern of posttransplant malignancies. Transplant Proc 1991;23: 1101–1103.

4 Swinnen LJ: Treatment of organ transplant-related lymphoma. Hematol Oncol Clin North Am 1997;11:963–973.

5 Ambinder RF: Human lymphotropic viruses associated with lymphoid malignancy: Epstein-Barr and HTLV-1. Hematol Oncol Clin North Am 1990;4:821–833.

6 Dunn SF, Krueger LJ: Immunosuppression of pediatric liver transplant recipients: Minimizing the risk of posttransplant lymphoproliferative disorders. Transplant Immunol Lett 1998;14:4–6, 10–11.

7 Minello-Franza A, Berjamy F, Bresson-Hadni S, Angonin R, Becker MC, Mantion G, Miguiet JP: Lymphoproliferative disorders in four orthotopic liver transplant patients. Transplant Proc 1995;27:1770–1773.

8 Armitage JM, Kormos RL, Stuart RS, Fricker FJ, Griffith BP, Nalesnik M, Hardesty RL, Dummer JS: Posttransplant lymphoproliferative disease in thoracic organ transplant patients: Ten years of cyclosporine-based immunosuppression. J Heart Lung Transplant 1991;10: 877–887.

9 Dharnidharka VR, Tejani A: Immunosuppression of pediatric kidney transplant recipients: Minimizing the risk of posttransplant lymphoproliferative disorder. Transplant Immunol Lett 1998;14:3, 7, 12.

10 Opelz G, Henderson R: Incidence of non-Hodgkin's lymphoma in kidney and heart transplant recipients. Lancet 1993;342:1514–1516.

11 Tsai DE, Porter DL, Schuster SJ, Tomaszewski JE, Montone KT, Luger S, Loh EY, Stadtmauer EA: Posttransplant lymphoproliferative disorder after organ transplantation: Long-term follow-up of 69 cases observed at a single center. Blood 1998;92(suppl 1):624A.

12 Savage P, Waxman J: Post-transplantation lymphoproliferative disease. Q J Med 1997;90: 497–503.

13 Basgoz N, Preiksaitis JK: Post-transplant lymphoproliferative disorder. Infect Dis Clin North Am 1995;9:901–923.

14 Harris NL, Ferry JA, Swerdlow SH: Posttransplant lymphoproliferative disorders: Summary of society for hematopathology workshop. Semin Diagn Pathol 1997;14:8–14.

15 Nalesnik MA, Jaffe R, Starzl TE, Demetris AJ, Porter K, Burnham JA, Makowka L, Ho M, Locker J: The pathology of posttransplant lymphoproliferative disorders occurring in the setting of cyclosporine A-prednisone immunosuppression. Am J Pathol 1988;133:173–192.

16 Knowles DM, Cesarman E, Chadburn A, Frizzera G, Chen J, Rose EA, Michler RE: Correlative morphologic and molecular genetic analysis demonstrates three distinct categories of posttransplantation lymphoproliferative disorders. Blood 1995;85:552–565.

17 Rickinson AB, Kieff E: Epstein-Barr virus; in Fields BN, Knipe DM (eds): Fields Virology, ed 3. Philadelphia, Lippincott-Raven, 1996, vol 2, pp 2397–2466.

18 Hanto DW, Sakamoto K, Purtilo DT, Simmons RI, Najarian JS: The Epstein-Barr virus in the pathogenesis of posttransplant lymphoproliferative disorders. Surgery 1981;90:204.

19 Riddler SA, Breinig MC, McKnight JLC: Increased levels of circulating Epstein-Barr Virus (EBV)-infected lymphocytes and decreased EBV nuclear antigen antibody responses are associated with the development of posttransplant lymphoproliferative disease in solid-organ transplant recipients. Blood 1994;84:972–984.

20 Zutter MM, Marin PJ, Sale GE, Shulman HM, Fisher L, Thomas ED, Durnam DM: Epstein-Barr virus lymphoproliferation after bone marrow transplantation. Blood 1998;72:520–529.

21 Lucas KG, Small TN, Heller G, Dupont B, O'Reilley RJ: The development of cellular immunity to Epstein-Barr virus after allogeneic bone marrow transplantation. Blood 1996;87: 2594–2603.

22 Walker RC, Marshall WF, Strickler JG, Wiesner RH, Velosa JA, Habermann TM, McGregor CG, Paya CV: Pretransplantation assessment of the risk of lymphoproliferative disorder. Clin Infect Dis 1995;20:1346–1353.

23 Manez R, Breinig MC, Linden P, Wilson J, Torre-Cisneros J, Kusne S, Dummer S, Ho M: Posttransplant lymphoproliferative disease in primary Epstein-Barr virus infection after liver transplantation: The role of cytomegalovirus disease. J Infect Dis 1997;176:1462–1467.

24 Kahan BD: Posttransplant lymphoproliferative disorder: The dark side of immunosuppression. Transplant Immunol Lett 1998;14:1.

25 Delecluse HJ, Rouault JP, French M, Dureau G, Magaud JP, Berger F: Post-transplant lymphoproliferative disorders with genetic abnormalities commonly found in malignant tumours. Br J Haematol 1995;89:90–97.

26 Klein G: Epstein-Barr virus strategy in normal and neoplastic B cells. Cell 1994;77:791–793.

27 Crawford DH, Sweny P, Edwards JM, Janossy G, Hoffbrand AV: Long-term T-cell-mediated immunity to Epstein-Barr virus in renal-allograft recipients receiving cyclosporin A. Lancet 1981;i:10–12.

28 Gaston JS, Rickinson AB, Epstein MA: Epstein-Barr-virus-specific T-cell memory in renal-allograft recipients under long-term immunosuppression. Lancet 1982;i:923–925.

29 Raab-Traub N, Flynn K: The structure of the termini of the Epstein-Barr virus as a marker of clonal cellular proliferation. Cell 1986;47:883–889.

30 Yates JL, Warren N, Sugden B: Stable replication of plasmids derived from Epstein-Barr virus in various mammalian cells. Nature 1985;313:812–815.

31 Randhawa PS, Jaffe R, Demetris AJ, Nalesnik M, Starzl TE, Chen YY, Weiss LM: Expression of Epstein-Barr virus-encoded small RNA (by the EBER-1 gene) in liver specimens from transplant recipients with post-transplantation lymphoproliferative disease. N Engl J Med 1992;327:1710–1714.

32 Liebowitz D: Epstein-Barr virus and a cellular signaling pathway in lymphomas from immunosuppressed patients. N Engl J Med 1998;338:1413–1421.

33 Lyons SF, Liebowitz DN: The roles of human viruses in the pathogenesis of lymphoma. Semin Oncol 1998;25:461–475.

34 Levitskaya J, Coram M, Levitsky V, Imreh S, Steigerwald-Mullen PM, Klein G, Kurilla MG, Masucci MG: Inhibition of antigen processing by the internal repeat region of the Epstein-Barr virus nuclear antigen-1. Nature 1995;375:685–688.

35 Wang D, Liebowitz D, Kieff E: An EBV membrane protein expressed in immortalized lymphocytes transforms established rodent cells. Cell 1985;43:831–840.

36 Kieff E: Epstein-Barr virus and its replication; in Fields BN, Knipe DM, Howley PM (eds): Fields Virology, ed 3. Philadelphia, Lippincott-Raven, 1996, vol 2, pp 2343–2396.

37 Lausoontornsiri W, Dizon EF, Liebowitz DN: Evolution of EBV-related post-transplantation lymphoproliferative disease. Blood 1998;92(suppl 1):315A.

38   Shapiro R, Chauvenet A, McGuire W, Pearson A, Craft AW, McGlave P, Filipovich A: Treatment of B-cell lymphoproliferative disorders with interferon-α and intravenous-γ globulin. N Engl J Med 1988;318:1334.

39   Faro A, Kurland G, Michaels MG, Dickman PS, Greally PG, Spichty KJ, Noyes BB, Boas SR, Fricker FJ, Armitage JM, Zeevi A: Interferon-α affects the immune response in post-transplant lymphoproliferative disorder. Am J Respir Crit Care Med 1996;153: 1442–1447.

40   O'Brien S, Bernert RA, Logan JL, Lien YHH: Remission of posttransplant lymphoproliferative disorder after interferon-α therapy. J Am Soc Nephrol 1997;8:1484–1489.

41   Cantarovich M, Barkun JS, Clarke Forbes RD, Kosiuk JP, Tchervenkov JI: Successful treatment of post-transplant lymphoproliferative disorder with interferon-α and intravenous immunoglobulin. Clin Transplant 1998;12:108–115.

42   Gross TG, Steinbuch M, DeFor T, Shapiro RS, McGlave P, Ramsay NKC, Wagner JE, Filipovich AH: B cell lymphoproliferative disorders following hematopoietic stem cell transplantation: Risk factors, treatment and outcome. Bone Marrow Transplant 1999;23:251–258.

43   Wood A, Angus B, Kestevan P, Dark J, Notarianni G, Miller S, Howard M, Proctor S, Middleton P: Alpha interferon gene deletions in post-transplant lymphoma. Br J Haematol 1997;98:1002–1003.

44   Birkeland SA, Hamilton-Dutoit S, Sandvej K, Andersen HMK, Bendtzen K, Moller B, Jorgensen KA: EBV-induced post-transplant lymphoproliferative disorder. Transplant Proc 1995;27:3467–3472.

45   Swinnen LJ, Gulley ML, Hamilton E, Schichman SA. EBV DNA quantitation in serum is highly correlated with the development and regression of post-transplant lymphoproliferative disorder in solid organ transplant recipients. Blood 1998;92(suppl 1):314A.

46   George D, Barnett L, Boulad F, Childs B, Castro-Malaspina H, Jakubowski A, Kernan NA, Papadopoulos E, Small TN, Szaboics P, Young J, Koulova L, O'Reilley RJ: Semi-quantitative PCR analysis of genomic EBV DNA post-BMT allows close surveillance of patients at risk for development of EBV-lymphoproliferative disorders allowing prompt intervention. Blood 1998;92(suppl 1):437A.

47   Green M, Cacciarelli TV, Mazariegos GV, Sigurdsson L, Qu L, Rowe DT, Reyes J: Serial measurement of Epstein-Barr viral load in peripheral blood in pediatric liver transplant recipients during treatment for posttransplant lymphoproliferative disease. Transplantation 1998; 66:1641–1644.

48   Crompton CH, Cheung RK, Donjon C, Miyazaki I, Feinmesser R, Hebert D, Dosch HM: Epstein-Barr virus surveillance after renal transplantation. Transplantation 1994;57: 1182–1189.

49   Alfieri C, Tanner J, Carpentier L, Perpete C, Savoie A, Paradis K, Delage G, Joncas J: Epstein-Barr virus transmission from a blood donor to an organ transplant recipient with recovery of the same virus strain from the recipient's blood and oropharynx. Blood 1996;87: 812–817.

50   Borisch B, Gatter KC, Tobler A, Theilkas L, Bunch C, Wainscoat JS, Fey MF: Epstein-Barr virus-associated anaplastic large cell lymphoma in renal transplant patients. Am J Clin Pathol 1992;98:312.

51   Frank D, Cesarman E, Liu YF, Michler RE, Knowles DM: Posttransplantation lymphoproliferative disorders frequently contain type A and not type B Epstein-Barr virus. Blood 1995;85: 1396–1403.

52   Sculley TB, Apollini A, Hurren L, Moss DE, Cooper DA: Coinfection with A- and B-type Epstein-Barr virus in human immunodeficiency virus-positive subjects. J Infect Dis 1990; 162:643.

53   Leblond V, Davi F, Charlotte F, Dorent R, Bitker MO, Sutton L, Gandjbakhch I, Binte JL, Raphael M: Posttransplant lymphoproliferative disorders not associated with Epstein-Barr virus: A distinct entity? J Clin Oncol 1998;16:2052–2059.

54   Leblond V, Sutton L, Dorent R, Davi F, Bitker MO, Gabarre J, Charlotte F, Ghoussoub JJ, Fourcad C, Fischer A, Gandjbakhch I, Binet JL, Raphael M: Lymphoproliferative disorders after organ transplantation: A report of 24 cases observed in a single center. J Clin Oncol 1995;13:961–968.

55   Wiesner RH, Marin E, Porayko M, Steers JL, Krom RA, Paya CV: Advances in the diagnosis, treatment and prevention of cytomegalovirus infections after liver transplantation. Gastroenterol Clin North Am 1993;22:351.

56   Chetty F, Biddolph S, Kaklamanis L, Cary N, Stewart S, Giatromanolaki A, Gatter K: Bcl-2 protein is strongly expressed in post-transplant lymphoproliferative disorders. J Pathol 1996; 180:254–258.

57   Tanner J, Tosato G: Impairment of natural killer functions by interleukin-6 increases lymphoblastoid cell tumorigenicity in athymic mice. J Clin Invest 1991;88:239–247.

58   Tosato G, Jones K, Breinig JK, McWilliams HP, McKnight JLC: Interleukin-6 production in posttransplant lymphoproliferative disease. J Clin Invest 1993;91:2806–2814.

59   Ye BH, Cattoretti G, Shen Q, Zhang J, Hawe N, de Waard R, Leung C, Nouri-Shirazi M, Orazi A, Chaganti RSK, Rothman P, Stall AM, Pandolfi PP, Dalla-Favera R: The BCL-6 proto-oncogene controls germinal-centre formation and Th2-type inflammation. Nat Genet 1997;16:161.

60   Cesarman E, Chadburn A, Liu UF, Migliazza A, Dalla-Faver R, Knowles DM: BCL-6 gene mutations in posttransplantation lymphoproliferative disorders predict response to therapy and clinical outcome. Blood 1998;92:2294–2302.

61   Mathur A, Kamat DM, Filipovich AH, Steinbuch M, Shapiro S: Immunoregulatory abnormalities in patients with Epstein-Barr virus-associated lymphoproliferative disorders. Transplantation 1994;57:1042–1045.

62   Swerdlow SH: Classification of the posttransplant lymphoproliferative disorders: From the past to the present. Semin Diagn Pathol 1997;14:2–7.

63   Cleary ML, Nalesnik MA, Shearer WT, Sklar J: Clonal analysis of transplant-associated lymphoproliferations based on the structure of the genomic termini of the Epstein-Barr virus. Blood 1998;72:349.

64   Shearer WR, Ritz J, Finegold MJ, Guerra IC, Rosenblatt HM, Lewis DE, Pollack MS, Taber LH, Sumaya CV, Grumet FC, Cleary ML, Warnke R, Sklar J: Epstein-Barr virus-associated B-cell proliferations of diverse clonal origins after bone marrow transplantation in a 12-year-old patient with severe combined immunodeficiency. N Engl J Med 1985;312: 1151.

65   Cleary ML, Sklar J: Lymphoproliferative disorders in cardiac transplant recipients are multiclonal lymphomas. Lancet 1984;ii:489–493.

66   Nelson BP, Locker J, Nalesnik MA, Fung JJ, Swerdlow SH: Clonal and morphological variation in a posttransplant lymphoproliferative disorder: Evolution from clonal T-cell to clonal B-cell predominance. Hum Pathol 1998;29:416–421.

67   Dusenbery D, Nalesnik MA, Locker J, Swerdlow SH: Cytologic features of post-transplant lymphoproliferative disorder. Diagn Cytopathol 1997;16:489–496.

68 Goral S, Felgar R, Shappell S: Posttransplantation lymphoproliferative disorder in a renal allograft recipient. Am J Kidney Dis 1997;30:301–307.

69 Drachenberg CB, Abruzzo LV, Klassen DK, Bartlett ST, Johnson LB, Kuo PC, Kumar D, Papadimitriou JC: Epstein-Barr virus-related posttransplantation lymphoproliferative disorder involving pancreas allografts: Histological differential diagnosis from acute allograft rejection. Hum Pathol 1998;29:569–577.

70 Haque T, Thomas JA, Falk KI, Parratt R, Hunt BJ, Yacoub M, Crawford DH: Transmission of donor Epstein-Barr virus (EBV) in transplanted organs causes lymphoproliferative disease in EBV-seronegative recipients. J Gen Virol 1996;77:1169–1172.

71 Mentzer SJ, Longtine J, Fingeroth J, Reilly JJ, DeCamp MM, O'Donnell W, Swanson SJ, Faller DV, Sugargaker DJ: Immunoblastic lymphoma of donor origin in the allograft after lung transplantation. Transplantation 1996;61:1720–1725.

72 Strazzabosco M, Corneo B, Iemmolo RM, Menin C, Gerunda G, Bonaldi L, Merenda R, Neri D, Poletti A, Montagna M, Del Mistro A, Faccioli AM, D'Andrea E: Epstein-Barr virus-associated post-transplant lympho-proliferative disease of donor origin in liver transplant recipients. J Hepatol 1997;26:926–934.

73 Lones MA, Lopez-Terrada D, Weiss LM, Shintaku IP, Said JW: Donor origin of posttransplant lymphoproliferative disorder localized to a liver allograft: Demonstration by fluorescence in situ hybridization. Arch Pathol Lab Med 1997;12:701–706.

74 Spiro IJ, Yandell DW, Li C, Saini S, Ferry J, Powelson J, Katkov WN, Cosimi AB: Brief report: Lymphoma of donor origin occurring in the porta hepatis of a transplanted liver. N Engl J Med 1993;329:27–29.

75 Le Frere-Belda MA, Martin N, Gaular P, Zafrani ES: Donor or recipient origin of post-transplantation lymphoproliferative disorders: Evaluation by in situ hybridization. Mod Pathol 1997;10:701–707.

76 Cheung ANY, Chan ACL, Chung LP, Chan TM, Cheng IKP, Chan KW: Post-transplantation lymphoproliferative disorder of donor origin in a sex-mismatched renal allograft as proven by chromosome in situ hybridization. Mod Pathol 1998;11:99–102.

77 Jones C, Bleau B, Buskard N, Magil A, Yeung K, Shackleton C, Cameron E, Erb S, Gascoyne R, Keown P: Simultaneous development of diffuse immunoblastic lymphoma in recipients of renal transplants from a single cadaver donor: Transmission of Epstein-Barr virus and triggering by OKT3. Am J Kidney Dis 1994;23:130–134.

78 Larson RS, Scott MA, McCurley TL, Vnencak-Jones CL: Microsatellite analysis of post-transplant lymphoproliferative disorders: Determination of donor/recipient origin and identification of putative lymphomagenic mechanism. Cancer Res 1996;56:4378–4381.

79 Weissmann DJ, Ferry JA, Harris NL, Louis DN, Delmonico F, Spiro I: Posttransplantation lymphoproliferative disorders in solid organ recipients are predominantly aggressive tumors of host origin. Hematopathology 1994;103:748–755.

80 Nagler A, Ilan Y, Amiel A, Eid A, Tur-Kaspa R: Systemic chimerism in sex-mismatched liver transplant recipients detected by fluorescence in situ hybridization. Transplantation 1994;57:1458–1461.

81 Hruban RH, Long PP, Perlman EJ, Hutchins GM, Baumgartner WA, Baughman KL, Griffin CA: Fluorescence in situ hybridization for the Y chromosome can be used to detect cells of recipient origin in allografted hearts following cardiac transplantation. Am J Pathol 1993;142:975–980.

82 Randhawa PS, Magnone M, Jordan M, Shapiro R, Demetris AJ, Nalesnik M: Renal allograft involvement by Epstein-Barr virus associated post-transplant lymphoproliferative disease. Am J Surg Pathol 1996;20:563–571.

83   Nalesnik MA: Posttransplant lymphoproliferative disease of donor origin. Arch Pathol Lab Med 1997;121:665–666.

84   Schouten HC, Hopman AHN, Haesevoets AM, Arends JW: Large-cell anaplastic non-Hodgkin's lymphoma originating in donor cells after allogenic bone marrow transplantation. Br J Haematol 1995;91:162–166.

85   Micallef INM, Chhanabhai M, Gascoyne RD, Shepherd JD, Fung HC, Nantel SH, Toze CL, Klingemann HG, Sutherland HJ, Hogge DE, Nevill TJ, Le A, Barnett MJ: Lymphoproliferative disorders following allogeneic bone marrow transplantation: The Vancouver experience. Bone Marrow Transplant 1998;22:981–987.

86   Hauke RJ, Greiner TC, Smir BN, Vose JM, Tarantolo SR, Bashir RM, Bierman PJ: Epstein-Barr virus-associated lymphoproliferative disorder after autologous bone marrow transplantation: Report of two cases. Bone Marrow Transplant 1998;21:1271–1274.

87   Shepherd JD, Gascoyne RD, Barnett MJ, Coghlan JD, Phillips GL: Polyclonal Epstein-Barr virus-associated lymphoproliferative disorder following autografting for chronic myeloid leukemia. Bone Marrow Transplant 1995;15:639–641.

88   Briz M, Fores R, Regidor C, Busto MJ, Ramon Y, Cajal S, Cabrera R, Diez JL, Sanjuan I, Fernandez MN: Epstein-Barr virus associated B-cell lymphoma after autologous bone marrow transplantation for T-cell acute lymphoblastic leukaemia. Br J Haematol 1997;98:485–487.

89   Spina M, Tirelli U, Zagonel V, Gloghini A, Volpe R, Babare R, Abbruzzese L, Talamini R, Vaccher E, Carbone A: Burkitt's lymphoma in adults with and without human immunodeficiency virus infection: A single-institution clinicopathologic study of 75 patients. Cancer 1998;82:766–774.

90   Hunt BJ, Thomas JA, Burke M, Walder H, Yacoub M, Crawford DH: Epstein-Barr virus associated Burkitt lymphoma in a heart transplant recipient. Transplantation 1996;62:869–872.

91   Van Gorp J, Doornewaard H, Verdonck LF, Klopping C, Vos PF, van den Tweel JG: Posttransplant T-cell lymphoma: Report of three cases and a review of the literature. Cancer 1994;73:3064–3072.

92   Grosso LE, Bee CS: T-cell rich Ki-1-positive post-transplant lymphoproliferative disorder: A previously undescribed variant following liver transplant. Pathology 1998;31:360–363.

93   Dockrell DH, Strickler JG, Paya CV: Epstein-Barr virus-induced T cell lymphoma in solid organ transplant recipients. Clin Infect Dis 1997;180–182.

94   Rostaing L, Tkaczuk J, Rigal-Huguet F, Lloveras JJ, Durand D: T-cell γδ lymphoproliferative disorders after renal transplantation. Transplant Proc 1995;27:1774–1775.

95   Schemankewitz E, Hammami A, Stahl R, Henderson JM, Check IJ: Multiple extramedullary plasmacytomas following orthotopic liver transplantation in a patient on cyclosporine therapy. Transplantation 1993;49:1019–1022.

96   Chucrallah AE, Crow MK, Rice LE, Rajagopalan S, Hudnall SD: Multiple myeloma after cardiac transplantation: An unusual form of posttransplant lymphoproliferative disorder. Hum Pathol 1994;25:541–545.

97   Fischer T, Miller M, Bott-Silverman C, Lichtin A: Posttransplant lymphoproliferative disease after cardiac transplantation. Transplantation 1996;62:1687–1690.

98   Bedrossian J, Metivier F, Jaccard A, Binet I, Pruna A, Idatte JM: Hodgkin's disease and cadaveric renal transplantation. Transplant Proc 1995;27:1783–1784.

99   Garnier JL, Lebranchu Y, Lefrancois N, Martin X, Dubernard JM, Berger F, Touraine JL: Hodgkin's disease after renal transplantation. Transplant Proc 1995;27:1785.

100 Meignin V, Devergie A, Brice P, Brison O, Parquet N, Ribaud P, Cojean I, Gaulard P, Gluckman E, Socie G, Janin A: Hodgkin's disease of donor origin after allogeneic bone marrow transplantation for myelogeneous chronic leukemia. Transplantation 1998;65:595–597.

101 Penn I: The effect of immunosuppression on pre-existing cancers. Transplantation 1993;55:742–747.

102 Gerritsen EJA, Stam ED, Hermans J, van den Berg H, Haraldsson A, van Tol MJD, Langlois van den Bergh R, Waaijer JLM, Kroes ACM, Kluin PM, Vossen JM: Risk factors for developing EBV-related B cell lymphoproliferative disorders after non-HLA-identical BMT in children. Bone Marrow Transplant 1996;18:377–382.

103 Cockfield SM, Preiksaitis JK, Jewell LD, Parfrey NA: Post-transplant lymphoproliferative disorder in renal allograft recipients. Transplantation 1993;56:88–96.

104 Pageaux GP, Bonnardet A, Picot MC, Perrigault PF, Coste V, Navarro F, Fabre JM, Domergue J, Descomps B, Blanc P, Michel H, Larrey D: Prevalence of monoclonal immunoglobulins after liver transplantation. Transplantation 1998;65:397–400.

105 Pham H, Lemoine A, Sol O, Azoulay D, Royer P, Samuel D, Charpentier C, Bismuth H, Debuire B: Monoclonal and oligoclonal gammopathies in liver transplant recipients. Transplantation 1994;58:253–257.

106 Touraine JL, Yafi SE, Bosi E, Chapuis-Cellier C, Ritter J, Blanc N, Dubernard JM, Pouteil-Noble C, Chevalier M, Creyssal R, Traeger J: Immunoglobulin abnormalities and infectious lymphoproliferative syndrome in cyclosporine-treated transplant patients. Transplant Proc 1983;15(suppl 1):2798–2804.

107 Touchard G, Pasdeloup T, Parpeix J, Hauet T, Bauwens M, Dumont G, Aucouturier P, Preud'homme JL: High prevalence and usual persistence of serum monoclonal immunoglobulins evidenced by sensitive methods in renal transplant recipients. Nephrol Dial Transplant 1997;12:1199–1203.

108 Bernardi M, La Rocca E, Castoldi R, Di Carlo V, Caldara R, Furiani S, Giudici D, Pozza G, Secchi A: Mono-oligoclonal immunoglobulin abnormalities in diabetic patients after kidney transplantation: Influence of simultaneous pancreas graft. Diabetologia 1998;41:1176–1179.

109 Niedobitek G, Mutimer DJ, Williams A, Whitehead L, Wilson P, Rooney N, Young LS, Hubscher SG: Epstein-Barr virus infection and malignant lymphomas in liver transplant recipients. Int J Cancer 1997;73:514–520.

110 Davis CL, Wood BL, Sabath DE, Joseph JS, Stehman-Breen C, Broudy VC: Interferon-α treatment of posttransplant lymphoproliferative disorder in recipients of solid organ transplants. Transplantation 1998;66:1770–1779.

111 Cacciarelli TV, Green M, Jaffe R, Mazariegos GV, Jain A, Fung JJ, Reyes J: Management of posttransplant lymphoproliferative disease in pediatric liver transplant recipients receiving primary tacrolimus (FK-506) therapy. Transplantation 1998;66:1047–1052.

112 Rea D, Fourcade C, Leblond V, Rowe M, Joab I, Edelman L, Bitker MO, Gandjbakhch I, Suberbielle C, Farcet JP: Patterns of EBV latent and replicative gene expression in EBV B-cell lymphoproliferative disorders after organ transplantation. Transplantation 1994;58:317–324.

113 Oertel S, Ruhnke M, Anagnostopolous I, Kahl A, Frewer A, Bechstein WO, Hummel M, Huhn D, Riess H: Treatment of Epstein-Barr virus-induced post-transplantation lymphoproliferative disorder with foscarnet alone in an adult after simultaneous heart and renal transplantation. Blood 1998;92(suppl 1):239B.

114 McDiarmid SV, Jordan S, Lee GS, Toyoda M, Goss JA, Vargas JH, Martin MG, Bahar R, Maxfield AL, Ament ME, Busutte RW: Prevention and preemptive therapy of posttransplant lymphoproliferative disease in pediatric liver recipients. Transplantation 1998;66:1604–1611.

115 Randhawa PS, Whiteside TL, Zeevi A, Elder EM, Rao AS, Demetris AJ, Weng X, Valdivia LA, Rakela J, Nalesnik MA: Effects of immunotherapy on experimental immunodeficiency-related lymphoproliferative disease. Transplantation 1998;65:264–268.

116 Clarke PA, Sharp NA, Arrand JR, Clemens MJ: Epstein-Barr virus gene expression in interferon-treated cells: Implications for the regulation of protein synthesis and the antiviral state. Biochim Biophys Acta 1990;172:1729.

117 Clemens M: Interferons and oncogenes. Nature 1985;313:531.

118 Kimchi A: Cytokine triggered molecular pathways that control cell arrest. J Cell Biochem 1992;50:1.

119 Swinnen LJ, Mullen GM, Carr TJ, Costanzo MR, Fisher RI: Aggressive treatment for postcardiac transplant lymphoproliferation. Blood 1995;86:3333–3340.

120 McCarthy M, Ramage J, McNair A, Gane E, Protmann B, Pagliuca A, Rela M, Heaton N, Mufti GJ, Williams R: The clinical diversity and role of chemotherapy in lymphoproliferative disorder in liver transplant recipients. J Hepatol 1997;27:1015–1021.

121 Garrett TJ, Chadburn A, Barr ML, Drusin RE, Chen JM, Schulman LL, Smith CR, Reison DS, Rose EA, Michler RE: Posttransplantation lymphoproliferative disorders treated with cyclophosphamide-doxorubicin-vincristine-prednisone chemotherapy. Cancer 1993;72:2782–2785.

122 O'Riordan JM, Molloy K, O'Briain DS, Corbally N, Devaney D, McShane D, Considine N, McCann SR: Localized, late-onset, high-grade lymphoma following bone marrow transplantation: Response to combination chemotherapy. Br J Haematol 1994;86:183–186.

123 Mahe B, Moreau P, Le Tortorec S, Hourmant M, Harousseau JL, Milpied N: Autologous bone marrow transplantation for cyclosporin-related lymphoma in a renal transplant patient. Bone Marrow Transplant 1994;14:645–646.

124 Cohen JI: Epstein-Barr virus lymphoproliferative disease associated with acquired immunodeficiency. Medicine 1991;70:137–160.

125 O'Reilly RJ, Small TN, Papadoupolos E, Lucas K, Lacerda J, Koulova L: Biology and adoptive cell therapy of Epstein-Barr virus-associated lymphoproliferative disorders in recipients of marrow allografts. Immunol Rev 1997;157:195–216.

126 Boyle TJ, Berend KR, DiMaio JM, Coles RE, Via DF, Lyerly HK: Adoptive transfer of cytotoxic T lymphocytes for the treatment of transplant-associated lymphoma. Surgery 1993;114:218–226.

127 DiMaio JM, Van Trigt P, Gaynor JW, Davis RD, Coveney E, Clary BM, Lyerly HK: Generation of tumor-specific T lymphocytes for the treatment of posttransplant lymphoma. Circulation 1995;92(suppl II):202–205.

128 Papadopoulos EB, Ladanyi M, Emanuel D, Mackinnon S, Boulad F, Carabasi MH, Castro-Malaspina H, Childs BH, Gillio AP, Small TN, Young JW, Kernan NA, O'Reilley RJ: Infusions of donor leukocytes as treatment of Epstein-Barr virus associated lymphoproliferative disorders complicating allogeneic marrow transplantation. N Engl J Med 1994;330:1185.

129 Heslop HE, Rooney CM: Adoptive cellular immunotherapy for EBV lymphoproliferative diseases. Immunol Rev 1997;157:217–222.

130 Rooney CM, Smith CA, Ng CYC, Loftin SK, Sixbey JW, Gan Y, Srivastava DK, Bowman LC, Krance RA, Brenner MK, Heslop HE: Infusion of cytotoxic T cells for the prevention and treatment of Epstein-Barr virus-induced lymphoma in allogeneic transplant recipients. Blood 1998;92:1549–1555.

131 Gustafsson A, Levitsky V, Zou J, Winiarski J, Frisan T, Ljungman P, Dalianis T, Ringden O, Ernberg I, Masucci JG: Adoptive transfer of Epstein-Barr virus specific cytotoxic T-cells to

patients at risk for posttransplant lymphoproliferative disease reduces the EBV DNA load in peripheral blood lymphocytes. Blood 1998;92(suppl 1):653A.

132 Li PKT, Tsang K, Phil M, Szeto CC, Wong TYH, To KF, Leung CB, Lui SF, Yu S, Lai FMM: Effective treatment of high-grade lymphoproliferative disorder after renal transplantation using autologous lymphocyte activated killer cell therapy. Am J Kidney Dis 1998;32: 813–819.

133 Benkerrou M, Jais JP, Leblond V, Durandy A, Sutton L, Bordigoni P, Garnier JL, Bidois JL, Le Deist F, Blanch S, Fischer A: Anti-B-cell monoclonal antibody treatment of severe post-transplant B-lymphoproliferative disorder: Prognostic factors and long-term outcome. Blood 1998;92:3137–3147.

134 Glotz D, Antoine C, Garnier JL, Anderson VA, Leong WS, Worth AT, Stevenson GT: Preliminary observations on the treatment of post-transplant lymphomas by multi-Fc chimeric antibodies. Tumor Target 1998;3:46–54.

135 Antoine C, Garnier JL, Duboust A, Bariety J, Stevenson G, Glotz D: Successful treatment of posttransplant lymphoproliferative disorder with renal graft preservation by monoclonal antibody therapy. Transplant Proc 1996;28:2825–2826.

136 Ben Hmida M, Mhiri C, Mnif J, Hachicha J, Kchaou MS, Riffle G, Binet JL, Jacobs C, Jarraya A: Primary brain lymphoma in a renal transplant patient: Unsuccessful intrathecal treatment with anti-B cell monoclonal antibodies (anti-CD21). Transplant Proc 1995; 27:1779–1780.

137 Reff ME, Carner K, Chambers KS, Chinn PC, Leonar JE, Raab R, Newman RA, Hanna N, Anderson DR: Depletion of B cells in vivo by a chimeric mouse human monoclonal antibody to CD20. Blood 1994;83:435–445.

138 Milpied N, Antoine C, Garnier JL, Parquet N, Vasseur B, Bouscary D, Carret AS, Faye A, Quartier P, Bourbigot B, Bourquard P, Hurault de Ligny B, Reguerre Y, Stoppa AM, Dubief F, Mathieu-Boue A, Leblond V: Humanized anti-CD20 monoclonal antibody (Rituximab) in B posttransplant lymphoproliferative disorders: A retrospective analysis of 32 patients. Ann Oncol 1999;10(suppl 3):5.

139 Oertel S, Krause D, Ruhnke M, Hummel M, Jonas S, Anagnostopoulos I, Huhn D, Riess H: A standardized approach for treatment of post-transplantation lymphoproliferative disorders after solid organ transplantation – A proposal. Blood 1998;92(suppl 1):239B.

140 Schaar CG, van Hoek B, van den Pyl JW, Veenendaal RE, de Fijter JW, Kluin PM, van Krieken JHJM, Hekman A, Terpstra WE, Lugtenburg PJ, Willemze R, Kluin-Nelemans JC: Successful outcome with a 'quintuple approach' of post-transplant lymphoproliferative disorder. Blood 1998;92(suppl 1):623A.

141 Khanna R, Sherritt M, Burrows SR: EBV structural antigens, gp350 and gp85, as targets for ex vivo virus-specific CTL during acute infectious mononucleosis: Potential use of gp350/gp85 CTL epitopes for vaccine design. J Immunol 1999;162:3063–3069.

142 Thomson SA, Sherritt MA, Medveczky J, Elliott SL, Moss DJ, Fernando GJP, Brown LE, Suhrbier A: Delivery of multiple CD8 cytotoxic T cell epitopes by DNA vaccination. J Immunol 1998;160:1717–1723.

143 Moss DJ, Suhrbier A, Elliott SL: Candidate vaccines for Epstein-Barr virus. BMJ 1998; 317:423–424.

M. Cantarovich, MD, Associate Professor of Medicine, Department of Medicine, Division of Transplantation, McGill University Health Center, 687 Pine Avenue West, Room C-682, Montreal, Quebec H3A 1A1 (Canada)
E-mail Marcelo.Cantarovich@MUHC.McGill.ca

Rüther U, Nunnensiek C, Schmoll H-J (eds): Secondary Neoplasias following Chemotherapy, Radiotherapy, and Immunosuppression. Contrib Oncol. Basel, Karger, 2000, vol 55, pp 347–362

Cytoprotection as a New Supportive Strategy in the Treatment of Solid Tumors

Jens Büntzel[a], Michael Glatzel[b], Dietmar Fröhlich[b], Klaus Küttner[a]

[a]Department of ORL, Head and Neck Surgery, and
[b]Department of Radiotherapy, Central Clinic Südthüringen, Suhl, Germany

Introduction

Radiotherapy and cytostatic treatment can induce various toxicities which may (1) be dose-limiting, and thus prognostically relevant, and (2) influence the quality of life of cancer patients. These two facts reflect the major problems of supportive care in cancer. For in addition to the basic antineoplastic therapy, the oncologist must deal with symptoms which affect patient comfort and treatment compliance. Whereas supportive care may be defined as interventional, the cytoprotective approach is prophylactic. Called cytoprotection, it seeks to protect normal tissue from therapeutic side effects – without decreasing antineoplastic efficacy [1]. Literature today discusses a number of such substances, and table 1 summarizes the current cytoprotective drugs that will be discussed in this article.

The concept of cytoprotection first came into being with the use of citrovorum factor (CV) or leucovorin (LV) as a cytoprotectant in conjunction with methotrexate (MTX). MTX blocks the dihydrofolate reductase enzyme, which is essential for the production of tetrahydrofolate and other types of reduced folates. Tetrahydrofolate and the cofactors are key to the transfer of carbon units in many biochemical reactions, such as in the conversion of deoxyuridylate to thymidylate in DNA synthesis. CV bypasses this block effectively by supplying tetrahydrofolate [2].

The murine leukemia experiments performed by Goldin et al. [3] showed increased survival times in animals receiving aminopterin (FA – folate antagonist) in conjunction with delayed administration of LV, compared to those treated with FA alone. The original clinical rescue concept was developed when Djerassi et al. [4] and Hryniuk and Bertino [5] used massive doses of MTX followed by LV to treat

Table 1. Potential cytoprotective agents and the toxic substances they target

Cytoprotectant	Target toxic substance	References
Glutathione	Platinum derivatives	6–9
Misoprostol	Radiotherapy (mucosa)	1, 10, 11
Amifostine	Platinum derivatives, radiotherapy	6, 12–14
Dexrazoxane	Anthracyclines (cardiotoxicity)	6, 15, 16
Selenium	Radiotherapy	17, 18
Mesna	Cyclophosphamide, ifosfamide	2, 19–21

human leukemia. In addition to this particular rescue approach, a series of further cytoprotective agents has been developed during the past few decades. Their pharmacology, preclinical data and clinical experience gained in their use are also described in this paper.

Selected Cytoprotective Agents

Amifostine

Therapy of cancer with irradiation or antineoplastic drugs involves a compromise between maximizing tumor eradication and minimizing normal tissue damage. This is why agents with sulfhydryl compounds, which have been shown to protect healthy tissue from these cytotoxic therapies and thus permit the delivery of higher doses of irradiation or cytotoxins, increase the therapeutic index and/or efficacy of multimodal treatment. Amifostine (WR-2721), a cytoprotective agent, was first developed as a radioprotective agent by the US Army to prevent damage from exposure to irradiation. It was found to protect a broad spectrum of normal tissues, and was subsequently investigated as a chemoprotective agent for toxicities induced by cisplatin, cyclophosphamide and other cytotoxic drugs.

Amifostine is a phosphorylated aminothiol prodrug activated by a membrane-bound alkaline phosphatase to its active form, WR-1065. WR-1065 acts as (1) a scavenger for active oxygen radicals; (2) a complex former for platinum derivatives, and (3) a donor of H atoms deployable in DNA repair [22]. Amifostine is not orally active. Once administered intravenously, it is rapidly cleared from the plasma compartment (clearance of 2.17 liters/min). It has a brief distribution half-life of about 0.9 min when administered as a bolus or as a brief intravenous infusion of about 15 min [23]. Amifostine thus has a low potential for drug interactions, as > 90% of amifostine is eliminated from plasma within 10 min. This cytoprotectant does not appear to undergo appreciable protein binding in patients, and is distributed to several tissues in experiments with rats and mice. Since pH values differ between normal and tumor tissue, so does the activity of membrane-bound alkaline phosphatase biodistribution. For this reason, experiments have been able to portray the logarithmic ratio of amifostine's activity in normal to tumor tissue (ratio 100:1) [24, 25].

In vitro studies indicate that adding amifostine to different cell lines treated by cisplatinum [26], paclitaxel [27] or cyclophosphamide derivatives [28] reduces the toxicity of these agents. In cells from leukemia patients, normal progenitor and stem cell recoveries were significantly increased by preincubation with amifostine before addition of perfosfamide or mafosfamide [29]. Amifostine and WR-1065 demonstrated protection against doxorubicin-, daunorubicin- and mitoxantron-induced damage, and enhanced intracellular glutathione levels in cardiomyocytes of rats in vitro [30].

The cytoprotective activity of amifostine has been reproduced in animal models. Dose-modifying factors of between 1.5 (carmustine) and 4.6 (chlormethine) were achieved for bone marrow protection in mice pretreated with amifostine prior to administration of carmustine, chlormethine, cisplatinum, cyclophosphamide, fluorouracil or melphalan [31, 32]. Additionally, greater doses of antineoplastic agents were administrable before severe toxicity occurred. Amifostine also reduced carboplatin-induced myelotoxicity when given at intervals from 30 min prior to 30 min after carboplatin administration. Protection was greatest when the cytoprotectant was injected 5 min before carboplatin [33]. Amifostine has also reduced cisplatin-induced nephrotoxicity in rats [34, 35]. Greater protection of the kidney was achieved against repetitive smaller doses of cisplatin than against a single dose [36]. In addition, the intestinal epithelium of mice given melphalan was also protected by amifostine [37], whereas amifostine was unable to reduce the intestinal side effects of fluorouracil [32].

The radioprotective properties of amifostine were also investigated in several in vitro experiments, in which the usual dose of 200–400 mg/kg amifostine was injected intraperitoneally to mice. In most of the studies, irradiation was derived from γ- (^{60}Co, ^{137}Cs), x-ray or neutron emissions, although an electron beam or β-irradiation was also used in a few investigations. Protection factors were calculated to quantify the degree of radioprotection (table 2) [22].

The cytoprotective potential of amifostine has been investigated in a number of clinical studies. One multinational, multicenter controlled clinical trial enrolled 242 patients with advanced (stages III and/or IV) ovarian cancer following staging and debulking surgery [38]. The women were randomized to receive either cyclophosphamide (1,000 mg/m^2) and cisplatin (100 mg/m^2) alone (120 women, control group), or a short-term 15-min infusion of 910 mg/m^2 of amifostine prior to the same two doses of cyclophosphamide and cisplatin (122 women; verum group). All of the women received appropriate antiemetics, intravenous hydration and mannitol

Table 2. Amifostine's factors of protection against radiation-induced toxicities for various normal mouse tissues (adapted from Spencer et al. [22])

Tissue	Amifostine dose, mg/kg	Protection factor
Bone marrow	200	1.8
Lung	400	1.2
Kidney	400	1.33
Parotid gland	400	1.9
Esophagus	400	1.21
Jejunum	200	1.21
Colon	400	1.4
Rectum	400	1.3
Spermatogonia	400	1.31
Vascular tissue	400	1.6
Skin	200	1.24
Hair follicles	400	1.33
Stroma	400	1.53

before receiving any of these drugs. Treatment was administered every 3 weeks for a total of 6 cycles. Toxicity of bone marrow was manifested as a nadir lowering of the neutrophile count to $< 500/mm^3$ (grade 4 neutropenia) which was associated with fever and/or signs of infection requiring hospitalization and treatment with broad-spectrum antibiotics. There was a cumulative increase in the frequency of such neutropenic events in the control group. Pretreatment with amifostine, however, reduced the episodes of neutropenic events by 55%. In the women pretreated with amifostine, the need for hospitalization and the number of days that the women required broad-spectrum antibiotics was reduced by 60%.

In addition, treatment with cisplatin is normally limited by its cumulative toxicity to the kidneys, peripheral nervous system and hearing. Pretreatment with amifostine significantly reduced these toxic effects that otherwise usually mean that basic treatment has to be stopped. Furthermore, the cumulative damage to the kidneys from repetitive doses of cisplatin – as evaluated by changes in the calculated creatinine clearance following the last cycle of treatment vs. baseline values – was reduced by 66% in the group treated with amifostine as compared to the controls. Amifostine pretreatment also significantly reduced cumulative neurotoxicity. At the same time, the antitumor impact of the chemotherapeutic regimen targeting the ovarian cancer was fully preserved, as was assessed by pathologic response rates (second-look surgery) and survival. This underscores the selective cytoprotective feature of amifostine.

Additional trials have tested whether amifostine's cytoprotective effect on normal organs enables patients to tolerate larger doses of cisplatin [39]. It was discovered that, following a 15-min infusion of amifostine (910 mg/m^2), patients with metastatic non-small-cell lung cancer (stage IV) were able to tolerate a larger dose of cisplatin (120 mg/m^2) administered every 4 weeks. These patients also received a weekly dose of vinblastine. Renal function, as assessed by calculated creatinine clearance, remained stable throughout 5 cycles of therapy. The overall response rate was 64% (25 patients), with a median survival time of 17 months, and 65% of these patients were alive at 1 year. These encouraging findings are undergoing tests in a multicenter, multinational randomized clinical trial.

Comparative effects of WR-2721 vs. G-CSF [40] were studied in patients with advanced non-small-cell lung cancer treated with high-dose carboplatin (AUC-9). Here, G-CSF and amifostine were found equipotent at preventing severe neutropenia (grade 3/4). In patients receiving G-CSF, grade 3/4 thrombocytopenia occurred in 2/9 and 5/9. All 7 of these patients required carboplatin dose reductions, and 3 of the 4 patients with grade 4 thrombocytopenia required platelet transfusions. In the 10 patients of the amifostine group, there were no patients with grade 3/4 thrombocytopenia. Amifostine protection of the megakaryocytic series was significantly superior to that of the controls.

Amifostine was originally developed as a radioprotector. A randomized trial conducted with patients with advanced, inoperable, nonresectable rectal cancer showed that pretreatment with amifostine significantly reduced the frequency of delayed radiation-induced toxicities to pelvic organs. Even so, the acute toxicity of pelvic irradiation could not be influenced by the cytoprotective agent [41].

Late and acute radiation-induced toxicities to oral mucosa and salivary glands in patients with head and neck cancer have been significantly ameliorated by amifostine. In a small randomized trial [42] for patients with advanced head and neck cancer who were treated with carboplatin and irradiation +/– amifostine, there was a significant reduction of dose-limiting grade 3/4 mucositis and thrombocytopenia. While 12 of the 14 patients of the control group developed severe side effects, no such adverse effects were observed among the 25 patients of the amifostine group.

In another phase I/II trial [43], patients with head and neck cancer were pretreated with 100–200 mg/m^2 per day of amifostine prior to each fractional dose of radiation. Nine to 12 months after radiation, stimulated parotid flow regenerated to > 60% of pretreatment values, although historical controls had predicted that these patients would normally achieve flow rates no better than 20% of baseline. These data are confirmed in a preliminary report of a recently finished multinational phase III trial [44]. Patients with head and neck cancer treated with curative radiation therapy and in whom 75% of both parotid glands were in the radiation field, were randomized to receive either radiotherapy or a 3-min injection of 200 mg/m^2 of amifostine 15–30 min before each daily fraction of 180–200 cGy of radiation. Both groups were administered a total dose of 63–70 Gy. The incidence of grade 2 xerostomia was significantly reduced in the amifostine-treated patients (p = 0.0004): incidence was 50% (n = 113) in the amifostine group vs. 77% (n = 121) in the patients given only radiation. Moreover, the median cumulative radiation dose at onset time of grade 2 xerostomia was significantly higher in the amifostine-treated patients than in those treated with radiation alone: 60 vs. 42 Gy (p = 0.0001). At the 12-month follow-up there was no difference in antitumor efficacy; 80% of patients in both groups showed no evidence of disease.

In the same vein, a recently published report on a phase II trial [45] shows that amifostine premedication can reduce the severe toxicities of radioiodine treatment for patients with thyroid cancer.

In summary, amifostine is the first broad-spectrum cytoprotective agent. It protects multiple organs from various cytotoxic drugs and radiation, while the antitumor effect of these cytotoxic agents is fully preserved [46].

Mesna

Mesna (sodium 2-mercaptoethanesulfonate) is a thiol compound that functions as a regional detoxifier of urotoxic ifosfamide metabolites such as acrolein, 4-hydroxyifosfamide, and chloroacetaldehyde. Once in the circulation, mesna is oxidized – by ethylenediaminetetra-acetic acid(EDTA)-inhibitable constituents – to dimesna, which is excreted by the kidneys [47]. 30–50% of the glomerularly excreted dimesna is then reduced in renal tubular epithelium by the glutathione reductase system. The free sulfhydryl groups of mesna resulting can interact directly with the double bond of acrolein, or with other toxic oxazaphosphorine metabolites in the bladder to form other stable and nontoxic compounds [48, 49].

Mesna is highly soluble in water and does not penetrate other tissues. It is readily excreted by the kidneys, so that it is concentrated in close apposition to the urothelium. The rapid urinary excretion of mesna leads to a real reduction of plasma concentration. Because of its high urothelial concentration, mesna is able to detoxify ifosfamide regionally in the urinary tract. What is more, neither the nonurinary toxic effects of ifosfamide nor, more importantly, its systemic antineoplastic effects are attenuated by the low levels of mesna in plasma [50, 51]. Because of its short half-life, the number of mesna administrations must be adapted to the half-life of the toxic alkylating agents.

Mesna can be administered intravenously or orally. Following administration of mesna tablets, bioavailability is 50–70%. The concentration of mesna in the urinary system is approximately half of that observed after intravenous administration, suggesting that the oral dose should be twice that of the usual intravenous dose. Peak mesna concentrations are seen 1–4 h after oral mesna application. Urinary excretion of the drug is nearly complete 4 h after intravenous injection, but continues up to 8 h after oral uptake. This is due to its delayed absorption by the gastrointestinal tract [50, 51].

Mesna is recommended as a uroprotector against the toxicities of ifosfamide and cyclophosphamide. In their review, Siu and Moore [50] described at least three randomized trials comparing the efficacy of mesna and/or placebo / no treatment for ifosfamide-induced urotoxicity [52–54]. In a placebo-controlled phase III trial, a significant reduction in micturition pain and in the sensation of residual urine was observed in the mesna group, as was a reduced incidence of moderate and severe hematuria. The (intravenous) dose of mesna administered was the equivalent of 60% of the ifosfamide dose divided into three parts daily.

Mesna's efficacy in reducing hemorrhagic cystitis – as the main toxic effect of high-dose cyclophosphamide – has recently been reviewed by Haselberger and Schwinghammer [55]. Even so, it has not yet been conclusively demonstrated to be superior to intravenous hyperhydration and/or bladder irrigation. However, mesna plus hyperhydration may soon become the standard in preventing cyclophosphamide-induced hemorrhagic cystitis.

Adverse effects are uncommon with mesna, although oral administration may be associated with gastrointestinal problems. Nausea and vomiting are most likely secondary to the unpleasant taste of oral mesna, which should be masked with juice or carbonated beverages. Adverse effects are generally even less pronounced with intravenous doses of mesna. There have been reports of diarrhea; abdominal pain; headache, limb and joint pain, and cardiac dysregulation, but these symptoms occurred with doses of 60 mg/kg or more given as a single bolus. Very rare allergic reactions have been described under mesna. In these cases, the patients responded to glucocorticoid therapy.

Dexrazoxane

The use of anthracyclines is significantly limited by their cardiac toxicity, which occurs in < 2% of patients given a cumulative dose of < 450 mg/m^2. If this dose is increased to > 600 mg/m^2, the risk of cardiotoxicity rises to 20–40%. Children react more cardiosensitively to anthracycline therapy than adults, although toxicity may not become apparent until years after cessation of therapy [56].

Cardiotoxicity principally occurs as a result of oxidative stress placed on myocytes by highly reactive oxygen species which are generated by the stable complex formed between iron and anthracyclines [57–59]. Consequently, the properties of free radical scavengers and metal-chelating agents have been investigated in the attempt to reduce cardiotoxicity of anthracyclines [59, 60].

Dexrazoxane is a cyclic derivative of edetic acid (EDTA), and provides cardiac protection from anthracyclines primarily through its metal-chelating activity. Its hydrolytic derivative has been shown to chelate both free and intracellular iron – including iron that is bound in anthracycline complexes – thereby preventing the generation of reactive oxygen species. It is these hydrolytic products which are probably responsible for most of the cardioprotective activity of dexrazoxane [61, 62].

The cardioprotective activity of the drug has been demonstrated in several animal models of anthracycline-induced cardiotoxicity. Here, its administration was associated with a significant reduction of cardiac lesions and with increased survival after toxic doses of anthracyclines. Dexrazoxane is most effective when given prior to, or simultaneously with, the cytostatic agent, as shown in experiments with beagles and rats. Delayed administration of dexrazoxane, however, seems to reduce its cytoprotective abilities [63, 64].

Human pharmacological studies with cancer patients have shown that the pharmacokinetics of dexrazoxane fit a two-compartment model with first-order elimination kinetics [65]. Absorption is linear with the dose ranging from 60 to 900 mg/m^2. After a 15-min i.v. infusion of dexrazoxane, the mean peak plasma concentration is 36.5 mg/l. Distribution half-life is 15 min, and the steady-state volume of distribution has been calculated to be about 1.1 liters/kg. The protein-binding part accounts for < 2% [56, 66]. Dexrazoxane is changed to its active form – the ring-opened hydrolytic derivative – by the dihydropyrimidine amidohydrolase enzyme (DHPase). Unchanged dexrazoxane has been detected in patients' urine, as have a diacid-diamide cleavage product and two monoacid-monoamide ring products. Total body clearance is about 0.29 liter/h/kg, primarily renally, and with an elimination half-life of 2–4 h [56, 67].

No pharmacokinetic data are available for patients with renal or hepatic impairment. A comparative pharmacological study investigated the differences between child and adult patients, and found that the steady-state volume of distribution was higher in younger patients, as was the total body clearance rate. Pharmacological characteristics of doxorubicin generally remain unchanged if it is administered 15–30 min after dexrazoxane. However, the properties of epirubicin can be altered by dexrazoxane doses of about >100 mg/m^2 [68, 69].

Clinical trials have shown that dexrazoxane can significantly reduce the incidence of cardiotoxicity in patients receiving anthracyclines for advanced breast cancer. Cardiac events indicative of cardiotoxicity include reduction in the resting left ventricular ejection fraction (LVEF) to < 45%, or a > 20% reduction compared to baseline; congestive heart failure (CHF), and/or a > 2-point increase in the Billingham biopsy score. In these studies, dosage ratio of dexrazoxane to doxorubicin was 10:1 or 20:1 [70, 71].

Two double-blind trials investigated the cardiotoxicity of doxorubicin with and without cytoprotection by dexrazoxane. While the incidence was 15 and 14% in the two protected groups, 31% of the controls without dexrazoxane developed cardiotoxicity. CHF occurred in 15% of the placebo recipients, but in no patients treated with dexrazoxane. Also, reduction of LVEF was greater in the control groups than in the dexrazoxane groups [72, 73].

In the majority of studies, dexrazoxane was started on the same day as the anthracyclines. However, the cytoprotectant also proved effective even when given after 300 mg/m^2 of doxorubicin had already been administered [56].

Dexrazoxane's cardioprotection is apparently not influenced by the presence or absence of cardiac risk factors in the patient [74], nor does it influence antitumor activity in the majority of studies [56]. However, in the largest study, tumor response in the dexrazoxane group was significantly lower than that in the placebo group (46.8 vs. 60.5%) [73]. Other studies (in part from the same study group) did not find any evidence of tumor protection by dexrazoxane.

The cardiac protection offered by dexrazoxane permits the administration of doxorubicin beyond the standard cumulative doses. However, it remains unclear whether this influences time to progression or survival rates. Only from small, uncontrolled studies have we obtained preliminary data which may indicate better survival with dexrazoxane adjunction in an anthracyline-based polychemotherapy regimen [56]. Further studies are necessary to fully understand dexrazoxane-induced cardioprotection in anthracycline-treated patients.

Data from several clinical trials on women with advanced breast cancer have shown that coadministration of dexrazoxane with anthracyclines does not compromise tolerability in the majority of patients. Hematologic toxicity was common in all treatment groups, but was generally more frequent in patients given dexrazoxane [72, 73]. Compared to placebo recipients, the incidence of severe leukocytopenia at nadir was significantly higher in the dexrazoxane group (78 vs. 68%). However, the degree of severe thrombocytopenia did not differ between the treatment groups. Incidence and nature of other side effects, including nausea, vomitus, mucositis, infection, fever, anemia, fatigue, alopecia, sepsis, stomatitis and diarrhea, were similar in both therapy groups. Pain on injection was more common in the dexrazoxane group, and was significantly higher than in the placebo group. There is only a small amount of data available that indicate that the drug has a tolerability in children and adolescents similar to that observed in women with advanced breast cancer [75, 76].

To protect against cardiotoxicity from anthracycline therapy, the dexrazoxane to anthracycline dosage ratio recommended is 10:1 in the USA or 20:1 in Europe. Dexrazoxane should be administered by short intravenous infusion starting approximately 30 min before anthracycline administration. In Europe, dexrazoxane should be started simultaneously with anthracycline treatment; whereas in the USA, a cumulative dose of 300 mg/m^2 of doxorubicin should be given before dexrazoxane is administered [56].

Selenium

Selenium (Se) was first associated with an increased cancer risk nearly 30 years ago. Since then, Se-containing drugs have demonstrated antineoplastic activity in a variety of experimental animal models and some epidemiologic chemopreventive

Table 3. Chemoprevention studies with selenium

Se characteristics	Cancer risk characteristics	Reference
Substitution of 200 µg Se as Na$_2$SeO$_3$ or Se-enriched yeast	Reduction of liver cancer risk in an area of prevalent hepatitis (Qidong, Shandong)	83
50 µg Se as enriched yeast plus vitamin E and β-carotene	Reduction of stomach cancer and of total cancer incidence in a high-risk population (Linxian)	84
200 µg Se as Na$_2$SeO$_3$	Reduction of secondary malignancies (lung, colorectal, prostate) after nonmelanomic skin cancer	85

studies that have linked Se status and individual human cancer risk. Two general hypotheses have been proposed to explain these relationships. The first is that Se seems to be necessary to express specific selenoproteins. Some of these function as main parts of the internal redox system, which is important for the prevention of radical-induced DNA damage and for regulating cell growth. The second hypothesis is that supplemental Se supports the production of Se metabolites that act directly to inhibit tumor cell growth and/or increase apoptosis [77].

Table 3 summarizes four chemopreventive trials which show, for a large number of patients, the importance of Se substitution in reducing cancer risk.

Recent literature notes that Se may also provide multilineage cytoprotection against toxicities from different kinds of antineoplastic therapy. The most surprising results were presented by Hehr et al. [78]. In a well-designed experimental study, they observed Se-related protection of human fibroblasts against toxicities from therapeutic irradiation. In the same experiments, moreover, adding Se did not protect human tumor cells (SCC). These experiments were thus the first to show Se's selective cytoprotection, a prerequisite if selenium is to be used in clinical practice. These findings on selectivity have gained support from the as yet unpublished data gathered by another group [79]. Hehr et al. [80] have already published preliminary clinical data on radioprotection with Se in rectal cancer patients (postoperative radiotherapy). These initial findings suggest a reduction in acute toxicities stemming from pelvic irradiation.

Other trials have observed chemoprotective effects of Se in patients receiving anthracycline-based chemotherapy [81], although all of these preliminary data are awaiting substantiation by larger phase III trials. Ongoing studies are investigating questions of dosage and administration modus involved in cytoprotection [82].

Conclusions

The clinical applications of the cytoprotectors and rescue agents described here are merely initial landmarks in a growing field of therapeutics. A number of strategies, involving the protection of normal tissues or the accumulation of cytotoxins in tumor tissue only, have already entered clinical use. Such strategies are increasingly the subject of preclinical investigations as well.

Our growing understanding of drug action and cellular targets has stimulated the development of cytoprotection as a new therapeutic strategy. The cytoprotective agents described herein and those already in clinical use underscore the validity of this approach. One advantage of this strategy is that once a drug has established its therapeutic efficacy, the foundations are laid for enhancing its results. In the next few years, the advantages of this concept may overcome the main obstacle to its clinical development; namely, the complexity of the studies required to demonstrate a therapeutic benefit unequivocally greater than the benefit offered by the antineoplastic agent alone. In any case, this strategy and the research efforts behind it are beginning to draw the attention of more and more members of the oncological community.

Closing Remarks

Because cytoprotection is a relatively new supportive approch, the longer-range outcome of clinical trials and experience is still under study. Several of the drugs discussed have clearly shown cytoprotective effects. For example, some studies report chemoprevention despite the reduction of acute and late toxicity. In addition, the early use of chemoprotective agents (such as mesna, amifostine and selenium) in primary therapy (chemo- and radiotherapy) may help reduce treatment-related secondary malignancies in the future.

References

1   Lee WR: Strategies to reduce acute and late morbidity associated with radiation therapy for the head and neck. ASTRO Refresher 411, 40th Annual Meeting, American Society for Therapeutic Radiology and Oncology, Phoenix, AZ, Oct 1998.
2   Klein P, Muggia FM: Cytoprotection: Shelter from the storm. Oncologist 1999;4:112–121.
3   Goldin A, Venditti JM, Kline I, et al: Eradication of leukemia cells (L1210) by MTX and MTX plus citrovorum factor. Nature 1966;212:1548–1550.
4   Djerassi I, Agir E, Roger GL Jr, et al: Long-term remissions in childhood acute leukemia: Use of infrequent infusions of MTX; supportive roles of platelet transfusions and citrovorum factors. Clin Pediatr 1966;5:502–509.
5   Hryniuk WM, Bertino JR: Treatment of leukemia with large doses of methotrexate and folinic acid: Clinical-biochemical correlates. J Clin Invest 1969;48:2140–2155.

6   Eisenhauer EA: Cytoprotection; in 23rd Congress European Society of Medical Oncology, Athens, Nov 6–10, 1998, pp 109–113.

7   Hamers FP, Brakkee JH, Cavaletti E, Tedeschi M, Marmonti L, Pezzoni G, Neijt JP, Gispen WH: Reduced glutathione protects against cisplatin-induced neurotoxicity in rats. Cancer Res 1993;53:544–549.

8   Di Re F, Bohm S, Oriana S, Spatti GB, Pirovano C, Tedeschi M, Zunino F: High dose cisplatin and cyclophosphamide with glutathione in the treatment of advanced ovarian cancer. Ann Oncol 1993;4:55–61.

9   Smyth JF, Bowman A, Perren T, Wilkinson P, Prescott RJ, Quinn KJ, Tedeschi M: Glutathione reduces the toxicity and improves quality of life of women diagnosed with ovarian cancer treated with cisplatin: Results of a double-blind, randomised trial. Ann Oncol 1997;8: 569–573.

10 Hanson WR, Thomas C: 16,16-Dimethylprostaglandin E_2 increases survival of murine intestinal stem cells when given before photon radiation. Radiat Res 1983;96:393.

11 Hanson WR, Marks JE, Reddy SP, Simon S, Mihalo WE, Tova Y: Protection from radiation-induced oral mucositis by a mouth rinse containing prostaglandin E_1 analog, misoprostol: A placebo-controlled double-blind clinical trial. Adv Exp Med Biol 1997;400B:811.

12 Spencer CM, Goa KL: Amifostine. A review of its pharmacodynamic properties, and therapeutic potential as a radioprotector and cytotoxic chemoprotector. Drugs 1995;50:1001–1031.

13 Wasserman TH, Chapman JD, Coleman CN, Kligerman MM: Chemical modifiers of radiation; in Perez CA, Brady LW (eds): Principles and Practice of Radiation Oncology, ed 3. Philadelphia, Lippincott, 1997, pp 685–704.

14 Tannehill SP, Metha MP: Amifostine and radiation therapy: Past, present and future. Semin Oncol 1996;23(suppl 8):69–77.

15 Speyer JL, Green MD, Kramer E, et al: Protective effect of the bispiperazinedione ICRF-187 against doxorubicin-induced cardiac toxicity in women with advanced breast cancer. N Engl J Med 1988;319:745–752.

16 Swain SM, Whaley FS, Gerber MC, Weisberg S, York M, Spicer D, Jones SE, Wadler S, Desai A, Vogel C, Speyer J, Mittelman A, Reddy S, Pendergrass K, Velez-Garcia E, Ewer MS, Bianchine JR, Gams RA: Cardioprotection with dexrazoxane for doxorubicin-containing therapy in advanced breast cancer. J Clin Oncol 1997;15:1318–1332.

17 Breccia A, Badiello R, Trenta A, Mattii M: On the chemical radioprotection by organic selenium compounds in vivo. Radiat Res 1969;38:483–492.

18 Patchen ML, MacVittle TJ, Weiss JF: Combined modality radioprotection: The use of glucan and selenium with WR-2721. Int J Radiat Oncol Biol Phys 1990;18:1059–1075.

19 Cervellino JC, Araujo CE, Pirisi C, Francia A, Cerruti R: Ifosfamide and Mesna for the treatment of advanced squamous cell head and neck cancer. Oncology 1991;48:89–92.

20 Goren MP: Oral administration of mesna with ifosfamide. Semin Oncol 1996;23(suppl 6):91–96.

21 Markman M, Kennedy A, Webster K, Kulp B, Peterson G, Belinson J: Continuous subcutaneous administration of mesna to prevent ifosfamide-induced hemorrhagic cystitis. Semin Oncol 1996;23(suppl 6):97–98.

22 Spencer C, Goa KL: Amifostine. A review of its pharmacodynamic and pharmacokinetic properties, and therapeutic potential as a radioprotector and cytotoxic chemoprotector. Drugs 1995;50:1001–1031.

23 Shaw LM, Turrisi AT, Glover DJ, Bonner HS, Norfleet AL, Weiler C, Kligerman MM: Human pharmacokinetics of WR-2721. Int J Radiat Oncol Biol Phys 1986;12:1501–1504.

24 Yuhas JM, Afzal SMJ, Afzal V: Variation in normal tissue responsiveness to WR-2721. Int J Radiat Oncol Biol Phys 1984;10:1537–1539.

25 Shaw LM, Glover DJ, Turrisi AT, et al: Pharmacokinetics of WR-2721. Pharmacol Ther 1988;39:195–201.

26 Mollman JE: Protection against cisplatin neurotoxicity in cultured dorsal root ganglion cells by WR-2721 (abstract). Neurology 1991;41(suppl 1):201.

27 Wang LM, Wang QW, Fernandes DJ, et al: Amifostine protects MRC-5 human lung fibroblasts from taxol toxicity without reducing its cytotoxic effect against human non-small cell lung cancer cells. Proc Am Assoc Cancer Res 1995;36:288.

28 Douay L, Hu C, Giarratana MC: Comparative effects of amifostine (ethyol) on normal hematopoietic stem cells versus human leukemic cells during ex vivo purging in autologous bone marrow transplants. Semin Oncol 1994;21(suppl 11):16–20.

29 Douay L, Hu C, Giarratana MC, Bouchet S, Conlon J, Capizzi RL, Gorin NC: Amifostine improves the antileukemic therapeutic index of mafosfamide: Implications for bone marrow purging. Blood 1995;86:2849–2855.

30 Dorr RT, Lagel KE: Anthracycline cardioprotection by amifostine (WR-2721) and its active metabolite (WR-1065) in vitro. Proc Am Soc Clin Oncol 1994;13:435.

31 Phillips TL, Yuhas JM, Wasserman TH: Differential protection against alkylating agent injury in tumors and normal tissues. Conference on Radioprotectors and Anticarcinogenes (1st: 1982: National Bureau of Standards); in Nygaard OF, Simic MG (eds): Radioprotector and Anticarcinogens. New York, Academic Press, 1983, pp 735–748.

32 Wasserman TH, Phillips TL, Ross G, Kane LJ: Differential protection against cytotoxic chemotherapeutic effects on bone marrow CFUs by WR-2721. Cancer Clin Trials 1981;4:3–6.

33 Treskes M, Boven E, van de Loosdrecht AA, Wijffels JF, Cloos J, Peters GJ, Pinedo HM, van der Vijgh WJ: Effects of the modulating agent WR-2721 on myelotoxicities and antitumour activity in carboplatin-treated mice. Eur J Cancer 1994; 30A:183–187.

34 Jordan SW, Yuhas JM, Glick J: Modulation of cis-platinum renal toxicity by the radioprotective agent WR-2721. Exp Mol Pathol 1982;36:297–305.

35 Yuhas JM, Culo F: Selective inhibition of the nephrotoxicity of cis-dichlorodiammineplatinum (II) by WR-2721 without altering its antitumor properties. Cancer Treat Rep 1980;64:57–64.

36 Yuhas JM, Spellman JM, Jordan SW, Pardini MC, Afzal SM, Culo F: Treatment of tumours with the combination of WR-2721 and cis-dichlorodiammineplatinum (II) or cyclophosphamide. Br J Cancer 1980;47:57–63.

37 Millar JL, McElwain TJ, Clutterbuck RD, Wist EA: The modification of melphalan toxicity in tumor-bearing mice by S-2-(3-aminopropylamino)ethylphosphorothioic acid (WR-2721). Am J Clin Oncol 1982;5:321–328.

38 Kemp G, Rose P, Lurain J, Berman M, et al: Amifostine pre-treatment for protection against cyclophosphamide-induced and cisplatin-induced toxicities: Results of a randomized control trial in patients with advanced ovarian cancer. J Clin Oncol 1996;14:2101–2112.

39 Schiller JH, Storer B, Berlin J, Wittenkeller J, Larson M, Pharo L, Larson M, Berry W: Amifostine, cisplatin, and vinblastine in metastatic non-small-cell lung cancer: A report of high response rate and prolonged survival. J Clin Oncol 1996;14:1913–1921.

40 Anderson H, Mercer V, Russell L, Oster W, Thatcher N: A phase III randomized study of carboplatin and amifostine vs. carboplatin and G-CSF in patients with operable non-small-cell lung cancer. Blood 1996;88:350.

41 Liu T, Liu Y, Zhang Z, Kligerman MM: Use of radiation with or without WR-2721 in advanced rectal cancer. Cancer 1992;69:2820–2825.

42 Büntzel J, Küttner K, Fröhlich D, Glatzel M: Selective cytoprotection with amifostine in concurrent radiochemotherapy for head and neck cancer. Ann Oncol 1998;9:505–509.

43   McDonald S, Meyerowitz C, Smudzin T, Rubin P: Preliminary results of a pilot study using WR-2721 before fractionated irradiation of the head and neck to reduce salivary gland dysfunction. Int J Radiat Oncol Biol Phys 1994;29:747–754.

44   Brizel D, Sauer R, Wannenmacher M, Henke M, Eschwege F, Wasserman T: Randomized phase III trial of radiation +/– amifostine in patients with head and neck cancer. Proc Am Soc Clin Oncol 1998;17:386a.

45   Bohuslavizki KH, Brenner W, Lassmann S, et al: Protection of salivary glands by amifostine in patients treated with high dose radioiodine. Eur J Cancer 1997;33(suppl 8):17.

46   Capizzi RL: Clinical status and optimal use of amifostine. Oncology (Huntington) 1999;13: 47–59.

47   Goren MP: Oral mesna: A review. Semin Oncol 1992;6(suppl 12):65–72.

48   Stofer-Vogel B, Cerny T, Borner M, Lauterburg BH: Oral bioavailability of mesna tablets. Cancer Chemother Pharmacol 1993;32:78–81.

49   Dorr RT: Chemoprotectants for cancer chemotherapy. Semin Oncol 1991;18(suppl. 2): 48–58.

50   Siu LL, Moore MJ: Use of mesna to prevent ifosfamide-induced urotoxicity, Support Care Cancer 1998;6:144–154.

51   Dechant KL, Brogden RN, Pilkington T, Faulds D: Ifosfamide/mesna: A review of its antineoplastic activity, pharmacokinetic properties and therapeutic efficacy in cancer. Drugs 1991;42: 428–467.

52   Fukuoka M, Negoro S, Masuda N, Furuse K, Kawahara M, Kodama N, Ikegami H, Nakamura S, Nishio H, Ohnoshi T: Placebo-controlled double-blind comparative study on the preventive efficacy of mesna against ifosfamide-induced urinary disorders. J Cancer Res Clin Oncol 1991;117:473–478.

53   Sakurai M, Saijo N, Shinkai T, Eguchi K, Sasaki Y, Tamura T, Sano T, Suemasu K, Jett JR: The protective effect of 2-mercapto-ethane sulfonate (MESNA) on hemorrhagic cystitis induced by high-dose ifosfamide treatment tested by a randomized crossover trial. Jpn J Clin Oncol 1986;16:153–156.

54   Bryant BM, Jarman M, Ford HT, Smith IE: Prevention of isophosphamide-induced urothelial toxicity with 2-mercaptoethane sulphonate sodium (mesnum) in patients with advanced carcinoma. Lancet 1980;ii:657–659.

55   Haselberger MB, Schwinghammer TL: Efficacy of mesna for prevention of hemorrhagic cystitis after high-dose cyclophosphamide therapy, Ann Pharmacol 1995;29:919–921.

56   Wiseman LR, Spencer CM: Dexrazoxane. A review of its use as a cardioprotective agent in patients receiving anthracycline-based chemotherapy. Drugs 1998;56:385–403.

57   Handa K, Sato S: Generation of free radicals of quinone group containing anti-cancer chemicals in NADPH-microsome system as evidenced by initiation of sulfite oxidation. Jpn J Cancer Res 1975;66:43–75.

58   Myers CE, McGuire WP, Liss RH, Ifrim I, Grotzinger K, Young RC: Adriamycin, the role of lipid peroxidation in cardiac toxicity and tumor response. Science 1977;197:165–167.

59   Weijl NI, Cleton FJ, Osanto S: Free radicals and antioxidants in chemotherapy-induced toxicity. Cancer Treat Rev 1997;23:209–240.

60   Legha S, Wang YN, Mackay B, et al: Clinical and pharmacological investigation of the effects of the α-tocopherol on Adriamycin cardiotoxicity. Ann NY Acad Sci 1982;393:411–418.

61   Buss JL, Hasinoff BB: The one-ring open hydrolysis product intermediates of the cardioprotective agent ICRF-187 (dexrazoxane) displace iron from iron-anthracycline complexes. Agents Actions 1993;40:86–95.

62 Hüsken BC, de Jong J, Beekman B, Onderwater RC, van der Vijgh WJ, Bast A: Modulation of the in vitro cardiotoxicity of doxorubicin by flavonoids. Cancer Chemother Pharmacol 1995;37:55–62.

63 Villani F, Galimberti M, Monti E, et al: Effects of ICRF-187 pretreatment against doxorubicin-induced delayed cardiotoxicity in the rat. Toxicol Appl Pharmacol 1990;102:292–299.

64 Herman EH, Ferrans VJ: Timing of treatment with ICRF-187 and its effect on chronic doxorubicin cardiotoxicity. Cancer Chemother Pharmacol 1993;32:445–449.

65 Holcenberg JS, Tutsch KD, Earhart RH, Ungerleider RS, Kamen BA, Pratt CB, Gribble TJ, Glaubiger DL: Phase I study of ICRF-187 in pediatric cancer patients and comparison of its pharmacokinetics in children and adults. Cancer Treat Rep 1986;70:703–709.

66 Vogel CL, Gorowski E, Davila E, et al: Phase I clinical trial and pharmacokinetics of weekly ICRF-187 (NSC 169780) infusion in patients with solid tumors. Invest New Drugs 1987;5:187–198.

67 Hasinoff BB: Pharmacodynamics of the hydrolysis activation of the cardioprotective agent (+)-1,2-bis(3,5-dioxopiperazinyl-1-yl)propane. J Pharm Sci 1994;83:64–67.

68 Robert L, Bellott R, Debled M, et al: Lack of interference of dexrazoxane on the pharmacokinetics of doxorubicin in cancer patients. Proc Am Soc Clin Oncol 1998;17:250a.

69 Jakobsen P, Sorensen B, Bastholt L, et al: The pharmacokinetics of high-dose epirubicin and of the cardioprotector ADR-529 given together with cyclophosphamide, 5-fluorouracil, and tamoxifen in metastatic breast cancer patients. Cancer Chemother Pharmacol 1994;35:45–52.

70 Speyer JL, Green MD, Kramer E, et al: Protective effect of bispiperazinedione ICRF-187 against doxorubicin-induced cardiotoxicity in women with advanced breast cancer. N Engl J Med 1988;319:745–752.

71 Speyer JL, Green MD, Zeleniuch-Jacquotte A, et al.: ICRF-187 permits longer treatment with doxorubicin in women with breast cancer. J Clin Oncol 1992;10:117–127.

72 Swain SM, Whaley FS, Gerber MC, Weisberg S, York M, Spicer D, Jones SE, Wadler S, Desai A, Vogel C, Speyer J, Mittelman A, Reddy S, Pendergrass K, Velez-Garcia E, Ewer MS, Bianchine JR, Gams RA: Cardioprotection with dexrazoxane for doxorubicin-containing therapy in advanced breast cancer. J Clin Oncol 1997;15:1318–1332.

73 Swain SM, Whaley FS, Gerber MC, Ewer MS, Bianchine JR, Gams RA: Delayed administration of dexrazoxane provides cardioprotection for patients with advanced breast cancer treated with doxorubicin-containing therapy. J Clin Oncol 1997;15:1333–1340.

74 Venturini M, Michelotti A, Del Mastro L, Gallo L, Carnino F, Garrone O, Tibaldi C, Molea N, Bellina RC, Pronzato P, Cyrus P, Vinke J, Testore F, Guelfi M, Lionetto R, Bruzzi P, Conte PF, Rosso R: Multicenter randomized controlled clinical trial to evaluate cardioprotection of dexrazoxane versus no cardioprotection in women receiving epirubicin chemotherapy for advanced breast cancer. J Clin Oncol 1996;14:3112–3120.

75 Schiavetti A, Castello MA, Versacci P, Varrasso G, Padula A, Ventriglia F, Werner B, Colloridi V: Use of ICRF-187 for prevention of anthracycline cardiotoxicity in children: Preliminary results. Pediatr Hematol Oncol 1997;14:213–222.

76 Wexler LH, Andrich MP, Venzon D, Berg SL, Weaver-McClure L, Chen CC, Dilsizian V, Avila N, Jarosinski P, Balis FM, Poplack DG, Horowitz ME: Randomized trial of the cardioprotective agent ICRF-187 in pediatric sarcoma patients treated with doxorubicin. J Clin Oncol 1996;14:362–372.

77 Combs GF Jr, Clark LC, Turnbull BW: Reduction of cancer mortality and incidence by selenium supplementation. Med Klin 1997;92(suppl III):42–45.

78 Hehr T, Bamberg M, Rodemann HP: Präklinische und klinische Relevanz der radioprotekti-
    ven Wirkung von Natriumselenit. InFo Onkol 1999;2(suppl 2):25–29.
79 Schleicher UM, Lopez Cotarelo C, Andreopoulos D, Handt S, Ammon J: Radioprotektion
    humaner Endothelzellen durch Natriumselenit. Med Welt 1999;94(suppl 3):35–38.
80 Hehr T, Hoffmann W, Bamberg M: Zur Rolle von Natriumselenit als Adjuvans in der Strah-
    lentherapie des Rektumkarzinoms. Med Welt 1997;92(suppl III):48–49.
81 Sill R: Stellenwert von Selen in der menschlichen Ernährung. EHK 1998;10:585–592.
82 Büntzel J: Erfahrungen mit Natriumselenit in der Behandlung von akuten und späten Neben-
    wirkungen der Radiochemotherapie von Kopf-Hals-Karzinomen. Med Welt 1999;94(suppl 3):
    49–53.
83   An P: Selenium and endemic cancer in China; in Whanger PM, Combs GF Jr, Yeh JY (eds):
    Environmental Bioinorganic Chemistry of Selenium. Beijing, Chinese Academy of Science,
    1995, pp 91–149.
84 Blot WJ, Li JY, Taylor PR, et al: Nutrition intervention trials in Linxian, China: Supplementa-
    tion with specific vitamin/mineral combinations, cancer incidence, and disease-specific mor-
    tality in the general population. J Natl Cancer Inst 1993;85:1483–1492.
85 Combs GF Jr, Clark LC, Turnbull BW: Cancer prevention by selenium: Evidence from a ran-
    domized clinical trial. InFo Onkol 1999;2(suppl 2):3–6.

Dr. Jens Büntzel, Hals-Nasen-Ohrenklinik, Zentralklinikum Südthüringen,
Albert-Schweitzer-Straße 2, D–98527 Suhl (Germany)
E-mail: dr.buentzel@t-online.de

Subject Index